Aggression and Adaptation
The Bright Side to Bad Behavior

Aggression and Adaptation
The Bright Side to Bad Behavior

Edited by

Patricia H. Hawley
Todd D. Little
University of Kansas

Philip C. Rodkin
University of Illinois, Urbana–Champaign

LAWRENCE ERLBAUM ASSOCIATES, PUBLISHERS
2007   Mahwah, New Jersey   London

Copyright © 2007 by Lawrence Erlbaum Associates, Inc.

Lawrence Erlbaum Associates, Inc., Publishers
10 Industrial Avenue
Mahwah, New Jersey 07430
www.erlbaum.com

Cover design by Tomai Maridou

Library of Congress Cataloging-in-Publication Data

Aggression and Adaptation: The Bright Side of Bad Behavior

ISBN 978-0-8058-5245-5 — ISBN 0-8058-5245-X (cloth)
ISBN 978-0-8058-6234-8 — ISBN 0-8058-6234-X (pbk)
ISBN 978-1-4106-1604-3 — ISBN 1-4106-1604-5 (e book)

Copyright information for this volume can be obtained by contacting the Library of Congress.

Books published by Lawrence Erlbaum Associates are printed on acid-free paper, and their bindings are chosen for strength and durability.

Printed in the United States of America
10 9 8 7 6 5 4 3 2 1

For Lorrie

Contents

Foreword

In 1817, the French Academy of Sciences offered a prize for anyone who could provide the best experimental demonstration and theoretical analysis of the diffraction of light by objects. Subtle aspects of diffraction were becoming something of a nuisance to the conventional scientific interpretation of the nature of light, a view that had served the scientific community with distinction for more than 100 years. That view, formalized a century earlier by Newton and substantiated by numerous subsequent experiments, was that light consisted of a continuous stream of tiny particles. Yet recent experiments by British prodigy Thomas Young had demonstrated that when light is passed through narrow, parallel slits in a barrier it produces light and dark bands on a receptor. Bands are a hallmark of interference of waves with one another, and wave-like interference is fundamentally inconsistent with the behavior of particles. Young's results were creating buzz in remote corners of the scientific community.

By all accounts (e.g., Gribbin, 1995), the Academy's prize was a gambit to bury this annoyance; deeply wedded to Newton's particle view, the Academy was confident that the larger scientific community would come forward with the evidence and argument necessary to bring Young's renegade results in line with a conventional understanding if not refute them entirely. The outcome was something very different. To the Academy's surprise, the competition attracted only two submissions—one from an anonymous crackpot and a second from the French engineer Augustin Fresnel. Fresnel's data and mathematical arguments concerning the shadows cast by objects at varying degrees of diffraction incontrovertibly confirmed the wave-like nature of light. But because it did not directly refute the incompatible particle interpretation, the Academy was left in the uncomfortable position of lending its imprimatur to two unassailable but seemingly irreconcilable views of the nature of light. Fresnel's bothersome submission, it is now appreciated, was the first significant step toward one of the best substantiated cornerstones of our contemporary, quantum mechanical understanding of physics (Gribbin, 1995): To understand light, it is necessary to embrace a foreign but fundamental duality. Like all matter, light is both a wave and a particle. The representations are opposing and appear incompatible, but each is valid, depending on the observer's point of view, purpose, and method.

Debates over light may seem a peculiar issue with which to foreshadow a volume on the psychology of aggression in children and adolescents, but the episode and context of Fresnel's submission to the Academy nearly two centuries ago is instructive. As Fresnel's did in its time and context, this submission appears at a point when scientific understanding of aggression is already well-developed. Few topics within developmental psychology can boast the same level of scientific interest as that currently enjoyed by study of aggression. Developmental interest in the topic is well over a century old and has produced a truly staggering number of books, edited volumes, comprehensive reviews, and individual articles (see Dodge, Coie, & Lynam, 2006). This level of interest is well placed. Aggression between children represents a special concern for society. Leaving aside the fear, injustice, and injury wrought upon its victims, aggressive behavior disrupts learning and other group activities in school classrooms. Aggressive children are at risk for school difficulties, constitute a large proportion of the individuals perpetrating delinquent and other criminal activities, and represent a significant toll on the resources of their families and psychological treatment facilities. Aggressive behavior rarely remits spontaneously, is resistant to change, and is extremely difficult to treat.

Developmentalists can also be justifiably proud of the robustness and rigor of their scientific understanding of the nature and origins of aggressive behavior in children. The topic has attracted some of psychology's best thinkers and the extant research includes–and in many cases unveiled–some of the most powerful and persuasive research designs and tools for statistical abstraction and interpretation. It has also produced broad generalizations about aggression that are replicable and as close as we are likely to come to psychological canons. Among others: The brains and biology of highly aggressive individuals are different. Unusually aggressive children reason in peculiar ways about social situations and have difficulty regulating emotions. Harsh and rejecting family environments, especially physically punitive or abusive ones, place growing children at risk for becoming excessively aggressive. Distortions of normal peer processes contribute to aggression and aggressiveness varies with circumstance, exposure to models, and cultural context.

At the same time, the literature hints at an approaching intellectual crossroads. From the start, models of aggression have been pessimistic, emphasizing pathology and maladjustment. Aggression, quite understandably, has been represented as a developmental failing–of individuals, socialization, culture, or biology and genetics. As noted, there has been little reason to question this perspective and abundant reason to accept it. Yet disquieting findings have also appeared, especially recently.

Some aggressive individuals reason in curiously sophisticated and skilled ways about social dilemmas, appear to come from seemingly appropriate homes, or do well in school and avoid broader trouble. Some are surprisingly popular with peers and aggression can bind children to one another in specific circumstances rather than repulse them. A closer reading of evolutionary theory also appears to suggest the important distinctions in form and function perhaps have been obscured. Like the puzzling bands of light and dark of Fresnel's time, these findings and musings hint at some messiness in our broad formulation of aggression. They suggest that the foundation of our understanding of aggression may be incomplete and, intriguingly, may require us to embrace the idea that aggression has incompatible but simultaneous adaptive and maladaptive faces. But these findings are easy to ignore in isolation.

This volume changes these findings; its contributors include many, even most, of the very authors whose work has separately contributed to the disquiet surrounding formulations of aggression. In bringing these arguments together, the volume promises to focus this discussion and insures that it will not go away. In this regard, the parallel to Fresnel is even more apt. Although Fresnel's contribution to understanding the wave-particle duality of matter is not well known outside of the discipline of physics, he is widely and duly recognized for the later invention of a specialized optical lens made up of series of concentric rings. This lens, still named after him and featured in lighthouses, is used to concentrate a beam of light on a subject. Although some chapters are frankly confrontational on occasion, most serve simply to identify square pegs that do not fit simply into the round holes of reigning theory. As appropriate at this stage, the reader will not encounter an overarching, common theoretical framework across chapters. Indeed, one strength of this collection is that the authors appear to have begun their inquiry from mostly distinctive theoretical perspectives or literatures. Further, the reader should not be disappointed to find that the collection lacks a coherent framework for overturning prevailing wisdom concerning the origins and function of aggression in children and adolescents. The evidence clearly falls far short of threatening to topple our current understanding of aggression and none of the contributions have this explicit or implicit aim. The collection should give us pause, however, and guard against complacency. Even at this early stage, this collection demonstrates that aggression, like material matter, resists classification as wholly one thing or another.

A further footnote to Fresnel bears mention in closing. History shows that Fresnel's submission to the Academy was met with some understandable resistance (Gribbin, 1995). The difficulty was that Fresnel did not posses sufficient mathematical skills to articulate all of the necessary arguments underlying his position. In view of their allegiance to the orthodox view, the Academy might have dismissed his contribution out of hand. In hindsight, doing so would only have long delayed an inevitable debate and conclusion. To their credit, the Academy did something remarkable and outside their original mandate. The judges turned the manuscript over to a highly skilled mathematician among their members, Simeon Poisson, who completed the calculations that Fresnel suggested but was not able to conduct himself. Further, when Poisson's calculations appeared to suggest an absurd and seemingly physically impossible event (a bright spot in the center of shadow cast by an object) the Academy responded by sponsoring the experiment necessary to test and confirm the effect. The authors and editors of this volume have suggested that their conclusions will challenge accepted wisdom concerning the adaptiveness of aggression. It will be a great interest to learn whether the collective of scholars who currently study aggression meet the challenge represented by this volume with the same curious outlook, generous spirit, and open mind that salvaged the prize for Fresnel.

REFERENCES

Dodge, K. A., Coie, J. D., & Lynam, D. (2006). Aggression and antisocial behavior in youth. In N. Eisenberg (Ed.), *Handbook of child psychology: Vol 3. Social, emotional, and personality development* (pp. 719–778). New York: Wiley.
Gribbin, J. (1995). *Schrodinger's kittens and the search for reality: Solving the quantum mysteries*. New York: Little Brown.

—Jeffrey G. Parker
The Pennsylvania State University

Preface

This book presents a true challenge for students of aggression. By "challenge," we do not mean to imply that material of this volume is particularly difficult to grasp, but rather it is challenging because it raises what for some might be disquieting questions about interpersonal functioning within human social groups that merit contemplation. Many chapters provoke the reader to ponder questions about "good" and "evil," for example, but the authors do not attempt to answer such questions. Instead, the authors offer alternate ways of viewing the complexities of human social behavior outside of explanations characteristic of human development textbooks. That is, the chapters within suggest that, rather than a problem to be solved, aggressive behavior offers avenues for personal growth, goal attainment, and positive peer regard.

Many students of aggression have read modern developmental theories of aggression (e.g., stemming from developmental psychopathology or clinical traditions) and found that they do not fully account for personal experiences with, or observations of, aggressive human behavior. Specifically, perspectives that seek to align aggressive behavior or trait aggressiveness closely with pathology cannot account well for those individuals who successfully execute aggressive tactics to gain status in the peer group despite (or maybe even because of) behavior that has been traditionally considered "antisocial."

The present volume offers alternative points of view to the prevailing orthodoxy that aggression equals pathology. Rather than seeking to triumph over the prevailing paradigm, however, each contributor seeks merely to challenge it by describing and explaining what have heretofore been considered incommodious exceptions to the aggression as pathology rules. We do not, however, claim that such cases constitute "moral goodness."

The book evolved from a symposium at the biennial meeting of the Society for Research in Child Development. William Bukowski served as the Discussant for what turned out to be a thought-provoking set of papers that addressed positive outcomes associated with aggressive behavior in several studies. The papers were unusual in that they claimed that the positive outcomes of aggression spread to the social sphere; namely, that aggression need not lead to social castigation, and may in fact bolster one's social standing. Those empirical papers appeared in a special volume of *Merrill-Palmer Quarterly*.

The dialog revved up within a panel discussion at the SRCD peer preconference in Tampa, Florida (*Is Aggression Always Maladaptive?*). The lively and friendly debate that carried on into the evening resulted in the framework of the present book.

OUTLINE OF THE BOOK

The title of the book, *Aggression and Adaptation* is purposefully broad because the authors herein address "adaptation" at multiple levels. The first level addresses ultimate causation or evolutionary history. Four chapters address the aggression–adaptation link from various evolutionary perspectives.

I (Hawley), for example, draw links between my theory of social dominance (resource control theory) and Maslow's hierarchy of needs (also with biological roots). I summarize a body of work that shows that highly aggressive socially dominant youths not only are supremely effective at resource control, but also enjoy positive personal and social outcomes that less aggressive youths do not (e.g., well-being, positive peer regard). Vaughn and Santos address the multiple levels of adaptation. Their chapter carefully distinguishes theoretical approaches that differentially focus on the proximate causation (e.g., social learning) versus ultimate causation (evolutionary biology) and makes clear how "adaptation" in the biological sense contrasts markedly to psychological views of aggression. By way of their review of work on inter- and intragroup aggression from an evolutionary bent, Vaughn and Santos remind us of the cohesive function of agonism, especially within the context of dominance relationships. Smith presents an ideological history of developmental approaches to aggression, and points out that the social engineering ethos of child psychology set it quite apart from co-developing evolutionary and sociological perspectives. Furthermore, he advises us that "socially undesirable" and "socially incompetent" are not in fact synonymous. Pellegrini rounds out these contributions with his view of social dominance, aggression and gender differences based on modern instantiations of Darwin's theory of sexual selection.

An important goal for the authors of this book is to open the way for fresh lines of empirical research based on an aggression as adaptation perspective. Here, Pellegrini's chapter bridges the conceptual and the empirical in that he tests his theoretical model of dominance and aggression longitudinally and draws connections to gender segregation, "rough and tumble," courtship, and adolescents' dating patterns. In contrast to the preceding chapters, Card and Little view adaptation as psychological adjustment. In their meta-analytic review, they show that while reactive aggression is associated with several indices of social and emotional maladjustment, instrumental aggression is not. Moreover, in some cases instrumental aggression is associated with improved adjustment. Similarly, defining adaptation in proximal terms, Cillessen and Mayeux review the popularity and aggression literatures and conclude that aggression in the peer system allows youth to achieve important social goals (i.e., status attainment). These authors close by outlining important pathways for future investigations. All three chapters successfully translate theoretical principles into empirical findings.

The next two chapters offer commentaries about the broader contexts in which these aforementioned peer systems occur. Sippola, Paget, and Buchanan, for example, refer to the classic work of Horney to argue that social aggression among girls can be at least partially understood by considering the North American context of competition-promoting "compulsory heterosexuality." In their view, girls' aggression can be viewed as resulting from attempts to cope with contradictory messages regarding femininity in a patriarchal society. In contrast, Bukowski and Abecassis draw on the self–other dialectic in addressing interpersonal competition, and point out that the seductive draw of reality television is due largely to its exaggerated depiction of the competitive processes that underlie many interpersonal relationships. The latter authors wonder if the path to social acceptance lies in one's ability to assert oneself and yet show concern for others. Both Sippola et al. and Bukowski and Abecassis note the influence of aggression in the media on children and connect how youth identify themselves with the agonistic interactions they read about or watch in popular fictional portrayals.

Our final two chapters from Farmer et al. and Rodkin and Wilson address the self–other dialectic in societal context by bringing forth the scholarship of the late Robert B. Cairns who, more than 20 years ago, understood that aggressive children were well-embedded in the social network. Farmer et al., for example, cast this tension (independent action vs. social synchronization) squarely into educational contexts. From this perspective, conflict and aggression can be seen as potential facilitators of social and personal growth. In addressing necessary efforts to control aggression, Farmer et al. urge school personnel to seek to understand the social dynamics underlying chronic aggression rather than responding to each episode independently. Finally, Rodkin and Wilson conclude that the view of aggression as maladaption stems from societal values and the linking of developmental science to political and power structures, rather than inconsistencies in theory per se. As far as improving the dispositions of peer ecologies, assertiveness training to ameliorate both aggression and passivity may be, these authors suggest, the highest road. Farmer et al. and Rodkin and Wilson draw out the implications of Cairns' original work by considering preventative interventions that concentrate on the social networks of aggressive children as a leverage point for behavioral change.

As the reader, you will doubtless find that a number of authors critique alternate (and predominant) approaches to aggression in no uncertain terms. Yet, the theoretical and empirical views expressed in the volume are morally agnostic regarding the "goodness" or "badness" of aggression. Instead, they offer thoughtful, reasoned reflections on aggression as one of the fundamental features of the human condition and entertain the perhaps seemingly counterintuitive notion that aggression and adaptation (ultimately and proximally) may not be an oxymoron after all.

My co-editors and I would first and foremost like to thank the contributors of the present volume for their thoughtful scholarship and personal investments in their chapters. We also extend our gratitude to Dorothy Espelage (University of Illinois, Urbana-Champagne), Amanda Rose (University of Missouri, Columbia), and three additional anonymous reviewers for aiding in setting us on the right track, as well as to Sarah Napientek and Paul Alderman of the University of Kansas for their technical assistance. Finally, we truly appreciate Debra Rieger, Sondra Guideman, and Rebecca Larsen (and the editorial staff) at Lawrence Erlbaum Associates for making this process smooth and utterly painless.

—*Patricia H. Hawley*

1

SOCIAL DOMINANCE IN CHILDHOOD AND ADOLESCENCE: WHY SOCIAL COMPETENCE AND AGGRESSION MAY GO HAND IN HAND

Patricia H. Hawley
University of Kansas

Evolutionary approaches to child behavior are rare breeds indeed. Certainly, the work of child ethologists (e.g., Bowlby, 1969) is often cited to exemplify the utility of applying (Darwinian) evolution to human behavior.[1] Theory development, however, was not a goal of old-school ethology (with attachment theory being a notable exception) because, according to its methodological philosophy (a legacy of Tinbergen, 1963), detailed observations and extensive behavioral catalogs (e.g., ethograms) take precedence over theory (Blurton Jones, 1972). Moreover, ethologists (like behaviorists), found intrinsic characteristics of individuals (e.g., intelligence, personality, and motivation) to be of dubious value. It thus comes as no surprise that ethology—although it is credited for bringing rigorous naturalistic observation to psychology—is better represented in historical overview sections of college texts than in later substantive chapters.

Nonetheless, ethological work has made sizable contributions to child development, especially on the topics of play, sex segregation,

---

[1]As a significant signal of the changing tide, however, see Bjorklund & Pellegrini, 2002.

1

and social dominance. In light of these contributions, it is surprising that the early work on social dominance in children failed to attract sustained attention in child psychology. One possible reason concerns methodology. Although social dominance has long been recognized by animal behaviorists to be an aspect of a relationship (Bernstein, 1981; Maslow, 1936; Scott, 1956), innovations in social psychology designed to explicitly explore relationship dynamics (e.g., the social relations model; Kenny & LaVoie, 1984) failed to cross disciplinary lines (but see Hawley & Little, 1999). Thus, dominance hierarchies involved the examination of interpersonal exchange only in a limited sense, and as such fell out of step with modern approaches (Vaughn, 1999). In addition, characteristics and developmental outcomes of the child participants (beyond gender, age, and size) were ignored: Ethologists never asked, "who are the players?" or "how do winning and losing impact the development of individuals?"

Furthermore, zoologists and descendent ethologists aligned social dominance not only with resource attainment and defense (material, social, territorial), but also with "struggles," "contests," and "agonism." Consequently, dominance explicitly involved elements of aggressiveness, threat, or fear (e.g., Brown & Hunsperger, 1963; Harlow & Yudin, 1933; Hinde, 1966; McGrew, 1972; Strayer & Strayer, 1976). Interpreting Darwin's mechanism for evolution (i.e., natural selection) in strictly overt competitive and therefore aggressive terms effectively closes out a good deal of human behavior that similarly arose out of inherently competitive forces; namely, reciprocal altruism (Trivers, 1971) and cooperation (Charlesworth, 1996; Kropotkin, 1902). Personal goals can be achieved not only directly and aggressively, but also indirectly with the aid of others.

In this chapter, I present an evolutionary metatheoretical perspective as an organizational framework for interpreting children's social and resource-directed behavior. In step with theoretical advances of the 20th century, I discuss interpersonal competition in terms of aggressive as well as cooperative strategies in the context of Resource Control Theory (Hawley, 1999). Modern evolutionary approaches challenge us to consider and clearly differentiate form and function of behavior; interpersonal transactions that appear on the surface (i.e., form) to be enacted for the good of another (e.g., reciprocation) may be effectively self-serving in function. Doing so regarding children's social behavior requires the turning of the logic we typically apply to child development slightly on its ear. In the present approach to social dominance I emphasize the importance of competition as a central organizing feature of children's (and adults') social organization, provide justification for (and evidence to suggest) that competitive males and females are more alike than different, and offer a theoretical rationale for why many aggressive youth not only are not rejected, but are socially central and liked. I also offer reasons to believe intervention programs would benefit by being informed by what may be a counterintuitive line of reasoning.

QUESTIONS ON HUMAN NATURE

In contrast to the turn of last century, the present views of human nature held by those currently involved in child development and education are largely dominated by the philosophies of Locke and perhaps more predominantly, Rousseau. Locke, one of the fathers of the empiricist movement (e.g., Locke; *An Essay Concerning Human Understanding*, 1690), denied the possibility of "innate ideas" and maintained that the identity of man and all knowledge is formed by experience. Locke's view on human nature meshed well with his political philosophy that is credited as the foundation of liberal democracy (Pinker, 2002) as well as the rise of behaviorism. From this view, negative behavior patterns are in large part consequent to inadvertent reinforcement or inappropriate modeling. Indeed, some of the most influential work in psychology on aggression stemmed from this philosophical bent (e.g., Bandura & Walters, 1959; Bandura, Ross, & Ross, 1961), and ultimately gave rise to effective interventions based on schedules of punishment and rewards and social learning principles (Bandura, 1969).

Contrasting to Locke's view though ultimately leading to similar conclusions, Rousseau's doctrine of the noble savage (*Émile*, 1762/1955) maintained that uncivilized man is peaceful, egalitarian, and in possession of inborn moral instincts. The darker side of humanity (e.g., competition, greed, violence) stemmed from the corrupting influence of modern civilization.[2] Rousseau was of course reacting to the treatise of Hobbes, who took an alternate extreme view that perpetual struggle results from man's natural propensity to behave out of self-interest and that societal controls were necessary to enforce a collective will (Hobbes, 1651/1885). Although Hobbes' philosophy no doubt was well on the mind of Freud (1930/1961), as well as many other turn-of-the-century natural philosophers favoring Darwin's work, developmentalists throughout the century tended to focus their attention on bettering

---

[2]These myths of the noble savage were maintained in anthropological circles through much of the 20th century, yet soundly debunked in recent decades. Even "peace-loving" chimpanzees (Pantroglodytes) were found to form male-aggressive coalitional bonds giving rise to raids and "panicide" (Wrangham & Peterson, 1996).

potentially corrupting environments so that children could enjoy the enhanced intelligence, self-control, and morality they so richly deserve (see Smith, this volume for an extended discussion).

Contemporary Views of Social Competence

Predominant modern views of child behavior and development largely assume, like Rousseau, that with proper care (e.g., minimal corruption), children will grow to be well behaved, other-oriented, and non-aggressive. Antisocial tendencies (broadly defined) are held to arise from unsuitable models, suboptimal parenting, misguided peers, or inappropriate media influences.

Moreover, youth aggression clearly imposes tremendous cost to society. Not only are costs borne by victims, but aggression and antisocial behavior are associated with maladjustment and psychopathology in the perpetrator as well. Aggressive youth are at higher risk for peer rejection (Coie & Dodge, 1998; Coie, Dodge, & Kupersmidt, 1990), risk-taking behavior (Brook & Newcomb, 1995), low educational achievement (Brook & Newcomb, 1995), and later unemployment (Kokko & Pulkkinen, 2000). These well-supported relationships (see Coie & Dodge, 1998, for review) have led to the observation, "insofar as aggression is positively linked to a measure of incompetence, it is seen as an index of incompetence itself" (Bukowski, 2003; p. 391).

Aggression as incompetence suits well prevailing models (e.g., in the developmental and risk literatures) that implicitly if not explicitly assume that positive and negative behaviors are at opposite ends of some unidimensional continuum; that is, there is a strong prevailing belief (in the absence of consistent data) that they will be strongly negatively correlated. Even the terms "prosocial" and "antisocial" (a lá Wispe, 1972) connote diametrical opposition. Adding to this impression of diametric division, prosociality and antisociality have long resided in distinct literatures (but see Krueger, Hicks, & McGue, 2001). Because of this disconnect, the theoretical and empirical relationship between these two broad categories invites rigorous examination.

At some level, however, this underlying message of aggression as maladaptation is confronted by common observation; namely, manipulation, deception, moderate hostility, and aggressive self-expression fit well our commonly held stereotypes of highly ambitious, successful, and powerful people (see also Christie, 1970; Feist, 1993; Hogan, Raskin, & Fazzini, 1990). Consistent with this casual observation, recent work has challenged expected relations between aggression and negative outcomes: Popular boys may be of the non-aggressive as well as aggressive varieties (Rodkin, Farmer, Pearl, & van Aker, 2000), aggressive children are no less socially central than non-aggressive children (Bagwell, Coie, Terry, & Lochman, 2000), and aggressive behavior has been related to status improvement (Sandstrom, 1999; see also Luthar & McMahon, 1996).

This body of work suggests that human social competence is not so uncomplicated that it may be described by an intuitive set of linear relationships. Morally laden approaches (e.g., victim-centered perspectives) may align competence solely with positive behaviors and traits that are assumed to support and attract others ("prosocial"), rather than those behaviors or traits assumed to undermine and repel others ("antisocial"). In contrast, broader approaches that define competence more in terms of social outcomes and social success pave the way for more complex possibilities and intriguing developmental questions; namely, what predicts social success in humans and do these predictors vary over the lifespan? And, importantly, what is the role of aggression? Inherent to many of these latter viewpoints is the notion that the competent self successfully pursues individual goals in the presence of others, presumably without excessively thwarting the goal attainment of other group members (e.g., Bost et al., 1998; Rubin & Rose-Krasnor, 1992). Multiple paths to social success are thus allowed, including those paths that may be characterized by aggressive self-expression.

Indeed the ultimate human quandary of balancing the needs of the self against those of the other preoccupied many founding fathers and mothers of psychology (e.g., Freud, McDougall, James, Maslow, Horney). Personality psychologist Robert Hogan (e.g., Hogan, 1982) reasoned that the most important differences across individuals involve affiliation and status striving, or, in his words, "getting along" (being liked, accepted) and "getting ahead" (effectiveness, power). Social competence may entail balancing the two (Hawley, 2002); that is, a type of social competence may entail competing successfully in ways that foster social acceptance. After following a novel line of inquiry, Bukowski (2003) recently pointed out that the words "competence" and "compete" share a common linguistic lineage that reveals that competence originally conveyed successful competition in the presence of others. Successful competition in the presence of others is the hallmark of social dominance, the topic to which we turn next.

ASCENDANCE AND SOCIAL DOMINANCE IN THE EARLY 20TH CENTURY

Indeed broader approaches to competence were embraced in the first decades of the 20th century in various independently developing disciplines. Social and personality psychologists addressed ascendance and submission in terms of "instincts" (McDougall. 1908) and what Allport referred to as a "prominent determining tendency in behavior" (Allport, 1928–1929; p. 119). Even early child developmentalists pursued ascendance in preschoolers in part because "the roles assumed by the children in the play groups were soon evident and distinctly apparent" (Jack 1934; p. 10).[3] Even though these approaches did not focus on aggression per se, forcefulness, punitiveness, self-interest, persistent pursuit of one's own goals—even if these goals conflicted with those of others—were central identifying features of the ascendant individual (Allport, 1928–1929; Jack, 1934).

Important for this developing argument, submissiveness, the behavioral opposite of ascendancy (i.e., yielding, suggestible, conciliatory, passive; Allport & Allport, 1921), originally heralded a certain level of social incompetence. Submissive individuals were observed to be guided more by the desires and behavior of others and were accordingly seen as being at risk for "lack of self-confidence" (e.g., evident by children's appeals to adults, fear of companions, etc.; Jack, 1934, p. 40; see also Bühler, 1927). Jack additionally observed a previously submissive child to behave more like an ascendant child after his or her experience (and therefore self-confidence) in the experimental play situation was enhanced. In the end, she concluded that ascendancy was a function of the individual–context interface and that ascendant behavior could be learned.

At the same time, though apparently independently (i.e., one finds very few cross-citations), animal behaviorists were zealously setting their sights on social dominance (i.e., ascendance). The concept of the linear social dominance hierarchy is most often credited to Schjelderup-Ebbe (1922) for his early work on the peck-order (literally) of domestic fowl. Shortly thereafter, Robert Yerkes energized primatologists by proclaiming that, "dominance and subordination are evident in every group of primates. Apparently there is no such thing as equality of status and opportunity … each individual secures in its social group the degree of opportunity for control and self expression to which its characteristics and stage of development entitle it" (Yerkes, 1925; p. 155).

Social dominance was (and continues to be) most typically assessed by the number and direction of physical attacks and/or threats directed at conspecifics or peers. In other words, "dominance is inferred whenever one individual is able to chastise another with impunity" (Klopfer, 1974; p. 154). Because the outcome of such contests was clearly related to priority access to resources, priority access was deemed the raison

---

[3]In light of Jack's observation that ascendant behavior of children was immediately evident even to the casual observer, it seems incongruous that influential ethologist, Blurton Jones, would suggest that the concept of dominance would not be useful for understanding the social organization of preschool children (Blurton Jones, 1967).

d'etre of social dominance. The work in the ensuing decades addressed the complexity of such hierarchies and how they were related to much more than material resources (e.g., sexual behavior, physical health, grooming patterns, social preference, etc.; see Hawley, 1999 for review; Maslow, 1936; Scott, 1956; Zuckerman, 1932) and as such, hierarchies were seen as a central organizing feature of group living primates. From this work, it is clear that dominant individuals (in humans and animals) play highly central and visible roles in groups and consequently are targets of others' gazes, attention, and imitation. I refer to this phenomenon here and elsewhere as the social centrality hypothesis (Hawley, 1999; see also Chance, 1976).

Although early-century child developmentalists worried about how to alter ascendant behavior (e.g., enhance it; Jack, 1934; Page, 1936), or reduce the aggression associated with it (e.g., Wooley, 1925), ethological approaches designed for studying animal behavior (and only later human behavior) were characteristically less judgmental and more objective in variable choice and interpretation (a hallmark of ethology; Hinde, 1982; Tinbergen, 1963). Furthermore, ethologists were far less reticent than early child developmentalists about linking dominance squarely with aggression: In fact, when ethology seized social dominance and claimed it as its own, aggression was clearly key and central (e.g., stuggles, fights, agonism). Yet at the same time, the psychologists would have agreed with the ethologists that characteristics associated with submissiveness (Allport, 1928–1929) or subordinance (Maslow, 1936) would be associated with poor psychological health. That is, socially dominant apes or monkeys, or ascendant humans might be annoying or frightening, but relative to lower ranking others, aggressive dominants fare quite well. In fact, it was from his early work on primate social dominance that Maslow developed his model of self-esteem and, ultimately, self-actualization.

The Work of Abraham Maslow

Maslow is primarily remembered for his hierarchy of needs (1943) and self-actualization (1950). Yet he started out as a student of Harry Harlow, the legendary primatologist who made the study of "mother–infant love" a respectable scientific endeavor (e.g., Harlow, 1958). During those early years under Harlow's tutelage, Maslow made some important contributions to the work on social dominance.

Social psychologists contemporary to Maslow regarded ascendance–submission either as dual instincts (McDougall, 1908) or independent "enduring dispositions" (e.g., Allport, 1928–1929). Maslow broke away from similar language used by his mentor (e.g., Harlow & Yudin, 1933) and argued for the terms dominance and subordinance to (a) characterize the hierarchical nature of a relationship rather than enduring attitudinal aspects of the individual, (b) explicitly make the case for a universal dominance drive, that is (c) expressed more or less successfully depending on the social context. As a consequence, he made subordinance less of a personal proclivity, but rather an unfortunate outcome of being in the presence of a dominant other. As such, Maslow put dominance and subordinance at opposite ends of a "common impulse" (Maslow, 1936).

In Maslow's observations of captive primates, the dominant animal first and foremost had priority access to resources (e.g., food and females; see also Zuckerman, 1932). Furthermore, he observed the dominant animal to be sexually assertive, by far the most aggressive (both proactively and reactively), more likely to initiate play, and to have freedom of movement. Interestingly, he found these characteristics to hold whether the dominant was male or female (see also Hawley, Little, & Card, 2005). Subordinance, in contrast, was evidenced by lack of access to food, passivity, withdrawal, and the absence of aggression (Maslow & Flanzbaum, 1936). Maslow further viewed the dominant animal as "one whose behavior patterns … are carried out without deference to the behavior patterns of his associates" (e.g., autonomy; Deci & Ryan, 1985). In contrast, subordinates were "… limited, or inhibited by the behavior patterns of its more dominant associates" (Maslow, 1936; p. 263). Furthermore, this dominant behavior was highly dependent on social context in that "subordinates" would repeatedly behave like dominants when the opportunity arose. Thus we can see already in Maslow's work, like Jack's, the understanding of dominance clearly being associated with individual-level characteristics, but also inherently highly context-dependent.

Maslow and Flanzbaum (1936) observed that dominance was less due to size and age, but rather an "attitude of aggression or confidence" (p. 308). In part, consequent to dominance status (a relationship) and dominance behavior (e.g., bursts of temper, hostility), dominant individuals were more likely to enjoy "dominance feeling" (or "self esteem"; 1942) which he viewed as the evaluation of the self in terms of feelings of capability or superiority. In terms of Maslow's hierarchy of needs, esteem needs (desire for strength, prestige, and autonomy) follow physiological, safety, and love needs (for most, but not all) and are followed by the need for self-actualization (striving to achieve one's unique potential). The thwarting of need fulfillment at any level, Maslow observed, is met with an emergency response and ultimately significant ill being. Continued chronic thwarting of prepotent needs inhibits the emergence of the higher need. Thus, in the case of thwarted self-esteem/dominance needs, self-actualization tends not to be pursued.

I outline Maslow not because I defer to him as the final authority on social dominance; he was ultimately guided by his desire to understand human motivation and psychological outcomes and was limited by the methods of his time. On the other hand, his view of human motivation and social organization had deep biological roots. Rather than resorting to simplistic genetically deterministic arguments and evolutionary implausibilities (e.g., postulating that subordinance is an adaptation in and of itself), he understood that human fulfillment, happiness, and autonomy were at least in part a function of hierarchical social organization, and that chronic subordinance would have clear negative psychological impact.

The psychological impact of a prolonged history of competitive losses should be borne in mind in the discussion below of "noncontrollers," a group of children that arise from a resource control theoretic perspective. Before introducing Resource Control Theory, however, the evolution of cooperation must be discussed because it bears directly on a proposed broad class of behavioral tactic; namely, prosocial strategies of resource control.

THE EVOLUTION OF COOPERATION

Historically, interpreters of natural selection have aligned it with overt aggressive competition (within and between species); that is, "the struggle for existence" (Darwin, 1859/1884, p. 48), and "… Creation's final law—Tho' Nature, red in tooth and claw …" (Tennyson, 1892. p. 256). This alignment is especially clear in the social dominance literature that delights in the splendid morphological characteristics of some dominant males where the forces of sexual selection (male–male competition for females; Darwin, 1871; Trivers, 1972) have resulted in a sexual dimorphism for size, strength, and morphological weaponry (e.g., horns, antlers, tusks, canine teeth). Such an interpretative stance has made the evolution of altruism one of the greatest quandaries in theoretical biology (but see Hamilton, 1964; Trivers, 1971).

Early minority views had far less impact. For example, Kropotkin (1902) contended that under some conditions, cooperation would be a naturally selected alternative to aggressive competition, especially under harsh conditions and low population density (such as those of Siberian Russia; Kropotkin, 1902). That is, the "struggle for existence" not only meant intra- and intergroup competition, but organism against environment. This latter struggle could best be won, Kropotkin wrote, via mutual aid. Thomas Huxley's gladiatorial view ("… the strongest, the swiftest, and the cunningest live to fight another day"; Huxley, 1888,

p. 200) carried far more weight with European naturalists and early popular writings solidified it in the public's imagination (e.g., Lorenz, 1967).

It was not until Robert Trivers's seminal work on reciprocal altruism (1971) that individual-level selection (cf. group selection; e.g., Lorenz, 1967; Wynne-Edwards, 1962) was united with a viable theory of "altruism" (see also Hamilton, 1964). Here, "altruistic" behavior, according to Trivers, is not particularly self-sacrificing when one considers delayed benefits. That is, within the context of group living, social individuals perform altruistic acts with the implicit expectation that favors will be returned in the long run; hence the moniker, reciprocal altruism. Many of our social emotional responses, according to Trivers, probably evolved to navigate the complex economics of such exchanges. Mistrust, for example, alerts us to a potential partner that is unlikely to reciprocate. Thus, we are disinclined toward those we do not trust to reciprocate, and so on. Similar themes can be found in the Social Exchange Theories of Social Psychology that also postulate that humans are sensitive to inequities and balances in exchange processes in our social relationships (e.g., Walster, Walster, & Bersheid, 1978; see also de Waal, 1982). Both theoretical orientations would predict, for example, that the appeal of a potential social partner is in part a function of what that partner can bring to the relationship as a commodity for exchange (e.g., status, information, or wealth). Even though social exchange theories have not as a rule adopted an evolutionary metatheoretical orientation, I nonetheless draw on social exchange perspectives in the following section when I discuss why socially dominant preschoolers and adolescents win positive peer regard (one of the ultimate key points of this chapter).

Theories operating under an evolutionary metatheoretical umbrella typically recognize that the structure of a behavior may not clearly reveal function. Developmentalists, in contrast, have not traditionally been of the opinion that reciprocation, cooperation, and indeed prosociality in general, are essentially selfish (in terms of individuals' reproductive success).[4] Here, cooperation, reciprocation, and prosociality in general are seen to be other-oriented and to naturally unfold in the absence of developmental insult (a Rousseau-inspired view). Exceptions are those rare theories that recognize that prosocial behavior or cooperation can be employed to achieve one's own goals rather than a way to help others achieve theirs. Bowlby (1969), for example, recognized that successful infants must elicit care from their caregivers, and they do this by smiling,

---

[4]Group life/communality is a self-serving strategy in that those who chose to live outside the group at best had a very hard time of it, and at worst were doomed to starve or be eaten. This is not to say group life is without cost. One may be at increased risk for pathogens, intragroup aggression, and competition.

gazing, and cooing in addition to the more urgent crying. Smiling has proven itself over human evolutionary history to be a good way to induce others to attend to you (and give you valued resources; Frederickson, 1998). This noncontroversial observation is not limited to infancy: Preschoolers, adolescents, and indeed adults more successfully enter reciprocal (resource-yielding) relationships (e.g., friendships) by being attractive to others via warmth, sociability, and willingness and desire to reciprocate. It should thus come as no surprise that these characteristics are typically viewed as indicators of social competence.

Dualism in Human Motivation and Behavior.   This dualism—that competitive forces give rise to both antagonistic and other oriented behavioral strategies—underlies the present theoretical perspective, Resource Control Theory (Hawley, 1999). Specifically, the present theoretical orientation assumes that aggression and prosociality are functionally similar, yet phenomenologically distinct. A cry and a coo evolved to similar ends (they serve the same function, i.e., decrease distance between infant and caregiver), even though they have very different structures (negative vs. positive affect, which, like prosocial and coercive strategies discussed in the following section, are structurally independent; see also Charlesworth, 1996).

RESOURCE CONTROL THEORY

Resource control theory (RCT) was born out of an attempt to reconcile the social dominance hierarchies of nonaggressive female Asian elephants (Hawley, 1994) with children's social development within hierachically organized peer groups. Unlike prevailing animal-based models of social dominance, RCT shifts the focus from the structure of behavior (i.e., form; "struggles," agonism, aggression), to the function of behavior (resource control; Hawley, 1999). Shifting the focus to function gives rise to questions about how resource control can be achieved. Although resource control is a common feature across species and within a species across the lifespan, how that control is achieved and/or maintained (i.e., strategies) may vary markedly across species, undergo significant transformation across developmental time (as Bowlby himself noted), and be sensitive to environmental cues.

The notion of resource has been given considerable attention in behavioral ecology (another legacy of Tinbergen). For our purposes, we consider resources broadly to be material, social, and informational (Hawley, 2006a). Organisms require material resources for growth (e.g., food), survival (e.g., nesting sites), and cognitive and behavioral development (e.g., environmental stimulants; White, 1959). Social resources serve as alliance partners (Pusey & Packer, 1997), mates (Darwin, 1871), and models for social learning (Giraldeau, 1997). Information facilitates the acquisitions of both social and material resources (Giraldeau, 1997).

Prosocial and Coercive Strategies of Resource Control

Some resource control strategies are rather peculiar (e.g., the blue-headed wrasse can morph from a female to a male and, as a result, enjoy much-improved reproductive outcomes) and thus fall outside of the present discussion. However, in light of the above sketch of agonism-based social dominance, but also considering cooperative behavior to be a viable strategy, the following line of reasoning is focused predominantly on two broad resource control strategies; coercive and prosocial.

Prosocial strategies and coercive strategies are related insofar as they are proposed to have a common function; namely, resource control. This implies that the two strategies may be positively correlated in contrast to negatively correlated as would be assumed by traditional developmental approaches that align prosociality with other-orientedness and antisociality with self-orientedness (i.e., that prosocial and antisocial behavior should be negatively correlated). Because all humans potentially have access to both strategy types, their relative employment is a source of important individual differences.

Within the context of my research program, we have assessed prosocial and coercive strategies observationally (Hawley, 2002), by way of self-report (Hawley, 2003a; Hawley, Little, & Pasupathi, 2002), peer nomination (Hawley, Card & Little, in press), and teacher report (Hawley, 2003b). Though the measurement tools have been evolving, prosocial strategies are generally indicated by goal attainment via socially acceptable behavior. Observationally, this means a toy is traded or politely requested, or unsolicited help is offered (the play material is thus effectively commandeered; Hawley, 2002). Questionnaire or rater items assess reciprocation, being nice, or promising friendship (Hawley, 2003b). Coercive strategies are indicated by taking, threatening, or bullying. These studies thus far have been based on children as young as 3 years through adolescence. Overall, we find that prosocial and coercive strategies vary from being mildly to strongly positively correlated, depending on how they were measured (the strongest relationship by way of observation of preschoolers was $r = .67$; Hawley, 2002). We have found no negative correlations between prosocial and coercive strategies. This state of affairs suggests common function (though not necessarily common origin; e.g., equifinality).

Variable Centered Approaches

Variable centered approaches, or those focusing on linear relationships among variables, generally find that "good things go together" to some degree. We have replicated these correlations as well (e.g., Hawley, 2003a, 2003b). For example, prosocial strategies are positively correlated with positive personality traits (e.g., agreeableness), social skills (e.g., attention to social cues), affirming self-evaluation (e.g., social self-concept), and positive peer regard (e.g., "liked most" nominations). Conversely, we would expect to find—and have found—coercive strategies to be associated with more negative characteristics such as hostility, aggression, and self-serving motives (e.g., extrinsic motives for pursuing relationships; power, popularity). These findings replicate others that are common in the literature thus are not considered a significant contribution of the present approach. We do not always find, however, significant negative relationships between prosocial strategies and less desirable traits such as hostility, cheating, and aggression (e.g., Hawley, 2003a). Nor were coercive strategies negatively related to positive traits such as agreeableness, conscientiousness, and social skill. This simply means that one cannot predict negative traits by the level of prosocial strategies employed by the individual, nor could one predict positive traits by the use of coercive stategies. To some, these patterns seem counterintuitive. We find that they are significantly illuminated and explained by adopting a person-centered approach derived from resource control theory.

Resource Control Subtypes: A Person-Centered Approach

Person-centered approaches are by no means unfamiliar to developmentalists (e.g., Ainsworth, 1967; Ainsworth, Blehar, Waters, & Wall, 1978). We have found a person-centered approach to social dominance to be highly and uniquely informative. Specifically, individuals can employ one or the other strategy, neither strategy, or both. We have defined being "high" on prosocial and coercive strategy employment as scoring in the top 33% of the respective distributions, and scoring "low" on said distributions to be in the lower 33%.

Some individuals clearly favor prosocial strategies over coercive strategies. In terms of measurement, they are evident behaviorally in a laboratory set-up, individuals report their endorsement of them, or others (teachers, peers, friends) describe participants in these terms. One earns the moniker "prosocial controller" when one scores in the upper 33rd percentile of prosocial strategies of resource control observed in agemates and the lower 66th percentile on coercive strategies. Others employ coercive strategies over prosocial: They become "coercive controllers" when they score in the upper 33rd percentile on coercive control and the lower 66th percentile on prosocial control. "Bistrategic controllers" (Machiavellians; Hawley, 2001, 2003a, 2006b), employ both strategies in the upper 33rd percentile, "noncontrollers" score in the lower 33rd percentile of both strategies. "Typical controllers," the largest group, comprise the remainder. Although the cut-offs for sub-group membership are arbitrary, results from the typology have proven to be well in line with what has been predicted from this evolutionary metatheoretical perspective.

Prosocial controllers, for example, are highly skilled, agreeable, and socially appealing. They report intrinsic motivations for pursuing friendships with others (e.g., joy, personal fulfillment; Hawley et al., 2002), and appear to enjoy friendships that are high in intimacy and low in conflict (Hawley, Card, et al., in press). They are above average on resource control that confers them (by definition) higher than average social dominance status.

Coercive controllers, although also higher than average on resource control, are aggressive, hostile, and unskilled relative to other youths (Hawley, 2003b). They do not win positive attention in preschool nor in adolescence. Their motivations for friendship are extrinsic (power and popularity) and their friendships are marked by high conflict and low intimacy. Their behavior, personalities, and social reception suggest that they are comparable to unskilled, socially rejected aggressors.

Bistrategic controllers have characteristics in common with both prosocial and coercive controllers. Like their coercively controlling counterparts, bistrategic preadolescents and adolescents cheat, have a very high desire for recognition of their accomplishments, and score among the highest on traditional measure of aggression (i.e., overt and relational; Hawley, 2003a). At the same time, like prosocial controllers, they attract peers, impress teachers, are socially skilled, open to experience, extroverted, and morally astute (Hawley, 2003a, 2003b). They are even rated as among the most physically attractive by teachers who know them (Hawley, Napientek, Mize, & McNamara, 2005). Not only do they appear to be extremely effective resource controllers in their own opinion and in the opinion of their peers (i.e., socially dominant), but they can also effectively achieve and maintain high-status reputations (e.g., Cillessen & Rose, 2005). Because they reign supreme in terms of resource control, they are considered highly socially dominant from this view.

Most developmental theories predict that such high levels of "antisocial" behavior would be associated with social skills deficits and, consequently, peer rejection (see Coie & Dodge, 1998, for a review). Indeed, such characteristics describe well coercive controllers. Children as young as 3 to 5 years old discriminate between these two types of aggressors in that they gravitate toward bistrategic controllers (e.g., choose them as friends) and away from coercive controllers (e.g., choose them as nonfriends; see also, Vaughn, this volume).

In stark contrast to bistrategic controllers, noncontrollers are the lowest by far on resource control thus earning them very low social dominance status. Overall they report feeling socially ineffective, lonely, and unable to attain goals. Noncontrolling preschoolers are described as the least assertive and aggressive by teachers, yet are among the lowest on positive peer regard (Hawley, Napientek, et al., 2006). Noncontrolling adolescents are among the lowest on positive affect, social self-concept, social skills, and, though low on aggression and hostility, are unpopular and perceived as rejected by their peers (Hawley, 2003a).

Thus, in summary, we, like others (e.g., Bierman, Smoot, & Aumiller, 1993; Coie, Dodge, Terry, & Wright, 1991; Newcomb, Bukowski, & Patee, 1993; Rodkin, Farmer, Pearl, & van Aker, 2000) find that aggressive children and youths (and likely adults) do not compose a homogenous group. Bistrategic controllers, despite their aggression, are socially skilled in ways coercive controllers (and noncontrollers) are not.

Social Centrality

In a review of the social dominance literature (Hawley, 1999), I suggested that, with the broadening of the social dominance construct to include prosocial strategies (in addition to traditional agonism-based notions of social dominance), human patterns of social organization would converge with those documented in animal groups; namely, that social dominants would attract positive attention from the group. As high-status individuals, the social centrality hypothesis suggests that bistrategic controllers should be well regarded by peers, sought out by them, and, for those who are less able to compete for their attention (e.g., because of their lower status), a target of their social aspirations. This hypothesis, however, faces competing hypotheses that would suggest that their aggressive behavior would be ultimately repellent to others, except perhaps for those drawn together by "common deviance" (e.g., Dishion, Andrews, & Crosby, 1995; Moffitt, 1993).

My colleagues and I have repeatedly found support for the social centrality hypothesis; bistrategic controllers are among the most sought out and socially prominent. Data gathered from thousands of participants from 3 to 17 years of age fails to support suggestions that the aggression employed by these children significantly negatively impacts their social standing among peers. On the contrary, it appears to enhance it (see also Cillessen & Mayeaux, 2004).

Are "Mean" Social Dominants *Liked*?

The term "status" currently holds multiple meanings, thus creating a vibrant yet somewhat confusing literature landscape. Ethnographic studies (e.g., Adler & Adler, 1995; Eder, 1995; Merten, 1997), for example, provide detailed accounts of adolescent "status hierarchies" characterized by competition for and defense of "popularity." Of the several contributions of this work, two are particularly relevant here. First, females' relational, social, or indirect aggression appears to be associated with popularity rather than unpopularity. Second, this literature highlights the fact that popularity and being liked (sometimes also referred to as sociometric status) are not identical. Thus, being socially prominent does not necessitate being beloved.

Currently, the relationship between social prominence (popularity) and social preference (being liked) is being explored to clarify these apparently overlapping yet distinct constructs (e.g., Cillessen & Mayeux, this volume). Recent work has shown that relational aggression appears to be positively associated with social prominence and becomes more so as children age. On the other hand, early positive associations between social preference and social prominence reduce over time. Thus, these two measures of peer status become more distinct as children grow older (Cillessen & Mayeux, 2004) suggesting that aggressive socially prominent adolescents are not in fact well liked.

This variable-centered work on social prominence, like the person-centered work stemming from resource control theory, attempts to address what we refer to as the peer regard–aggression paradox[5] (Hawley, Little, et al., 2005; Hawley & McNamara, 2006) by teasing apart two dimensions of status (social preference and social prominence) and exploring their relationship longitudinally (e.g., Cillessen & Mayeux, 2004; Rose, Swenson, & Waller, 2004). The distinction between social prominence and social preference is critical because socially preferred youth enjoy present and future positive outcomes such as emotional adjustment and high quality friendships. It is not presently clear from these variable centered approaches, however, whether socially prominent youths also enjoy these outcomes, or whether immediate status advantages are followed by long-term adjustment difficulties because of the lower quality friendships these children are believed to bear (Cillessen & Rose, 2005).

In contrast, our work from resource control theory arrives at very different conclusions. Recent work has shown (Hawley, Card, et al., in

---

[5]The apparent social attractiveness of aggressive individuals which, from some perspectives, is unexpected.

press) that bistrategically controlling adolescents enjoy as many reciprocal best friendships as the other resource control groups, but receive
more nominations for best friendship than average (that is, they are
named by their peers as being the peers' "best friend"). Moreover,
detailed analyses of their bidirectional relationship processes (i.e.,
where both parties of the reciprocal best friendship describe the quality of that relationship) showed that the friendships of bistrategic controllers are among the highest in terms of positive features (i.e., high on
intimacy, companionship, and fun). These same relationships, however,
also have high levels of conflict. Where such a relationship stands on
the "quality continuum" when characterized by positive and negative
features is open to debate. It is useful to note, however, that prominent
marital researchers as well as primatologists have made the case that
the amount of conflict is less important than the ways this conflict is
resolved (de Waal, 2000; Gottman, 1994; but see Brendgen, Markiewicz,
Doyle, & Bukowski, 2001). At this time, however, we have little reason
to believe that bistrategic controllers suffer from poor quality relationships. Thus, we do not believe they necessarily carry any long-term risk
associated with low-friendship quality.

In the end, we come to similar conclusions as those early ascendancy and dominance researchers; individuals with very high social
dominance status appear to fare quite well.

GENDER DIFFERENCES AND SIMILARITIES

Because we align social dominance with competitive success, we, in
contrast to those who align social dominance more closely with agonism and physical aggression, expect fewer gender differences because
we do not believe competition for resources is any less important for
females than males. Indeed, resource competition may well be more
important and have more long-term, cross-generational implications for
females (Hawley, Little, et al., 2005, Hrdy, 1999). Although my colleagues
and I have documented that males overall report higher levels of dominance motivations and aggression than females (Hawley, Little, et al.,
2005), we find that by comparing males and females within the resource
control types, gender differences reduce considerably and in some cases
disappear altogether. For example, there are as many bistrategic girls as
there are bistrategic boys, even though they are derived by identical
criteria (i.e., girls were not normed separately from boys). Like bistrategic boys, bistrategic girls report high levels of motivations associated
with social dominance, as well as high levels of overt and relational
aggression (a finding anticipated by Maslow). Also like bistrategic boys,

bistrategic girls are liked more than average, their aggressive behavior (both overt and relational) notwithstanding. Likewise, bistrategic boys exhibit behaviors typically associated with girls (emotion-decoding skills, high levels of relational aggression). Thus it appears to us that high status individuals utilize all manner of behaviors associated with status pursuit rather than operating solely within gender normative expectations.

Not only do gender differences reduce considerably when looking at within status gender variability, we find that differences even reverse in direction from that which is predicted from other perspectives. For example, high-status/aggressive females experience social backlash in occupational contexts where they are punished socially (i.e., judged negatively) for their agency (e.g., Rudman & Glick, 1999). Resource control theory would predict that high-status females in general would be highly socially attractive for the same reason that high status males would be (i.e., the social centrality hypothesis); namely, they have demonstrated competency with material, social, and informational resources and as such make for highly valued alliance partners (Walster et al., 1978). In this work, bistrategic females were found to be equally socially attractive as bistrategic males and more socially attractive than prosocially controlling males. Additionally, those not already friends with bistrategic females aspired to be (Hawley, Little, et al., 2005). This suggests that others recognize that these high status individuals bring much to relationships and wish to engage in reciprocal exchange with them (i.e., forge a friendship). In other words, we generally wish to affiliate with those of higher status, if only we could compete successfully for their attention.

SOCIAL DOMINANCE: A FUNCTION OF GENES AND ENVIRONMENT

Contextual factors are fundamental to social dominance from the present approach. First, from the previous discussion, we see that aggressiveness alone is a suboptimal strategy. The bistrategic profile encourages us to broaden our understanding of context to include other characteristics of the individual such as the presence of social skills and proclivities: Aggression coupled with more positive qualities make for social and material success in ways that aggression alone does not.

Second, social dominance (i.e., competitive superiority) is an aspect of a relationship asymmetry. Though recognized early on, this point was not adequately addressed by ethological studies of social dominance that emphasized hierarchies over complex dyadic relationships (Vaughn, 1999). We now know that social behavior, including that involving a contested resource, is highly dependent on the identities of the players, their personal characteristics, and the unique history of their interactions. By employing a social relations paradigm (i.e., Kenny & Lavoie, 1984), for example, and observing multiple dyadic interactions in a controlled laboratory setting, my colleagues and I (Hawley & Little, 1999) found high ranking preschoolers more likely to engage in social play (see also Maslow, 1936) and issue directives (see also Jack, 1934), whereas social subordinates were more likely to defer to dominants and imitate them (see also Bühler, 1927). Importantly, like Jack and Maslow, we found children of middle rank to modify their behavior according to the rank of their social partner. In the presence of social dominants, middle-ranking children deferred and imitated. In the presence of subordinates, however, they confidently engaged the play material. When given the opportunity, subordinates behaved like dominants.

It follows then that social dominance cannot be solely a genetically encoded trait because competition transcends the individual to encompass relationships. Thus, it would be inappropriate to speak of a "gene for dominance." Resource-directedness is very likely the underlying evolutionary adaptation of which we speak. It would not be a stretch to claim that those who were not resource directed are not our ancestors.

Yet there is clearly variability in the manner in which resource directedness is expressed and, accordingly, the genetic underpinnings of several traits predicting social dominance can also be considered. For example, in defining social dominance in terms of competition rather than agonism, we have not found social dominance to be strongly related to size or gender. Instead, we find stronger associations with temperament, personality, and motivational features. In preschoolers, for example, we have found social dominance to be predicted by persistence, extroversion, and openness to experience, all of which may be heritable to some extent.

Furthermore, in addition to the well-substantiated fact that aggressive behavior can be learned (e.g., Bandura et al., 1961), there is also undoubtedly a conditioned component to relative success or failure at competition and therefore also the form and intensity of future attempts (see also Pusey & Packer, 1997). When there are "winners" of competition, there sadly must also be "losers." Experiencing early losses repeatedly in competitive interactions could intensify individual differences in persistence or effectance motivation. For Maslow (1937), this feature was "dominance feeling" or later, "self-esteem" (Maslow, 1942). Some might call it "hope" (e.g., Snyder, 2002), others, "agency" (e.g., Hawley & Little, 2002; Skinner, Chapman, & Baltes, 1988). Because the noncontrolling strategy can be created experientially, genetic mechanisms need not be invoked for explaining losing strategies. Deferring to others can be considered simply making the best of a bad situation.

Patterns of deferring to social dominants emerge already before preschool (Bühler, 1927; Hawley & Little, 1999). Indeed, it is the possibility of a persistent pattern of deference that raises concern for the development of social subordinates, those who employ neither coercive nor prosocial strategies (i.e., noncontrollers). What if a socially subordinate child seldom has the opportunity to play the dominant role or to behave like dominants (a lá Maslow and Jack)? Anecdotally, I have observed nonverbal and withdrawn noncontrollers blossom into agentic extroverts within weeks of dominant peers graduating to kindergarten. What of the noncontroller who enjoys no such contextual transformation; is his or her learning opportunities thusly restricted? Are they learning they can have little effect on the world? From the present perspective, these noncontrolling youths are most at risk for psychopathology because, as just described, they apparently make few control attempts, do not know their impact on the social world, and find themselves rejected, victimized, and depressed.

IMPLICATIONS FOR INTERVENTION

The material and social success of bistrategics resource controllers are due at least in part to their elevated levels of aggression because this feature sets them apart from prosocial controllers. By virtue of the fact that they are well-regarded by many in the peer group, it appears that developing humans do not find aggression quite as repellant as conventional wisdom might suggest.

On the other hand, every act of aggression presumably has a victim. We should bear in mind, however, the distinction between repeated victims of aggression (e.g., whipping boys, etc.; Olweus, 1993) from those who are aggressed against by their powerful peers within their friendship circles. In our studies, we have seen no evidence that bistrategic controllers wantonly wound others for pleasure, or even repeatedly target those weaker than themselves (i.e., they do not appear to be the classic "schoolyard bullies"). Indeed, the targets of their aggression appear to be their very own best friends (Hawley, Card, et al., in press; see also Vaughn, this volume).

Coercive controllers, in contrast to bistrategic controllers, are undercontrolled, have poor social skills, and low peer acceptance. These characteristics presumably bring these aggressive children to the attention of school personnel for referral to interventions targeting aggressive behavior (Burke, Loeber, & Birmaher, 2002). Teachers even rate these children as the least physically attractive, perhaps consequent to dealing with these deficits on a daily basis (Hawley, Napientek, et al., 2005). Therapeutic interventions could be viewed as a form of skill-building whereby these children are taught the prosocial skills they need to balance their shortcomings that emerge from purely coercive attempts (e.g., Fraser et al., 2005).

Interventions that have proven effective for unskilled aggressors like coercive controllers are likely to be less effective with bistrategic controllers. Recall that despite their high levels of aggression (relational and overt), they are socially attuned and morally developed (and in adolescence, their aggression may not be detected by teachers; Hawley, 2003a). Thus, the moral education, skill-building, perspective taking enhancements, and sensitivity training would likely be of little value to youths who are already excelling in these domains. Does this work suggest the targets of our interventions should be noncontrollers and they should be taught to behave more like bistrategics? A related question was similarly posed by Helen Woolley (1925) in her description of Agnes, a 4-year-old girl who stood out her "desire to manage," her "intense interest in her fellowmen," an ability to anticipate the needs and emotions of others (including adults), persistence, sympathy towards other children, as well as her capacity for aggression. Woolley asked whether we should extinguish the "executive skills" of a developing girl or nurture them. The answers are far from clear and are unlikely to draw consensus.

CONTROVERSY AND MORALITY

Resource control theory gives rise to testable predictions about profiles of strategy employment in social groups. Specifically, we would expect that social dominance (i.e., successful resource control) to be well served by aggression balanced with social skills and, moreover, that such effective balancing would win both material and social rewards. Yet our expectations and findings about socially dominant bistrategic males and females strike some as "controversial" and "unexpected." Why? Perhaps, because Rousseauian philosophies and derivative theoretical perspectives generally consider aggression to be a key marker of incompetence and pathology. To claim that such "psychopathology" can be beneficial and therefore "good" would be controversial indeed. However, these claims have not been made anywhere.

First, it is not at all clear that aggressive self expression is "pathological," particularly when accompanied by prosocial skills and strategies. The bistrategic profile has made this point abundantly clear. They are extroverted and open to experience, have well-developed social skills, and experience friendships more than most. Rather than being limited by few behavioral options for a given situation (e.g., "only defer," or "only recip-rocate"), they appear to have more options than most (e.g., reciprocate, dominate, retaliate). Additionally, they may stand superior in their ability to size up situations and predict the behaviors, goals, and motivations of others (Sutton, Smith, & Swettenham, 1999a, 1999b; see also Hawley, 2006b, for an extended discussion from evolutionary and game theoretic perspectives). The concern about the bistrategic profile appears to be one of relative values derived ultimately from moral treatises.

By taking an evolutionary stance and pointing out that aggression appears to be employed effectively with benefit by some, do we con-clude that "aggression is good"? Beginning students of evolutionary theory commonly fall into the trap of concluding that what is "natural" is "good." Infanticide is "natural" insofar as it occurs with great regu-larity in many taxa, including humans. Do we therefore conclude that "infanticide is good"? Of course not. The issue is not merely academic. Some of the most mean-spirited and inhumane social policies derived from this naturalistic fallacy (e.g., Spencer, 1855).

For centuries, natural scientists struggled to see God's benevolence in nature (to "… infer God's essence from the products of his creation"; Gould, 1983, p. 38). Nature, it was recognized offered profound beauty and evidence of design. Yet on closer inspection, nature also proved to be extremely cruel. Nature in fact is amoral and therefore cannot give rise to ethical principles (Gould, 1983; Moore, 1903). I am no theologian, philoso-pher, or ethicist and thus am ill-qualified to comment on the nature of "goodness." Suffice it to say that one should not simplistically conclude that "aggression is good" based on the preceding presentation.

CONCLUSIONS

Those wishing to align social competence with "goodness" are unlikely to find solace in these final comments. Just as Freud did not see happiness as a realistic outcome of societal constraints, Darwin did not imply that the successful group-living individual would embody moral righteous-ness. I agree with Bukowski (2003) who pointed out that "univariate claims" linking positive behavior with positive outcomes and negative behavior with negative outcomes are not likely to adequately capture the complexity of human behavior. Though we are by nature gregarious, we are also acquisitive. A unique brand of social competence may very well be found where these two independent forces collide.

REFERENCES

Adler, P. A., & Adler, P. (1995). Dynamics of inclusion and exclusion in preadolesent cliques. *Social Psychology Quarterly, 58*, 145–162.

Ainsworth, M. D. S. (1967). *Infancy in Uganda; infant care and the growth of love.* Baltimore: Johns Hopkins Press.

Ainsworth, M. D. S., Blehar, M. C., Waters, E., & Wall, S. (1978). *Patterns of attachment: A psychological study of the strange situation.* Hillsdale, NJ: Lawrence Erlbaum Associates.

Allport, G. W. (1928–1929). A test for ascendance-submission. *Journal of Abnormal and Social Psychology, 23*, 118–136.

Allport, F. H., & Allport, G. W. (1921). Personality traits: Their classification and measurement. *Journal of Abnormal and Social Psychology, 16*, 6–40.

Bagwell, C. L., Coie, J. D., Terry, R. A., & Lochman, J. E. (2000). Peer clique participation and social status in preadolescence. *Merrill-Palmer Quarterly, 46*, 280–305.

Bandura, A. (1969). *Principles of behavior modification.* New York: Holt, Rinehart, & Winston.

Bandura, A., Ross, D., & Ross, S. A. (1961). Transmission of aggression through imitation of aggressive models. *Journal of Abnormal and Social Psychology, 63*, 575–582.

Bandura, A., & Walters, R. H. (1959). *Adolescent aggression.* New York: Ronald Press.

Bernstein, I. S. (1981). Dominance: The baby and the bathwater. *Behavioral and Brain Sciences, 4*, 419–457.

Bierman, K. L., Smoot, D. L., & Aumiller, K. (1993). Characteristics of aggressive-rejected, aggressive (non-rejected), and rejected (non-aggressive) boys. *Child Development, 64*, 139–151.

Bjorklund, D. F., & Pellegrini, A. D. (2002). *The origins of human nature: Evolutionary developmental psychology.* Washington DC: American Psychological Association.

Blurton Jones, N.G. (1967). An ethological study of some aspects of social behaviour of children in nursery school. In D. Morris (Ed.), *Primate ethology* (pp. 347–368). Chicago, IL: Aldine.

Blurton Jones, N. (1972). Characteristics of ethological studies of human behaviour. In N. Blurton Jones (Ed.), *Ethological studies of child behaviour* (pp. 3–33). Cambridge, UK: Cambridge University Press.

Bost, K. K., Vaughn, B. E., Washington, W. N., Cielinski, K. L., & Bradbard, M. R. (1998). Social competence, social support, and attachment: Demarcation of construct domains, measurement, and paths of influence for preschool children attending Head Start. *Child Development, 69*, 192–218.

Bowlby, J. (1969). *Attachment and loss (Vols. 1 and 2).* New York: Basic Books.

Brendgen, M., Markiewicz, D., Doyle, A. B., & Bukowski, W. M. (2001). The relations between friendship quality, ranked-friendship preference, and adolescents' behavior with their friends. *Merrill-Palmer Quarterly, 47*, 395–415.

Brook J. S., & Newcomb, M. D. (1995). Childhood aggression and unconventionality: Impact on later academic achievement, drug use, and workforce involvement. *Journal of Genetic Psychology, 156*, 393–410.

Brown, J. L., & Hunsperger, R. W. (1963). Neuroethology and the motivation of agonistic behavior. *Animal Behavior, 11,* 439–448.

Bühler, C. (1927). Die ersten socialen Verhaltungsweisen des Kindes [The first social behavior of the child]. In C. Bühler, H. Hetzer, & B. Tudor-Hart (Eds.), *Soziologische und psychologische studien über das erste Lebensjahr* (Social and psychological studies of the first year of life] (pp. 1–202). Jena, Germany: Gustav Fischer.

Bukowski, W. M. (2003). What does it mean to say that aggressive children are competent or incompetent? *Merrill-Palmer Quarterly, 49,* 390–400.

Burke, J. D., Loeber, R., & Birmaher, B. (2002). Oppositional defiant disorder and conduct disorder: A review of the past 10 years, part II. *Journal of the American Academy of Child and Adolescent Psychiatry, 41,* 1275–1293.

Chance, M. R. A. (1976). Attention structures as the basis of primate rank orders. *Man, 2,* 503–518.

Charlesworth, W. R. (1996). Co-operation and competition: Contributions to an evolutionary and developmental model. *International Journal of Behavioral Development, 19,* 25–38.

Christie, R. (1970). Why Machiavelli? In R. Christie & F. Geis (Eds.), *Studies in Machiavellianism* (pp. 1–9). New York: Academic Press.

Cillessen, A. H. N., & Mayeux, L. (2004). From censure to reinforcement: Developmental changes in the association between aggression and social status. *Child Development, 75,* 147–163.

Cillessen, A. H. N., & Rose, A. J. (2005). Understanding popularity in the peer system. *Current Directions in Psychological Science. 14,* 10–105.

Coie, J. D., & Dodge, K. A. (1998). Aggression and antisocial behavior. In W. Damon (Series Ed.) & N. Eisenberg (Vol. Ed.), *Handbook of child psychology: Vol. 3. Social, emotional, and personality development* (5th ed., pp. 779–862). New York: Wiley.

Coie, J. D., Dodge, K. A., & Kupersmidt, J. (1990). Peer group behavior and social status. In S. R. Asher & J. D. Coie (Eds.), *Peer rejection in childhood* (pp. 17–59). New York: Cambridge University Press.

Coie, J. D., Dodge, K. A., Terry, R., & Wright, V. (1991). The role of aggression in peer relations: An analysis of aggression episodes in boys' play groups. *Child Development, 62,* 812–826.

Darwin, C. (1859/1884). *On the origin of species by means of natural selection* (7th ed.). New York: Appleton & Co.

Darwin, C. (1871). *The descent of man and selection in relation to sex.* London: Murray.

Deci, E. L., & Ryan, R. M. (1985). *Intrinsic motivation and self determination in human behavior.* New York: Plenum.

Dishion, T. J, Andrews, D. W., & Crosby, L. (1995). Antisocial boys and their friends in early adolescence: Relationship characteristics, quality, and interactional processes. *Child Development, 66,* 139–151.

Eder, D. (1995). *School talk: Gender and adolescent culture.* New Brunswik, NJ: Rutgers University Press.

Feist, G. J. (1993). A structural model of scientific eminence. *Psychological Science, 4,* 366–371.

Fraser, M. W., Galinsky, M. J., Smokowski, P. R., Day, S. H., Terzian, M. A., Rose, R. A., et al. (2005). Social information-processing skills training to promote social competence and prevent aggressive behavior in the third grades. *Journal of Consulting and Clinical Psychology, 73*, 1045–1055.

Fredrickson, B. L. (1998). What good are positive emotions? *Review of General Psychology, 2*, 300–319.

Freud, S. S. (1930/1961). *Civilization and its discontents.* New York: Norton.

Giraldeau, L. A. (1997). The ecology of information use. In J. R. Krebs & N. B. Davies (Eds.), *Behavioural ecology: An evolutionary approach* (4th ed., pp. 42–68). Malden, MA: Blackwell.

Gottman, J. M. (1994). *What predicts divorce? : The relationship between marital processes and marital outcomes.* Hillsdale, NJ: Lawrence Erlbaum Associates.

Gould, S. J. (1983). *Hen's teeth and horse's toes.* New York: Norton.

Hamilton, W. D. (1964). The genetical evolution of social behaviour I and II. *Journal of Theoretical Biology, 7*, 1–52.

Harlow, H. F. (1958). The nature of love. *American Psychologist, 13*, 573–685.

Harlow, H. F., & Yudin, H. C. (1933). Social behavior of primates: I. Social facilitation of feeding in monkeys and its relation to attitudes of ascendance and submission. *Journal of Comparative Psychology, 16*, 171–185.

Hawley, P. H. (1994). *On being an elephant: A quantitative intraindividual analysis of the behavior of Elephas maximus.* Unpublished doctoral dissertation, University of California, Riverside.

Hawley, P. H. (1999). The ontogenesis of social dominance: A strategy-based evolutionary perspective. *Developmental Review, 19*, 97–132.

Hawley, P. H. (2001, April). Coercive strategies of resource control in pre/adolescents: *Maladaptation vs. Machiavellianism.* Symposium presentation at the Biennial Meeting of the Society for Research in Child Development, Minneapolis, MN.

Hawley, P. H. (2002). Social dominance and prosocial and coercive strategies of resource control in preschoolers. *International Journal of Behavioral Development, 26*, 167–176.

Hawley, P. H. (2003a). Strategies of control, aggression, and morality in preschoolers: An evolutionary perspective. *Journal of Experimental Child Psychology, 85*, 213–235.

Hawley, P. H. (2003b). Prosocial and coercive configurations of resource control in early adolescence: A case for the well-adapted Machiavellian. *Merrill-Palmer Quarterly, 49*, 279–309.

Hawley, P. H. (2006a). *Resource control strategies inventory–revised.* Unpublished questionnaire. University of Kansas, Lawrence, KS.

Hawley, P. H. (2006b). Evolution and personality: A new look at Machiavellianism. In D. Mroczek & T. Little (Eds.), *Handbook of personality development* (pp. 147–161). Mahwah, NJ: Lawrence Erlbaum Associates.

Hawley, P. H., Card, N. A., & Little, T. D. (in press). The allure of the mean friend: Relationship quality and processes of aggressive adolescents. *International Journal of Behavioral Development.*

Hawley, P. H., & Little, T. D. (1999). Winning some and losing some: A social relations approach to social dominance in toddlers. *Merrill-Palmer Quarterly, 45,* 185–214.

Hawley, P. H., & Little, T. D. (2002). Evolutionary and developmental perspectives on the agentic self. In D. Cervone & W. Mischel (Eds.), *Advances in personality science, Vol. 1* (pp. 177–195). New York: Guilford.

Hawley, P. H., Little, T. D, & Card, N. A. (2005). *The myth of the alpha male: A new look at dominance-related beliefs and behaviors among adolescent males and females.* Manuscript under review.

Hawley, P. H., Little, T. D., & Pasupathi, M. (2002). Winning friends and influencing peers: Strategies of peer influence in late childhood. *International Journal of Behavioral Development, 26*, 466–474.

Hawley, P. H., & McNamara, K. A. (2006, April). *Machiavellianism and emotional competence: Addressing the peer regard—aggression paradox.* Paper presented at the Biennial Meeting of the Society for Research on Adolescence. San Francisco, CA.

Hawley, P. H., Napientek, S. E., Mize, J. A., & McNamara, K. A. (2006). *Beauty and power: The social and visual appeal of aggressive social dominants.* Manuscript under review.

Hinde, R. A. (1966). *Animal behaviour: A synthesis of ethology and comparative psychology.* New York: McGraw-Hill.

Hinde, R. A. (1982). *Ethology: Its nature and relations with other sciences.* New York: Oxford.

Hobbes, T. (1651/1885) *Leviathan, or the matter, form and power of a commonwealth, ecclesiastical and civil.* London: Routledge & Sons.

Hogan, R. (1982). A socioanalytic theory of personality. *Nebraska Symposium on Motivation, 30,* 55–89.

Hogan, R., Raskin, R., & Fazzini, D. (1990). The dark side of charisma. In K. E. Clark & M. B. Clark, (Eds.), *Measures of leadership* (pp. 343–354). West Orange, NJ: Leadership Library of America, Inc.

Hrdy, S. B. (1999). *The woman that never evolved.* Cambridge, MA: Harvard University Press.

Huxley, T. (1888). The struggle for existence in human society. *The Nineteenth Century, 23,* 195–236.

Jack, L. M. (1934). An experimental study of the ascendant behavior in preschool children. Behavior of the preschool child. In G. D. Stoddard (Ed.), *University of Iowa Studies in Child Welfare, 9,* 9–65.

Kenny, D., & LaVoie, L. (1984). The social relations model. In L. Berkowitz (Ed.), *Advances in experimental social psychology* (Vol. 18, pp. 142–182). New York: Academic Press.

Klopfer, P. H. (1974). *An introduction to animal behavior: Ethology's first century.* Englewood Cliffs, NJ: Prentice-Hall.

Kokko, K., & Pulkkinen, L. (2000). Aggression in childhood and longterm unemployment in adulthood: A cycle of maladaptation and some protective factors. *Developmental Psychology, 36,* 463–472.

Kropotkin, P. (1902). *Mutual aid: A factor of evolution.* London: Doubleday.

Krueger, R. F., Hicks, B. M., & McGue, M. (2001). Altruism and antisocial behavior: Independent tendencies, unique personality correlates, distinct etiologies. *Psychological Science, 12,* 397–402.

Locke, J. (1690/1975). *An essay concerning human understanding.* Oxford, UK: Clarendon Press.

Lorenz, K. (1967). *On aggression.* New York: Bantam.

Luthar, S. S., & McMahon, T. J. (1996). Peer reputation among inner-city adolescents: Structure and correlates. *Journal of Research on Adolescence, 6,* 581–603.

Maslow, A. (1936). The role of dominance in the social and sexual behavior of infra-human primates: I. Observations at Vilas Park Zoo. *Journal of Genetic Psychology, 48,* 261–277.

Maslow, A. (1937). Dominance-feeling, behavior, and status. *Psychological Review, 44,* 404–429.

Maslow, A. (1940). Dominance-quality and social behavior in infra-human primates. *Journal of Social Psychology, 11,* 313–324.

Maslow, A. (1942). Self-esteem (dominance-feeling) and sexuality in women. *The Journal of Social Psychology,, 16,* 259–294.

Maslow, A. (1943). A theory of human motivation. *Psychological Review, 50,* 370–396.

Maslow, A. (1950). *Self-actualizing people: A study of psychological health. Personality Symposium: Symposium #1 on values.* New York: Grune & Stratton.

Maslow, A., & Flanzbaum, S. (1936). The role of dominance in the social and sexual behavior of infra-human primates: II. An experimental determination of the dominance behavior syndrome. *Journal of Genetic Psychology, 48,* 278–309.

McDougall, W. (1908). *An introduction to social psychology.* Boston: John W. Luce.

McGrew, W. C. (1972). *An ethological study of children's behavior.* New York: Academic Press.

Merten, D. (1997). The meaning of meanness: Popularity, competition, and conflict among junior high school girls. *Sociology of Education, 70,* 175–191.

Moffitt, T. E. (1993). Adolescence-limited and life-course-persistent antisocial behavior: A developmental taxonomy. *Psychological Review, 100,* 674–701.

Moore, G. E. (1903). *Principia ethica.* Cambridge, UK: Cambridge University Press.

Newcomb, A. F., Bukowski, W. M., & Pattee, L. (1993). Children's peer relations: A meta-analytic review of popular, rejected, neglected, controversial and average sociometric status. *Psychological Bulletin, 113,* 99–128.

Olweus, D. (1993). *Bullying at school.* Oxford, UK: Blackwell.

Page, M. L. (1936). The modification of ascendant behavior in preschool children. *Iowa Studies in Child Welfare, 12.*

Pellegrini, A. D. (2004). Sexual segregation in childhood: A review of evidence for two hypotheses. Animal Behaviour, *68,* 435–443.

Pinker, S. (2002). *The blank slate: The modern denial of human nature.* New York: Viking.

Pusey, A. E., & Packer, C. (1997). The ecology of relationships. In J. R. Krebs & N. B. Davies (Eds.), *Behavioural ecology: An evolutionary approach* (4th ed., pp. 254–283). Malden, MA: Blackwell.

Rodkin, P. C., Farmer, T. W., Pearl, R., & Van Acker, R. (2000). Heterogeneity of popular boys: Antisocial and prosocial configurations. *Developmental Psychology, 36,* 14–24.

Rose, A. J., Swenson, L. P., & Waller, E. M. (2004). Overt and relational aggression and perceived popularity: Developmental differences in concurrent and prospective relations. *Developmental Psychology, 40*, 378–387.

Rousseau, J. J. (1762/1955). *Emile.* New York: Dutton.

Rubin, K. H., & Rose-Krasnor, L. (1992) Interpersonal problem solving and social competence in children. In V. B. Van Hasselt & M. Hersen (Eds.), *Handbook of social development: A lifespan perspective* (pp. 283–323). New York: Plenum.

Rudman, L. A., & Glick, P. (1999). Feminized management and backlash toward agentic women: The hidden costs to women of a kinder, gentler image of middle managers. *Journal of Personality and Social Psychology, 77*, 1004–1010.

Sandstrom, M. J. (1999). A developmental perspective on peer rejection: Mechanisms of stability and change. *Child Development, 70*, 955–966.

Scott, J. P. (1956). The analysis of social organization in animals. *Ecology, 37*, 213–221.

Schjelderup-Ebbe, T. (1922). Beiträge zur Sozialpsychologie des Haushuhns [Contributions to the social psychology of domestic chickens]. *Zeitschrift für Psychologie, 88*, 225–252.

Skinner, E. A., Chapman, M., & Baltes, P. B. (1988). Children's beliefs about control, means-ends, and agency: Developmental differences during middle childhood. *International Journal of Behavioral Development, 11*, 369–388.

Snyder, C. R. (2002). Hope theory: Rainbows in the mind. *Psychological Inquiry, 13*, 249–275.

Spencer, H. (1855). *The principles of psychology.* London: Longman, Brown, Green, and Longman.

Strayer, F. F., & Strayer, J. (1976). An ethological analysis of social agonism and dominance relations among preschool children. *Child Development, 47*, 980–989.

Sutton, J., Smith, P. K., & Swettenham, J. (1999a). Bullying and "theory of mind": A critique of the "social skills deficit" view of anti-social behaviour. *Social Development, 8*, 117–127.

Sutton, J., Smith, P. K., & Swettenham, J. (1999b). Social cognition and bullying: Social inadequacy or skilled manipulation? *British Journal of Developmental Psychology, 17*, 435–450.

Tennyson, A. L. (1892). *In memoriam A. H. H.* New York: Grosset & Dunlap.

Tinbergen, N. (1963). On aims and methods of ethology. *Zeitschrift fur Tierpsychologie, 20*, 410–433.

Trivers, R. L. (1971). The evolution of reciprocal altruism. *Quarterly Review of Biology, 46*, 35–57.

Trivers, R. L. (1972). Parental investment and sexual selection. In B. Campbell (Ed.), *Sexual selection and the descent of man: 1871–1971* (pp. 136–179). Chicago: Aldine.

Vaughn, B. E. (1999). Power is knowledge (and vice versa): A commentary on "On winning some and losing some: A Social relations approach to social dominance in toddlers. *Merrill-Palmer Quarterly, 45*, 215–225.

de Waal, F. B. M. (1982). *Chimpanzee politics: Power and sex among apes.* New York: Harper & Row.

de Waal, F. B. M. (2000). The first kiss: Foundations of conflict resolution research in animals. In F. Aureli & F. B. M. de Waal (Eds.), *Natural conflict resolution* (pp. 15–33). Berkeley, CA: University of California.

Walster, E., Walster, G. W., & Berscheid, E. (1978). *Equity: Theory and research.* Boston: Allyn & Bacon.

White, R.W. (1959). Motivation reconsidered: The concept of competence. *Psychological Review, 66*, 297–333.

Wispe, L. G. (1972). Positive forms of social behavior: An overview. *Journal of Social Issues, 28*, 1–19.

Woolley, H. T. (1925). Agnes: A dominant personality in the making. *Pedagogical Seminary, 32*, 569–598.

Wrangham, R., & Peterson, D. (1996). *Demonic males: Apes and the origins of human violence.* New York: Houghton Mifflin.

Wynne-Edwards, V. C. (1962). *Animal dispersion in relation to social behaviour.* London: Oliver & Boyd.

Yerkes, R. M. (1925). *Almost human.* New York: Century.

Zuckerman, S. (1932). *The social behavior of monkeys and apes.* New York: Harcourt, Brace.

2

AN EVOLUTIONARY/ECOLOGICAL ACCOUNT OF AGGRESSIVE BEHAVIOR AND TRAIT AGGRESSION IN HUMAN CHILDREN AND ADOLESCENTS

Brian E. Vaughn
Auburn University

Antonio José Santos
Instituto Superior de Psicologia Aplicada

> Competition does not invariably result in aggression, but the existence of aggression is evidence for competition ... Competition is not necessarily the proximate cause of all conflict, nor does the winner of a contest necessarily gain immediate benefits; ultimately, aggression must pay off or long ago the meek would have inherited the earth.
>
> —Donald Symons, *Play and Aggression* (1978, p. 156).

That aggressive behavior and/or trait aggressiveness is considered a critical social, personal, and public health "problem" is evidenced by the 14,100 article and chapter titles retrieved in a Google Scholar search on the phrase "the problem of aggressive behavior in children" that was run in preparation for this chapter. The lengthy catalogue of published papers on aggressive behavior and trait aggression reflects a deep and abiding interest in these topics in the social and behavioral sciences. Indeed the problems of conflict and aggression have been of central interest in sociology (e.g., Marx & Engels, 1848; Parsons, 1947), psychiatry (e.g., Freud, 1961), and psychology (e.g., Baldwin, 1911; Darwin, 1871; James, 1890) since these academic and professional disciplines were established more than a century ago. Although the analyses offered from different disciplines tended to explain aggression and conflict from the perspectives of varying disciplinary matrices (e.g., sociological explanations tended to emphasize class, status, power, and authority rather than instinct or sexual selection), each attempted to explain why people frequently don't get along. Because aggressive behavior appears to disrupt the social fabric connecting individuals to others at all levels of social organization (e.g., dyads, families, classrooms, communities, societies), programmatic attempts to prevent the expression of aggressive behavior and/or to reduce its impact have been requested by parents, teachers, and governing agencies with some urgency.

From the perspective of this chapter, Freud's (1961) observations concerning civilization and its discontents is a reasonable starting point because he was the first theorist to discuss aggressive behavior and trait aggression from a developmental perspective. For Freud, the aggressive instinct is aroused from the inevitable conflicts between desire and possibility within intimate relationships and is observable from the earliest months of infancy. In his view, civilization and socialization have the containment of this instinct and regulation of its expression as both a goal and a function. Although Freud's hydraulic metaphor and his notion of destructive instincts are no longer credible as science, his insights about the necessity of social and self-regulation of aggressive behavior are as fresh today as they were in 1930. Indeed, many authors have reiterated his sentiment (usually without attribution) since *Civilization and Its Discontents* was published (e.g., Lorenz, 1966).

Behaviorally oriented psychologists found Freud's instinct model unacceptable and also rejected his pessimistic view concerning the inevitability of conflict and aggression (see Baron & Richardson, 1994, for a discussion). However, these learning theorists had not extinguished their own belief in drives and they attempted to recast the causal matrix leading to aggressive behavior in their own drive terminology. In the early social learning model, frustration motivated the expression of aggression (e.g., Dollard, Doob, Miller, Mowrer, & Sears, 1939; Miller, Sears, Mowrer, Doob, & Dollard, 1941). Although the initial formulation of the frustration–aggression hypothesis suggested both that the observation of aggressive behavior was sufficient to assume prior frustration and that frustration inevitably induces aggressive behavior (Dollard et al., 1939), this position was modified by Miller et al. (1941). They acknowledged that, sometimes, aggressive behavior does not occur after frustration because other response tendencies instigated by frustration may inhibit or be incompatible with aggressive behavior. Eventually, even the initial assumption to the effect that aggressive behavior was necessarily preceded by frustration was shown to be too broad (e.g., Zillman, 1979) and it is now understood that many aggressive acts need not imply prior frustration (Baron & Richardson, 1994).

A second-generation social learning approach to aggressive behavior moved further from Freud than did Dollard et al. (1939), eschewing drives and instincts altogether (e.g., Bandura, 1969, 1973). On this view, observing (certain) others engaged in aggressive behavior is, in some circumstances, sufficient both to learn those behaviors and to instigate them in children. In this model, observational learning can be more potent than is direct experience because experimenting with aggressive may put the individual at some risk of injury (Bandura, 1973). Aggressive behavior, once acquired, is maintained in the repertoire as an operant. As originally proposed, the motivation to acquire, express, and maintain aggressive behavior (no traits required) could all be located outside the organism. As a consequence, the "problem" of aggression should, in principle, be solvable without much active participation of the organism. Bandura revised his initial views considerably to include major roles for the cognitive and emotional activity of the person (e.g., Bandura, 1986) and now refers to his approach as "cognitive-social learning theory." This general framework has been applied and extended by many scientists studying aggressive behavior and trait aggression and now includes assumptions and propositions about contexts as organizing influences (e.g., Cairns & Cairns, 1995, Patterson, DeBaryshe, & Ramsay, 1989) and about cognitive structures for the processing of social information relevant to aggressive behavior (e.g., Crick & Dodge, 1994; Dodge & Crick, 1990; Dodge & Somberg, 1987).

Psychoanalytic and learning-based explanations of aggressive behavior and trait aggressiveness are diverse with regard to process, mechanisms, motivation, and characterizations of function associated with aggression. Nevertheless, regardless of whether an approach locates the source of aggressive behavior in the person, outside the person, or in the processes connecting the person to his or her context, such explanations have in common the underlying notion that aggressive behavior and trait aggressiveness are disruptive, undesirable, maladaptive, (probably) evil, and require remediation. Given that aggressive behavior and trait aggression have such bad reputations and given that scientists have been engaged in explaining these phenomena (and proposing relevant interventions) for more than a century, it is surprising to find that levels of aggressive behavior in society has not declined much, except as a function of population demography (i.e., when the supply of young males is in decline). Not only are aggressive behavior and aggressive individuals common across age, time, and social group, but also many socially successful individuals behave very aggressively and/or exhibit relatively high trait aggression (e.g., Hawley, 2003; Hawley & Vaughn, 2003; Prinstein & Cillessen, 2003; Rodkin, Farmer, Pearl, & Van Acker, 2000). How can this be?

Without rejecting insights generated from psychoanalytic and social learning traditions and without denying that aggressive behavior is often disrupts the status quo, we suggest that most questions regarding aggression have been narrowly posed and that they neglect (to a greater or lesser extent) general understandings about behavior arising from evolutionary biology. For example, early (e.g., until about 1986) social learning formulations tended to focus on the factors or conditions immediately antecedent to aggressive acts and/or on status relations between a model and the learner. More current social learning approaches consider family interaction histories from early childhood forward as contextual antecedent factors (e.g., Patterson, 1982) and some, (e.g., Crick & Dodge, 1994; Dodge & Crick, 1990) add social information processing parameters to the list of causal antecedents to aggression. These issues of proximal causes for aggression are important but they do not allow for other sources of influence from development and phylogeny that are also pertinent and relevant (Tinbergen, 1951). From an evolutionary perspective, these other sources of influence refer to ultimate, rather than proximal, sources of influence.

To address questions about ultimate causes, it is necessary to consider the adaptive functions of the behavior and social-ecological contexts in which the behavior is expressed in addition to describing its emergence during development. Adopting an ethological and evolutionary framework affords a morally neutral stance on aggressive behavior and trait aggressiveness, thereby allowing them to be considered as normal and normative rather than deviant. This framework also allows us to pose questions about whether aggressive behavior makes it possible for some individuals to successfully attain short or long-term goals that would have otherwise been unattainable and, finally, whether attainment of these goals contributes to variability in reproductive success or inclusive fitness. If the answers to these questions are "yes, even if only by a small margin," we can be confident that aggressive behavior and traits supporting this behavior are an aspect of human nature shaped by natural selection, and need not imply a defective or deviant social history or a genetic anomaly. Furthermore, this perspective suggests positive associations between measures of aggressive behavior, trait aggressiveness, and indices of social competence and social status, but only for those individuals who apply aggressive tactics and strategies successfully.

Continued aggression without attainment of goals need not signify either competence or status in relevant social groups.

An evolutionary approach also demands consideration of aggression from a developmental perspective; a point that Freud appreciated but could not explain empirically. Life-course considerations of aggressive behavior and trait aggressiveness recently have become central to research concerning pathologies of aggression (e.g., Cairns & Cairns, 1995; Huesmann, Eron, Lefkowitz, & Walder, 1984; Moffit, Caspi, Diskson, Silva, & Santon, 1996; Tremblay, 2000; Tremblay, Nagin, Ségun, Zoccolillo et al., 2004). For the most part, these studies focus on rank-order stabilities of aggression as behavior or trait. This is not a trivial problem, if the central research purpose is to identify future criminals or persons likely to require mental health services or to propose preventive interventions to redirect at-risk children to more productive social paths. Nevertheless, this work (again, in general) has not examined the functional role of aggressive behavior and/or trait aggressiveness across the lifespan. That is to say, does aggression pay off for the aggressor in terms of resource acquisition supporting reproductive success or inclusive fitness? Significant exceptions to this generalization are found in Cairns's work (e.g., 1979; Cairns & Cairns, 1995) and, in recent papers by Tremblay (e.g., 2000). They have considered both life-course and individual difference questions regarding aggression and related these to relevant functional outcomes. Cairns's theoretical and empirical work, especially, was informed by an appreciation of evolutionary and epigenetic insights (e.g., Gottlieb, 1992, 1997). More than most other investigators from the social learning tradition, Cairns considered social and physical ecologies as contingent facts favoring (or not) aggressive behavior and trait aggressiveness.

A final distinction between evolutionary–ecological approaches to the topics of aggressive behavior and trait aggressiveness is an emphasis on comparative study, both cross-cultural and cross-species. There are no more than a handful of cross-cultural comparison studies in this area and the boldest of these have been led by ethologists, rather than by developmental or clinical psychologists (e.g., Smith, Cowie, Olafsson, & Liefooghe, 2002). Although there are relevant cross-cultural and historical/archaeological studies of aggressive and violent behavior among adults (see Ghiglieri, 1999 or LeBlanc, 2003 for popular treatments) reported by anthropologists, these do not, as a rule, provide useful information about development. Perhaps because many primatologists were trained as physical anthropologists, cross-species reports (e.g., Wrangham & Peterson, 1996) also tend to focus on the aggressive behavior of adults (often males) and provide rather scant discussion of development (but see Pereira, 1992, 1995; Symons, 1978;

and chapters in Pereira & Fairbanks, 2002a). Even without a serious discussion of development, a sampling of reports in the ethnographic and primatology literatures is sufficient to convince fair-minded readers that aggressive behavior, trait aggressiveness, and even violence is not necessarily evidence of deviance or mental disorder. Rather, aggression is a normal, predictable means by which individuals (perhaps especially males) resolve conflicts of interest in certain times, in certain places, and under certain circumstances. Furthermore, many aggressive episodes between familiar partners are followed by reparation through reconciliation (de Waal, 1986a, 1989a). Thus, as long as aggression does not result in permanent physical or psychological damage, the cycle of aggressive behavior/reconciliation may serve to promote or even strengthen the bonds between individuals in a specific social dyad or group.

These interpretations do not imply that aggressive behavior is socially desirable or any less disruptive to the agendas of group members and leaders; they simply suggest that aggressive behavior and trait aggressiveness are normal aspects of human nature and must be understood as a part of a nexus of other normal social behaviors and traits. In the next section of this chapter, a brief and selective review of studies concerning primate and human aggression and violence is presented in support of the notion that aggressive behavior and trait aggressiveness are normal and expectable primate (both human and nonhuman) activities and traits that are exhibited and are relevant in contexts where every individual cannot do or have everything he or she wants.

AGGRESSION AND VIOLENCE AMONG NON-HUMAN PRIMATES

For a variety of philosophical, political, and religious reasons, the "state of nature" had been romanticized and idealized in Western thought since renaissance times. This view was, however, challenged decisively in the 18th and 19th centuries in the realms of philosophy (e.g., Hobbes), economics (Malthus), and evolution (Darwin). By the late 19th century, the notion that "nature" was competitive was so widespread that it influenced poets such as Tennyson who wrote of "nature, red in tooth and claw," to refer to the fact that many species make their "livings" by preying on the old and weak in other species. The recognition that resource competition between species is never ending also changed views on intraspecies competition, aggression, and violence, but even as astute an observer as Konrad Lorenz (e.g., 1966) was convinced that aggressive struggles within (nonhuman) species were resolved without serious injury or death of contestants, when one contestant signaled submission or otherwise indicated defeat by leaving the contest.

Lorenz (1966) was very concerned by human aggression and violence. In his view, the use of weapons over great distances makes it impossible to perceive and respond to submissive signals between combatants, thus increasing the likelihood of a lethal outcome. We know now that Lorenz was too optimistic about intraspecies relations among animals; as among humans, nonhuman animals also violently attack, kill, and occasionally eat their own kind (e.g., Goodall, 1977, 1991; de Waal, 1986b; Manson & Wrangham, 1991; Nashida, Hiraiwa-Hasegawa, Hasegawa, & Takahata, 1985; Nashida & Kawanaka, 1985; Watts, 1989; Watts & Mitani, 2000; Wrangham, 1999; Wrangham & Peterson, 1996). By now, the evidence documenting capacities of nonhuman primates, to attack and slaughter conspecifics is incontrovertible (see Wilson & Wrangham, 2003). Nevertheless, the vast majority of competitions and conflicts between members of an established social group (or between two groups) concerning resources are resolved without resorting to violent aggression. Rather, priority of access to resources (with the definition of "resources" being extremely broad) is usually settled with reference to the intra- or intergroup dominance structure, more or less in the manner suggested by Lorenz (1966). The phenomena of dyadic social dominance and hierarchical dominance structures have been recognized and studied by ethologists and other animal behaviorists since the 1920s (e.g., Schjelderup-Ebbe, 1922). The preponderance of evidence suggests that dyadic dominance and group dominance structures are found in the majority of group-living animals, including humans (see Hawley, 1999, for a review).

An evolutionary account of social dominance should consider both developmental and adaptive significance of the behaviors and traits underlying dyadic dominance and group dominance structures. For the most part, such an evolutionary account would explain the ontogenetic and phylogenetic bases for the phenomenon in terms of relations with reproductive success and inclusive fitness (where "inclusive fitness" is understood as the reproductive success of the both the individual and closely related kin e.g., [Hamilton, 1964; Oli, 2003; Wilson, 1975]). That is to say, social dominance should be clearly related to the acquisition of resources contributing meaningfully to variations in reproductive success or inclusive fitness of more vs. less socially dominant group members. Evidence favoring this interpretation has been documented for nonhuman primate species (e.g., Altmann et al., 1996; Bercovitch & Numberg, 1997; Gust et al., 1998; Mitani, Watts, & Muller, 2002) and for humans as well (see Low, 2000, chaps. 6–9). In addition to reproductive benefits, social dominance has also been found to be associated with a range of health domains. Sapolsky (e.g., 2004) suggests that social rank in a group can influence health, especially with regard to stress-related diseases. Although relations to health outcomes are complex and not invariably linear or positive (Sapolsky, 2004), on balance it's good to be the king (Brooks, *History of the World, Part I,* 1981).

It should come as no surprise that individuals strive for social dominance within their groups or that exchanges between groups reflect variations of group superiority (see Wrangham & Peterson, 1996, for extended discussion of consequences associated with marked imbalances of social power between groups of chimpanzees). It is important to keep in mind, however, that "dominance" is a description of a social relationship between members of a dyad or group and is not, as such, a "trait" that will be transmitted through normal biological processes, even if suites of behaviors and traits that may contribute to social dominance are heritable. Social dominance is a social construction that must be assembled ontogenetically within the "social lifetime" of a relevant group on a dyad-by-dyad basis (family, age-sex class, residential community, etc.). Describing the mechanisms and processes by which individuals establish dominance has also proved to be a time-consuming and controversial task (e.g., Gauthier & Strayer, 1986; Hawley, 1999; Vaughn, 1999).

For group-living old-world monkeys, it is common to find that juveniles occupy dominance positions that are just below that of their mothers (e.g., Goldman & Loy, 1997; Koyama, 2003; Kuester, 1988). For species in which females remain in their natal groups (which includes most of the ground-dwelling monkeys and some ape species, but conspicuously not chimpanzees or, typically, humans, Harcourt, 1978; Wrangham & Peterson, 1996), this means that the social position of females is largely determined by the matriline into which they are born. For these species, it is common that males leave their natal groups and the privileges (or inequities) of rank do not necessarily follow them to their new social group. They must compete, frequently aggressively, for a position in the dominance hierarchy in their new group and the outcome of those competitions is significant both from proximal and ultimate perspectives. Not surprisingly, young males who are able to find and form coalitions with male kin in the new groups tend to have greater luck breaking into the existing hierarchy. In any event, transition to a new group tests the strength and aggressive skills of the young male. Given the inevitable male–male dominance competition in rheseus monkey society, it should come as no surprise that much of the playful activity of juvenile rheseus monkeys looks like practice for aggressive fighting (Symons, 1978).

Male–male competition is no less significant among chimpanzees, even though adolescent males are not necessarily encouraged to leave their natal groups by other males. Rather, it is more common that maturing females move on. Among wild chimpanzees, both males and females compete (within sex) for status in the group (Goodall, 1968; Pusey, Williams, & Goodall, 1997). Mitani et al. (2002) reviewed evidence suggesting that the stakes in these competitions are significant as more dominant males and females in chimpanzee societies tend to enjoy greater reproductive success than do lower status (less dominant) peers. Among chimpanzees, male dominance depends on both physical prowess and political skill (e.g., de Waal, 1982). Central among the these political skills is coalition building; that is to say, two or more individuals form a (relatively) enduring relationship and support each other across a range of contexts such as meat-sharing and patrolling of territorial boundaries (e.g., Mitani & Watts, 2001; Nashida, 1983; Nashida & Hosaka, 1996; Watts & Mitani, 2000; Wrangham, 1999). Furthermore, coalitions of two or more lower status males may, on occasion, threaten and defeat individuals of higher dominance rank (Mitani et al., 2002). Perhaps interestingly, in light of their relevance to human activities, coalitions of male chimpanzees do not necessarily reflect genetic relatedness (e.g., Goldberg & Wrangham, 1997; Mitani, Merriwether, & Zhang, 2000).

Intragroup aggression serves both to create and maintain the dominance hierarchy in chimpanzee society. Aggression can also, on occasion, destabilize and reorganize the dominance structure, as when a coalition defeats and (perhaps) dismembers a more dominant male (e.g., Riss & Goodall, 1977; de Waal, 1986b). Moreover, chimpanzees have adopted a habit, shared by many human groups, of engaging in intergroup aggression and violence. The attacks on and destruction of neighboring groups are well described (e.g., Goodall et al., 1979; Manson, & Wrangham, 1991; Watts, 2004; Wilson, Hauser, & Wrangham, 2001; Wrangham, 1999) and seem to have functions similar to comparable exchanges among humans; namely the acquisition (by the victorious group) of resources (previously) controlled by the losing group (e.g., LeBlanc, 2003; Wrangham & Peterson, 1996). Violent intergroup conflicts leading to the dissolution of one group (usually due to chimpicide inflicted on most or all adult males and sometimes on females and infants) are conditioned on many parameters and are not everyday occurrences, even if they make headlines when observed. Wrangham and Peterson (1996) summarize arguments suggesting that access to resources is a precipitating factor but only when a relatively marked imbalance is found between neighboring groups. That is, when one social unit has appreciably more adult males than a neighbor and some valuable resource is noticeably rare, the probability of violent intergroup exchanges increases.

This brief overview of the presence and functional role of aggressive behavior and trait aggressiveness among primates, perhaps especially the apes, is not comprehensive. For example, Bonobos are not discussed and these cousins to chimpanzees may not be as aggressive as their relatives; nor have we discussed sex differences in aggressive behavior or male–female aggression, and these are marked in many primate species. Rather, our review is intended to suggest that aggressive behavior and trait aggressiveness are integral to what is meant by a "normal" primate individual and "normal primate society." Aggression is not a sign of deviance or disorder among our primate relatives. Of course, this discourse does not imply that aggressive behavior is the primary mode of behavioral exchange among primates or that social dominance is the only important dimension structuring the interactions and relationships among group members. As de Waal's (and others) basic and popular scientific writings suggest (e.g., Strayer, Bovenkert, & Koopman, 1975; de Waal, 1982, 1986a, 1989b, 2000, 2001; de Waal & Yoshihara, 1983; Weaver & de Waal, 2003), intragroup aggressive episodes serve also to bring group members together through reconciliation, even if the immediate consequence is to drive them apart. Indeed, de Waal argues that the social order of primate societies is largely organized around patterns of reconciliation and reparation of relationships by group members, especially when these relationships are highly valued (Aureli & de Waal, 2000; de Waal, 2000).

AGGRESSION AND VIOLENCE AMONG HUMAN PRIMATES

Discussion of evolved solutions to the problems of life, especially life in groups, is often discomforting and even disorganizing for developmental and clinical child psychologists trained in cognitive social-learning and/or biological psychiatry traditions (e.g., chapters by social psychologists in Groebel & Hinde, 1989). If aggressive behavior is normal and isn't evil or evidence of a behavioral/mental deficit or disorder, why are we "treating" and "preventing" its expression? What about bullies, violent spouses, murderers, suicide bombers, and rogue states with access to weapons of mass destruction? And what about intergroup violence, whether at the level of family/tribe, local teen youth organization, or nation states; what about war? Surely, aggression and violence at these levels cannot be "evolved solutions" for conflicts of interest among humans. Or, can they (and, if they are, were Freud and Lorenz right)?

There may be a certain comfort in the notion that human kind once lived in near perfect harmony with nature and with each other.

Unfortunately, there is no evidence in history or prehistory to support this myth, and, as noted above, our common ancestor with chimpanzees was probably not so very peaceful either. LeBlanc (2003) summarized evidence from the prehistory of every continent inhabited by the genus Homo and concluded that intergroup wars have been part and parcel of human societies from our beginnings. Furthermore, from evidence available on present-day hunting/gathering and non-industrial agricultural societies, LeBlanc concluded that intergroup warfare was such a major facet of the lives of prehistoric peoples that upwards of 40%–60% of adult males of any group could expect to die as a result of war over the course of their adult lives. Ironically (by LeBlanc's estimate), in this age of global wars, weapons of mass destruction, and rogue states, only about 2–4% of adult males suffer a similar fate.

More interesting than the simple fact that prehistoric groups did not always just get along is LeBlanc's (2003) discussion of the timing of intergroup aggression and violence. Ancestral populations were not necessarily in a constant state of war; rather, conflict and warfare tended to occur primarily in times of climate changes or environmental degradation resulting in scarcity of nutritional resources. He argued that the primary resources contested in prehistory were food and territory (to grow or hunt for food). Evidence from currently extant hunter/gatherer and primitive agricultural societies (e.g., Chagnon, 1997, 2000) suggests that reproductive resources are also at issue when groups of men engage in violent conflict. Chagnon estimated that 50% of adult males among the Yanomamo tribes die in conflicts concerning nutritional and reproductive resources. These kinds of observations suggest that the ultimate causes (and perhaps effects) of intergroup aggression and violence have not changed much since our species shared a common ancestor with chimpanzees (indeed, if the story being spun about the relatively peaceful and sexually egalitarian Bonobos [Sannen, Heistermann, van Elsacker, Mohle & Eens, 2003; de Waal, 1995] holds up, we may be compelled to conclude that the evolutionary changes are occurring in the Pan line rather than in Homo). Fundamentally, intergroup conflicts concern group level conflicts of (self) interest.

A BRIGHT SIDE OF BAD BEHAVIOR

Developmental scientists and clinical child psychologists are so used to interpreting children's aggressive behavior as a sign of maladjustment that studies of the positive consequences of aggressive behavior and trait aggressiveness have not, until rather recently, been published in leading developmental journals. A few provocative papers describing social dominance structures among children and adolescents were published in the 1970s and 1980s, but interest in this topic declined for a variety of reasons (see Vaughn, 1999) until the past few years. Nevertheless, if we are to explain the persistence of aggressive behavior and trait aggressiveness among children, in the face of a social learning tradition insistent on the inherent incompetence of aggression (e.g., Crick, 2003), we must explore the possibility that aggressive behavior has beneficial outcomes for at least some children, some of the time.

Several studies indicate that aggressive behavior can be associated with successfully attaining social goals and, more importantly, that some very socially successful children are highly aggressive. Vaughn, Vollenweider, Bost, Azria-Evans, & Snider (2003) examined the social competence correlates of negative behavior rates (a category that included aggressive episodes) for preschool children and found that negative behavior was positively and significantly correlated with an index of social competence in two separate samples. Subsequent analyses decomposed the social competence index into interactive, adult-rated, and peer sociometric components. Initiating negative interactions was positively correlated with the interactive and adult rated facets social competence, but not with the sociometric components. Further analyses examined aspects of child aggressive behavior from adult ratings (called "coercive," "brittle," and "dominant" in this study). Only scores for aggressive behavior characterized as "dominant" were positively associated with the social competence indices (this score was even a significant correlate of sociometric acceptance). In both samples, initiation of negative interactions also was modestly, but significantly, associated with negative sociometric nominations, as would be anticipated from most existing literature on children for this age. Nevertheless, the data suggest that aggressive behavior per se is not unequivocally maladaptive.

Hawley and associates (e.g., Hawley, 2002, 2003; Hawley & Little, 1999; Hawley, Little, & Pasupathi, 2002) have used person-centered approaches in their studies of resource control in samples of toddlers, children, and adolescents. Hawley (e.g., 1999) argued that access to and use of valued resources is desirable and may serve as a proxy for "fitness" among human juveniles. Although the measures of resource acquisition and control differ from toddlerhood to adolescence, her data show that aggressive strategies of resource control can pay off for some group members. More interesting, however, are data showing that older children and adolescents who use a mixture of prosocial and coercive strategies to acquire and control resources tend to be the most successful (e.g., Hawley, 2003; Hawley et al., 2002). Not only are bi-strategic children more successful than other types (i.e., single strategy, no dominant strategy) in controlling valued resources, but also they are (for the most part) not distinguishable from prosocial mono-strategists in terms of desirable qualities; for example, bi-strategic children are perceived to be popular in the peer group, nominated as liked, and enjoy high-quality relationships with best friends (Hawley, 2003). Peers (but not teachers) recognized the high levels of aggressive and coercive behavior among bi-strategists, but apparently did not punish them to control their aggression. By way of comparison, coercive mono-strategists tend to be less successful at controlling resources than either bi-strategists or prosocial mono-strategists. Hawley's studies demonstrate convincingly that aggressive behavior can, when exhibited by some individuals in certain contexts, be an asset in children's social repertoires.

Taking a somewhat different approach to acquisition of social resources, Cairns, Farmer, Rodkin, and their associates have looked at friendships of aggressive children (especially boys). In their work (e.g., Cairns, Cairns, Neckerman, Gest, & Gariepy, 1988; Estell, Farmer, Pearl, Van Acker, & Rodkin, 2003; Farmer & Rodkin, 1996; Rodkin et al., 2000), aggressive children have as many reciprocated friends as do their non-aggressive peers and aggressive children are seen as equally "central" in social networks as their less aggressive peers. Furthermore, some more aggressive children are strategically aggressive in the pursuit of dominance (Farmer, 2000). Like Hawley, these investigators argue for within-group heterogeneity and suggest that there are multiple pathways to social success and social integration in children's groups. Their analyses of popular children (e.g., Rodkin et al., 2000) indicate that some boys achieve popular status in their groups as a consequence of their aggressive behavior and are not handicapped or socially rejected by virtue of their aggression. Pellegrini and associates (e.g., Pellegrini, 2003; Pellegrini & Bartini, 2001; Pellegrini & Long, 2003) extended this line of research to cross-sex relationships. They reported that adolescent boys who use aggression to establish dominance among males in the peer group were preferred as (hypothetical) dating partners by same-age girls. For early adolescent girls, (hypothetical) dating popularity was positively related to their use of social (or relational) styles of aggression.

Taken together, the studies reviewed in this section suggest that it is not the fact of aggressive behavior or trait aggressiveness per se that supports social success but rather the strategic use of aggression to attain specific goals in specific contexts. Put somewhat more bluntly, aggressive children who are otherwise socially competent seem to fare well in their peer groups at all ages. They do not attain their social goals solely on the basis of aggressive behavior but they can call on their aggressive skills when warranted. These conclusions are consistent with the interpretations of aggressive behavior in primate groups and with an abundance of historic and anthropological evidence demonstrating associations between social power (based on aggressive behavior or the threat of such behavior) and reproductive success and inclusive fitness for human males (e.g., reviews by Gangestad & Simpson, 2000; Sapolsky, 2004; Wrangham & Peterson, 1996).

AGGRESSIVE BEHAVIOR AND SOCIAL DOMINANCE IN CHILDREN'S GROUPS

Relations between aggressive episodes and social dominance are complicated for adult primates (e.g., Kappeler, 1993; Rowell, 1974; de Waal, 1989a) and it is not always the case that individuals initiating the most agonistic episodes are also the most dominant in the group (e.g., Altmann, Sapolsky, & Licht, 1995). In principle (if not practice), an individual introduced to an established group need only defeat decisively the current alpha member (in the presence of other group members) to become top-ranked. Nevertheless, in most group-living primates, it is relatively easy to determine dyadic dominance relationships on the basis of directed agonism and to infer from these the group hierarchy. This fact served to justify the study of the social organization in children's groups from the perspective of social ethology in the 1970s (e.g., Abramovitch, 1976; Missakian, 1976; Sluckin & Smith, 1977; Strayer, Chapeskie, & Strayer, 1978; Santos & Winegar, 1999; Strayer & Strayer, 1976). These studies demonstrated that dyads could be characterized reliably in terms of dominance status and that group structures inferred from dyadic exchanges suggested linear hierarchies (e.g., Missakian, 1980; Strayer & Strayer, 1976).

Such hierarchies also characterize adolescent groups (e.g., Pellegrini & Bartini, 2001; Weisfeld, Omark, & Cronin, 1980), although dyadic dominance relations tend to be established/observed in terms of peer nominations or ratings and/or on verbal as well as physical attempts at social control (see Weisfeld et al., 1980). Direct observation of physical aggression is not common among adolescents, perhaps because the risks involved are much greater than for younger children. Weisfeld et al. (1980) suggested that dominance based on agonistic exchanges are likely to be seen at younger ages, but that the residual effect is that children (boys in their study) who establish dominance on the basis of aggression when young are advantaged in terms of peer recognition and access to resources in the social group as adolescents, even though their rates of physical conflict may be reduced during adolescence. Pellegrini and Bartini (2001) reach a similar conclusion, but suggest that when the peer group is reorganized, as when children transfer from elementary to middle or junior high schools, aggressive exchanges become, once again, the currency of social dominance.

With evidence that dominance orders could be reliably observed in groups across childhood and adolescence, child ethologists turned to functional questions (see Santos & Winegar, 1999). One such question focused on the assumption from the primate literature to the effect that dominance orders, once established, serve to constrain the overall level of aggression in the group, because outcomes of such encounters are predictable and the subordinate animal will avoid them. Although studies of children have not provided unequivocal evidence that reduction of aggressive behavior at the group level follows the establishment of group hierarchies, some indirect evidence consistent with this functional explanation has been reported. Strayer (e.g., Strayer, 1989; Strayer & Trudel, 1984) found that the agonistic episodes show and initial increase but then decline as a proportion of the total social interaction profiles of children from 1 to 5 years of age. Over this same time period, the stability of status rankings increased from about 70% for 1-year-olds to more than 90% for 3- and 5-year-old children. These increased proportions were found even though the proportion of relationships that were observed to engage in agonistic exchanges declined from 75% of 1-year-olds to only 40% of 5-year-olds. These findings were based on cross-sectional evaluations; nevertheless, they may be interpreted as evidence that the establishment of a dominance order within a group leads to a reduction in aggression at the group.

Other studies examined relations between dominance and other structural features of children's groups. Several investigators probed the arguments by Chance and Jolly (1976) to the effect that dominance and social attention should be strongly associated, on the assumption that dominant individuals were central members of the larger group. Some observational studies suggested a relation between dominance and receiving visual attention from peers (Abramovitch, 1976; Abramovitch & Strayer, 1978; Hold, 1977) but these findings were not fully supported in later studies (e.g., Vaughn & Waters, 1980, 1981). Vaughn and Waters (1980, 1981) reported that visual regard showed a moderate association with dominance rank based on resource control but not with dominance rank based on initiated agonism. In their studies, visual attention was more strongly associated with sociometric preference than with dominance. Vaughn and Waters (1981) concluded that peer attention was attracted by peer social competence, rather than to dominance per se, and that relations between visual regard both measures of dominance and sociometric preference were mediated by peer social competence.

Recent studies of social dominance (e.g., Hawley, 1999, 2003; Hawley & Little, 1999; Hawley et al., 2002; LaFreniere & Charlesworth, 1983, 1987) have emphasized resource control rather than directed agonism leading to submission as the most relevant dimension of social dominance from early childhood through adolescence. Defined as resource control, distinctions between social dominance and social competence become blurred (Vaughn, 1999); this most likely accounts for the positive associations between aggression and indices of social skills/social competence reviewed in the previous section. Nevertheless, however dominance is defined, evidence of a social status hierarchy based on aggressive exchanges (or the threat thereof) can be found in the peer groups of children and adolescents. Behavioral and psychological correlates of dominance status may differ across developmental stages, but we can conclude that this dimension is salient and relevant to the functioning of most human groups, including those of adults. To the extent that aggressive behavior organizes aspects of social structure, we conclude also that aggressive behavior is an adaptive element of the human social behavioral repertoire.

AGGRESSION, DOMINANCE, AND AFFILIATION

Although de Waal (e.g., 1986a) is often credited with calling attention to the cohesive function of aggressive behavior among primates, this phenomenon had been studied and described by F. F. Strayer and associates in groups of captive primates (e.g., Strayer et al., 1975; Strayer & Harris, 1978) and in groups of children (e.g., Strayer, 1980a, 1980b; Strayer & Noel, 1986) prior to de Waal's discussion of the issue (e.g., 1982). Among children (e.g., Strayer, 1980a, 1992; Strayer & Noel, 1986), dominance status was socially attractive. That is, more socially dominant children were targets of their peers' affiliative initiations at higher than chance levels and were preferred as play partners by peers, whereas less socially dominant children were not so strongly preferred. In Strayer's work, preference for socially dominant play partners is most clearly evident among older preschool children (i.e., 4- and 5-year-olds in their studies) and is generally absent for groups under 2 years of age. Pellegrini and Bartini (2001) reported similar findings in a sample of preadolescent boys, although positive relations between dominance and social preferences were seen only after the transition to middle school. Hawley (e.g., 2003) also reported, for a sample of 5th- to 10th-grade-level children, that individuals who report using both prosocial and coercive strategies for controlling valued resources (bi-strategic) were described as socially central, agreeable, and liked by peers and teachers. Taken together, these findings suggest that children's aggressive behavior and trait aggressiveness are not a priori signs of deviance or maladaptation. Rather, in certain contexts and with certain peers, aggressive behavior can serve to establish and maintain structural aspects of groups that provide both affordances and constraints on the behavioral transactions of group members.

Although the traditional views on aggressive behavior and trait aggressiveness from both the social learning and evolutionary/ecological perspectives suggested that aggression is disruptive and dispersive (e.g., Coie & Dodge, 1998, Lorenz, 1966; McGrew, 1972), investigators from both traditions have recognized that many (perhaps most) conflicts between familiar children are resolved satisfactorily (or at least to the degree that dyadic interaction continues). For example, Hartup, Laursen, Stewart, and Easton (1988) observed conflicts among preschool children and found that friends engaged in conflict as often as did neutral associates but some friends were more likely to resolve the conflict equitably and some were more likely to continue interaction after the conflict. Although they do not use de Waal's terms, the Hartup et al. (1988) results suggest that reconciliation is most common in valued relationships. Verbeek and de Waal (2001) also reported on reconciliation among preschool children and suggested several social and contextual parameters associated with reconciliation. Verbeek and de Waal found reconciliation to be more common among friends than nonfriends. They also reported that preconflict interaction between opponents was a positive predictor of reconciliation.

Butovskaya and Kozintesev (1997) studied primary schoolchildren (6–7 years old) and found that most children tended to initiate reconciliation within a minute after the conflict ended (similar to reports for nonhuman primates). They also found that dyads with relatively high numbers of friendly contacts also had higher numbers of aggressive conflicts and dyads with few friendly interactions also had fewer aggressive conflicts. Interviews with study participants indicated that children viewed reconciliation between friends as both more likely and more important than between nonfriends. Butovskaya and Kozintsev (1997) showed that aggressive conflict was followed by reconciliation more frequently than by dispersion of the conflicted pair. Interestingly, the successful aggressor was more likely to initiate reconciliation than was the victim. They note that among nonhuman primate species with more rigid dominance hierarchies it is more common for a dominant animal to initiate reconciliation than for a subordinate to do so (e.g., York & Rowell, 1988). It will be most interesting to examine children's groups with varying degrees of rigidity for dominance rank with regard to the initiation of reconciliation to determine whether dominance constrains these activities for children as for patas monkeys.

Studies of adolescent peer conflicts and their resolution are quite rare and have not been much influenced (to date) by the interests or methods of primatologists. This may be due to the difficulty involved with direct observation of conflicts for adolescents and may also be due to reliance on interview methods among developmental scientists studying adolescent development. Raffaelli (1997) did assess conflicts and resolutions for adolescents and their friends (siblings' conflicts were also considered) and her results also suggest that resolution/reconciliation is common following adolescent conflicts. Raffaelli interviewed adolescents and queried them about the onset of the conflict, its course, and the outcome of conflict. In these interviews, marked sex differences were apparent in terms of both the incidence and the means of conflict resolution. More than 60% of boys reported that conflicts with friends were resolved and the mean conflict resolution time was under 17 minutes. On the other hand, girls reported that more than 70% of conflicts were not resolved and the time to resolution of conflicts took more than 60 minutes. More than 76% of boys reporting on conflicts with friends resolved their conflicts at the time of the dispute and did not adopt specific relationship repair strategies postconflict. By comparison, only 42% of girls reporting friend conflicts repaired their relationship without some specific strategy such as making amends after the conflict. It is important to note that the conflicts studied by Raffaelli (1997) tended to center on psychological (as opposed to physical) disputes. Conflicts between female friends tended to focus on relationship betrayal, whereas conflicts between male friends tended to focus on dominance relations. Even so, her results are easily assimilated to the framework just discussed in relation to preschool and school age children's reconciliation after aggressive exchanges.

Considering results of studies just reviewed, it is clear that conflicts between friends are relatively common across childhood and adolescence, and many (if not most) conflicts result in attempts to repair the relationship. This is consistent with de Waal's (e.g., 1989a) notion that the conflict–reconciliation cycle is observed most clearly in valued relationships. It is inevitable that conflicts of interest will arise within a human dyad because their psychological and genetic interests will never be completely isomorphic. On occasion, what is best for one partner will not be in the best interests of the other and in most such instances, the dyad member exerting the greatest physical or social power prevails. Nevertheless, when the relationship is valued by both members, it is in their interests to resolve the conflict and continue the relationship; hence an evolved capacity (and associated motivation) to reconcile. Among nonhuman primates, dyadic relationships serve many supportive functions including physical maintenance (e.g., grooming), emotional support, and defense of self or resources against others (both inter- and intragroup contestants). Studies of human children have documented similar support functions for friends, but have not progressed so far as to relate these functions to frequency or success of postconflict reconciliations. Such studies could now be initiated, on the basis of current knowledge and could provide evidence of prosocial outcomes contingent on aggressive exchanges and their resolution.

IS AN EVOLUTIONARY/ECOLOGICAL PERSPECTIVE INCOMMENSURATE WITH THE CURRENT BIOCOGNITIVE-SOCIAL LEARNING PERSPECTIVE ON AGGRESSIVE BEHAVIOR AND TRAIT AGGRESSIVENESS?

There can be no doubt that aggression has been an element of the adaptive behavior repertoires and personalities of nonhuman and human primates for as long as these taxa have existed. Prehistoric, historical, and current observations indicate that humans routinely use aggression and violence to resolve conflicts of interest relevant to reproductive success and inclusive fitness, even though these means are not the only, and likely not primary, means for resolving such conflicts. How can this be reconciled with the prevailing social and developmental science insistence on interpretations of aggressive behavior as manifestations of evil? To investigators with a background in evolutionary thinking, this is a trick question based on the assumption that proximal and ultimate factors explaining any class of activity or the traits supporting that activity are conceptually separable. That these factors are not separable has been taken for granted for more than half a century by ethologists, sociobiologists, and ecologists (e.g., Tinbergen, 1951; Wilson, 1975). From this perspective, consideration of ultimate causes and meanings of aggressive behavior and trait aggressiveness should enrich, rather than compete with, considerations of the proximal causes offered by traditional social, clinical, and developmental scientists. Such an integrative approach also enriches interpretations at the ultimate level as well, insofar as individual differences and development remain relatively peripheral in discussions of ultimate causes of aggressive behavior and trait aggressiveness.

One way to initiate the integration to which we just alluded would be to assume that aggressive behavior, including violence, and trait aggressiveness are neither good nor bad, a priori, but constitute tactics (and their underlying motivations) that can be used successfully (or not) to resolve conflicts of interest that are salient to interactants. Taking this stance leads to an immediate rejection of main effects, reductionist explanations of aggressive behavior, whether based on biological (e.g., genes "for" aggressiveness) or social (e.g., cycles of coerciveness) factors, as too simple for the observed phenomena. At the same time, the evolutionary/ecological perspective provides a succinct description of maladaptive aggressive strategies; to wit, repeated initiation of aggressive tactics for resolving conflicts of interest that do not lead to resolutions favoring the initiator across both shorter and longer time frames. Such children would be properly identified as incompetent aggressors.

One prototype of this sort of maladaptation would be Harlow's isolation-reared rhesus infants who, as adults, tended to show high levels of (apparently inappropriate) aggressive behavior when attempts were made to insert them into established groups. Males of this sort "disappeared" from the group and typically were not subsequently found (alive). Female isolation-reared monkeys did not necessarily "disappear" from the group but tended to be very aggressive toward offspring, if they managed to become impregnated (e.g., Harlow, Harlow, Dodsworth, & Arling, 1966). For obvious reasons, studies like this are never conducted with humans at any developmental period, although anecdotal reports of the disappearance or mysterious death of hyperaggressive men appear on occasion (e.g., Galliher, Kunkel, & Hobbs, 1986). Boehm (e.g., 1999) suggested that pre-agriculturalist societies used just this sort of strategy (or threatened to do so) to control the dominance aspirations of physically powerful or talented (e.g., superior hunter) men. For children, victims of bullies who are themselves aggressive (even bullying) towards other peers might constitute another prototypic example (e.g., Juvonven, Graham, & Schuster, 2003; Pellegrini, 1998; Pellegrini, Bartini, & Brooks, 1999; Salmivalli & Nieminen, 2002).

Although persistent but incompetent aggressors are generally recognized as being poorly adapted to their social context, the proportion of aggressive children with this profile may not be large (about 6% in the sample reported on by Juvonen et al., 2003). Of perhaps greater concern are children, adolescents, and adults who default to aggression or violence as their preferred social tactic when faced with conflicts of interest and who routinely win in such contests. An evolutionary/ecological perspective suggests that damaging aggressive behavior is both costly and risky to all combatants and should (all other things being equal) be avoided when possible (see discussion in Pellis, Pellis, & Foroud, 2005). The relevant questions focus on the relative benefits (vs. energetic costs) of aggressive acts and on the risks of injury associated with aggression. When cost and risk values are low (independent of the reasons these might be low), aggression and even violence are likely to be elevated. This may be one reason why rates of angry, aggressive-like behaviors are highest among toddlers (low risk of retaliation by targets) and why homicidal violence peaks in late adolescence/early adulthood (failing to attain signs of status or dominance at the transition to adulthood may reduce the desirability of a male in the eyes of potential mates, Tremblay & Nagin, 2005). Not surprisingly, rates of aggressive acts tend to decline from toddlerhood as children interact more frequently with peers (who may be less restrained than caregivers in their reactions to aggressive behavior) and homicide rates decline when young men acquire status, jobs, and mates (they have something important to lose).

Viewing variations in rates and types of aggressive behavior in terms of energetic costs and risks of injury contextualizes aggression in ways that perspectives locating individual differences within the person (in terms of either genes or socialization history) do not. Developmentally, constraints on aggressive behavior are expected to be low when the risk is low (either because the likelihood of retaliatory aggression is low or because opponents really cannot hit hard enough to cause more than superficial damage). To the extent that juvenile play activities are practiced (Symons, 1978), the low-cost, low-risk aggressive behavior of children can be viewed as practice for "serious" conflicts that will arise in the future. An evolutionary/ecological perspective does not assume that children are prescient concerning future competitions, it only requires that their behavior is consistent with such a future. As peer opponents become stronger and more skilled, the incidence of high-intensity aggression should decrease, if only because the risk of damage increases. As just discussed, one consequence of the establishment of dyadic dominance relationships may be reducing the probability of damaging aggression between dyad members.

Adults, on the other hand, are aware of social and physical facts that their offspring or caregiving charges cannot imagine and they often estimate the costs/benefits and risks of damage for aggressive behavior differently than do children (Trivers, 1974). This may be why adults seem more intent on constraining children's aggressive behavior than on maximizing the beneficial practice effects such activities offer, and, conversely, why children seem to have greater tolerance for peers' aggression than do parents and other adult supervisors. Even so, adults generally prefer that children in their care keep aggressive behavior to a minimum and, as a result, usually monitor the interactions of young children closely enough to intervene in aggressive episodes before serious damage to either the initiator or target occurs. Strategies of monitoring and intervention may vary across classes of caregivers (e.g., parents may be more inclined to monitor and intervene in favor of their own child than are care providers unrelated to their charges) and across developmental time (e.g., perhaps less attention is devoted to monitoring and intervening as children become more physically and socially skilled). Monitoring and intervention are common as well among group-living primates, although Pereira (1992) suggests that species differences exist in terms of which juveniles are monitored most closely, and, when monkeys intervene, kin tend to be favored.

Another adult strategy for limiting the display of aggressive behavior is the manipulation of children's age-class groups. It is common practice to group children according to age and caregivers/teachers and institutional administrators routinely separate children who fight with each other as groups are reorganized from the end of one "academic" session to the beginning of the next. Drawing on the insight from the evolutionary-ecological perspective concerning the selective advantage of avoiding damaging aggressive encounters, teachers/caregivers might also consider transferring a young, hyperaggressive child from her or his age-class to a group of children 1–2 years older, who would likely be larger, more physically powerful, and more willing to socialize by consequences than the child's same-age peers. Evidence from non-human primate studies (e.g., de Waal & Johanowicz, 1993) suggests that even highly aggressive individuals can learn new (and transferable) patterns of relating to peer group members when given the proper tutoring environment. We are unaware of a systematic study of this sort with children, but anecdotal reports from teachers/care providers we have consulted suggest that this intervention produces the desired results.

To sum up this section, we suggest that the two broad approaches to explaining aggressive behavior and trait aggressiveness arising from the biocognitive-social learning and the evolutionary-ecological traditions are not incommensurate, but rather complement and inform each other. Adopting this more catholic perspective requires jettisoning notions such as an instinctual basis for aggressive behavior as well as the presumption that aggressive behavior is, a priori, evidence of immaturity or depravity; even though human children (like their nonhuman cousins) are evolved to behave aggressively in certain contexts and may be incompetent in their selection and execution of aggressive tactics when resolving conflicts of interest. This integrative approach also demands that explanations and interpretations of aggressive behavior and trait aggressiveness must address both intra and interpersonal sources of influence. That is to say, some individuals may be more disposed to choose and use aggressive tactics for the resolution of conflicts of interest, but the targets of these tactics are rarely chosen at random, except by the least socially competent and/or youngest aggressors. Put another way, the social context is as much a determinant of aggressive behavior as genetic background or socialization history.

WHY AGGRESSIVE BEHAVIOR WON'T JUST GO AWAY

At the outset, we argued that the dominant conceptual framework in the developmental sciences (i.e., biocognitive-social learning) had failed to satisfactorily account for the presence and maintenance of aggressive behavioral tactics and trait aggressiveness in the repertoires (and personalities) of children and adolescents. We further suggested that the dominant framework characterized aggressive behavior in children as a sign of immaturity, social incompetence, or deviance that put children at risk of becoming social pariahs, delinquents, or criminals (see Coie & Dodge, 1998). We acknowledge that these characterizations of childhood aggressive behavior and trait aggressiveness are grounded in a plethora of data revealing significant associations between frequencies and rates of various categories of aggressive behavior and a broad range of life, observation, self-report and test data indicative of personal and social maladaptation; nevertheless, we believe that these associations are misleading, for a number of reasons.

First, we find long-standing and enduring lines of evidence from both nonhuman and human primate literatures suggesting that aggressive behavior and trait aggressiveness are adaptations to competitive social environments at both intra- and intergroup levels. Human and nonhuman primates evolved in environments in which resources necessary for growth, maintenance, and reproduction were not super-abundant and that gave rise to many real and potential conflicts of interest. Evidence from prehistoric sites (e.g., LeBlanc, 2003), from observations of presently living hunter–gatherer societies (e.g., Chagnon, 1997), and from the nightly news suggests that aggressive behavior and trait aggressiveness were instrumental in resolving those conflicts. Put somewhat differently, presently existing humans would not be alive if their ancestors had failed to behave aggressively and even violently from time to time. At the very least, it must be true that aggressive behavior is adaptive some of the time.

Second, our reviews of literature on aggressive behavior and its correlates in both nonhuman and human primates indicate that the capacity for and the expression of aggressive behavior can have beneficial consequences and lead to largely positive outcomes for individuals in social groups. Furthermore, to the extent that nonlethal, within-group aggressive encounters promote reconciliation between contestants (de Waal, 1989b, 1992), we can characterize some aggressive behavior as leading to increased coherence and positive sociality at the dyadic and group levels. Related to this is the notion that established dominance orders may be a precursor to reduced levels of (potentially damaging) aggressive exchanges between group members. We do not argue that aggressive behavior is largely seen in the service of prosocial motives or goals, but findings from these studies suggest that aggressive behavior need not be viewed as motivated solely by antisocial feelings. Again, we draw the inference that aggressiveness may be adaptive (healthy) for individuals and for the groups in which they exist, at least some of the time.

Finally, we have argued that adopting a an evolutionary-ecological perspective, with its dual emphases on understanding all classes of behavior and the underlying tendencies or traits motivating the behavioral exemplars of those classes as evidence of adaptation and on the phylogenetic history of the class (as revealed by comparisons with related species), can complement (rather than supplant) the dominant conceptual framework with its emphases on proximal determinants of individual behavior and the developmental assembly of behaviors through ontogenetic time. Integrating these perspectives is not a simple matter (as we hope our discussion has illustrated), but it should be very rewarding in terms of both explaining and changing the frequency with which interpersonal conflicts of interest are resolved using aggressive behavioral tactics. This chapter was prepared, in part, as an invitation to representatives from both empirical traditions to attempt such collaborations.

CONCLUSIONS

The problem of interpersonal aggression and trait aggressiveness has festered within the social and behavioral sciences as well as in psychiatry for more than a century. Whether the source of the problem is located in the person, as external to the person, or in the contexts that relate the person to environments, most clinical and/or developmental explanations of aggressive behavior and trait aggression have in common the underlying beliefs that aggressive behavior and trait aggressiveness are undesirable, bad, maladaptive, and probably evil. Those beliefs are challenged in this chapter and an account of aggressive behavior and trait aggressiveness that considers the ecological and evolutionary contexts of aggressive behavior and trait aggressiveness is offered as an alternative explanation for these phenomena. On this account, both aggressive behavior and trait aggressiveness are characterized as adaptive solutions to a range of challenges faced by human (and primate) ancestors. As such, aggressive behavior and trait aggressiveness can be considered as normal and expectable in many interpersonal contexts across the human lifespan. Successful aggression will likely be associated with a wide range of positive outcomes and will also likely be observed among the most competent and successful of individuals. However, unsuccessful aggression is likely associated with a range of negative outcomes and will frequently be observed as characteristic of less competent individuals. A selected review of human and nonhuman primate literatures supports these speculative hypotheses, although we acknowledge that arguments supporting the adaptive significance of aggressive behavior and trait aggressiveness do not reduce the potential for disruptive consequences in family, classroom, or community life contingent on the expression of trait aggression in these contexts. Some principles concerning the management of children's aggressive behavior deriving from ecological, evolutionary, and social developmental psychology are presented and discussed.

ACKNOWLEDGMENT

Support for the preparation of this chapter has been provided in part by NSF grants BCS 99-83391, and BCS 01- 26163.

REFERENCES

Abramovitch, R. (1976). The relation of attention and proximity rank in preschool children. In M. Chance & R. Larsen (Eds.), *The social structure of attention.* (pp. 154–176). London: Wiley.

Abramovitch, R., & Strayer, F. F. (1978). Preschool social organization: Agonistic spacing and attentional behaviors. In P. Pliner, T. Kramer, & T. Alloway (Eds.), *Recent advances in the study of communication and affect* (Vol. 6, pp. 197–217). New York: Plenum.

Altmann, J., Alberts, S. C., Haines, S. A., Dubach, J., Muruth, P., et al. (1996). Behavior predicts genetic structure in a wild primate group. *Proceedings of the National Academy of Science, USA. 93*, 5797–5801.

Altmann, J., Sapolsky, R., & Licht, P. (1995). Baboon fertility and social status. *Nature, 377*, 688–690.

Aureli, F., Das, M., Verleur, D., & van Hooff, J. A. R. (1994). Postconflict social interactions among barbary macaques *(Macaca sylvanus)*. *International Journal of Primatology, 15*, 471–484.

Aureli, F., & de Waal, F. B. M. (2000). *Natural conflict resolution.* Berkeley, CA: University of California Press.

Baldwin, J. M. (1911). Social competition and individualism. In J. M. Baldwin, *The individual and society or psychology and sociology* (pp. 77–117). Boston: Richard G. Badger.

Bandura, A. (1969). *Principles of behavior modification.* Holt, Rinehart, & Winston, Inc.

Bandura, A. (1973). *Aggression: A social learning analysis.* Edgewood Cliffs, NJ: Prentice-Hall.

Bandura, A. (1986). *Social foundations of thought and action: A social cognitive theory*. Englewood Cliffs, NJ: Prentice-Hall.

Baron, R. A., & Richardson, D. R. (1994). *Human aggression* (2nd ed.). New York: Plenum.

Bercovitch. F. B., & Numberg, P. (1997). Genetic determination of paternity and variation in male reproductive success in two populations of rheseus macaques. *Electrophoresis, 18*, 1701–1705.

Berkowitz, L. (1989). Frustration-aggressive hypothesis: Examination and reformulation. *Psychological Bulletin, 106*, 59–73.

Boehm, C. (1999). *Hierarchy in the forest: The evolution of egalitarian behavior*. Cambridge, MA: Harvard University Press.

Brooks, M. (1981). *The History of the World. Part 1*. Los Angeles, CA: Film distributed by Twentieth Century Fox.

Butovskaya, M., & Kozintsev, A. (1997). Aggression, friendship, and reconciliation in Russian primary schoolchildren. *Aggressive Behavior, 25*, 125–139.

Cairns, R. B. (1979). *Social development. The origins and plasticity of social interchanges*. San Francisco, CA: Freeman.

Cairns, R. B., Cairns, B. D., Neckerman, H. J, Gest, S. D., & Gariepy, J. L. (1988). Social networks and aggressive behavior: Peer support or peer rejection? *Developmental Psychology, 24*, 815–823.

Cairns, R. B., & Cairns, B. D. (1995). *Lifelines and risks: Pathways of youth in our time*. New York: Cambridge University Press.

Chagnon, N. A. (1997). *Yanomamo: The fierce people* (6th ed.). New York: Holt, Rinehart, and Winston.

Chagnon, N. A. (2000). Manipulating kinship rules: A form of male Yanomamo reproductive competition. In L. Cronk, N. Chagnon, & W. Irons (Eds.), *Adaptation and human behavior: An anthropological perspective* (pp. 115–132). Hawthorne, NY: Aldine de Gruyter.

Chance, M. R. A., & Jolly, C. J. (1970). *Social groups of monkeys, apes and men*. London: Jonathan Cape.

Crick, N. R., & Dodge, K. A. (1994). A review and reformulation of social information-processing mechanisms in children's social adjustment. *Psychological Bulletin, 115*, 74–101.

Crick, N. R. (2003, March). *Aggressive behavior is never adaptive*. Paper presented to the SRCD Peer Pre-Conference, Tampa, FL.

Dodge, K. A., & Crick, N. R. (1990). Social information-processing bases of aggressive behavior in children. *Personality & Social Psychology Bulletin, 16*, 8–22.

Dodge, K. A., & Somberg, D. R. (1987). Hostile attributional biases among aggressive boys are exacerbated under condition of threats to the self. *Child Development, 58*, 313–224.

Dollard, J., Doob, L. W., Miller, N. E., Mowrer, O. H., & Sears, R. R. (1939). *Frustration and aggression*. New Haven: Yale University Press.

Estell, D. B., Farmer, T. W., Pearl, R., Van Acker, R., & Rodkin, P. C. (2003). Heterogeneity in the relationship between popularity and aggression: Individual, group, and classroom influences. *New Directions for Child and Adolescent Development, 101*, 75–85.

Farmer, T., & Rodkin, P. C. (1966). Antisocial and prosocial correlates of class-room social positions. *Social Development, 5,* 174–188.

Farmer, T. W. (2000). The social dynamics of aggressive and disruptive behavior in school: Implications for behavioral consultation. *Journal of Educational and Psychological Consultation, 11,* 299–321.

Freud, S. (1961). *Civilization and its discontents.* New York: Norton.

Galliher, J. F., Kunkel, K. R., & Hobbs, D. J. (1986). Media explanations of small-town vigilante murder: Limitations and alternatives. *Crime, Law, and Social Change, 10,* 125–136.

Gangestad, S. W., & Simpson, J. A. (2000). The evolution of human mating: Trade-offs and strategic pluralism. *Behavioral and Brain Sciences, 23,* 573–644.

Gauthier, R., & Strayer, F. F. (1986). Empirical techniques for the identification of dominance. In D. M. Taub & F. A. King (Eds.), *Current perspectives in primate social dynamics* (pp. 120–133). New York: Van Nostrand Reinhold.

Ghiglieri, M. P. (1999). *The dark side of man.* New York: Basic Books.

Goldberg, T., & Wrangham, R. (1997). Genetic correlates of social behavior in wild chimpanzees: Evidence from mitochondrial DNA. *Animal Behavior, 54,* 559–570.

Goldman, E. N., & Loy, J. (1997). Longitudinal study of dominance relations among captive Patas monkeys. *American Journal of Primatology, 42,* 41–51.

Goodall, J. (1968). The behaviour of free-living chimpanzees in the Gombe Stream Reserve. *Animal Behavior Monograph, 1,* 165–311.

Goodall, J. (1977). Infant killing and cannibalism in free-living chimpanzees. *Folia Primatologica, 22,* 259–282.

Goodall, J. (1991). Unusual violence in the overthrow of an alpha male chim-panzee at Gombe. In T. Nashida et al. (Eds.), *Topics in Primatology, Vol 1: Human Origins* (pp. 131–142). Tokyo: University of Tokyo Press.

Goodall, J., Bandura, A., Bergmann, E., Busse, C., Matama, H., et al. (1979). Intercommunity interactions in the chimpanzee population of the Gombe National Park. In D. Hamburg & E. McCown, (Eds.), *The great apes* (pp. 13–54). Menlo Park: Benjamin/Cummings.

Gottlieb, G. (1992). *Individual development and evolution: The genesis of novel behavior.* New York: Oxford University Press.

Gottlieb, G. (1997). *Synthesizing nature-nurture: Prenatal roots of instinctive behavior.* Malwah, NJ: Lawrence Erlbaum Associates.

Groebel, J., & Hinde, R. A., (1989). *Aggression and war: Their biological and social bases.* Cambridge, UK: Cambridge University Press.

Gust, D. A., McCaster, T., Gordon, T. P., Gergits, W. F., Casna, N. J., & McClure, H. M. (1998). Paternity in Sooty Mangabeys. *International Journal of Primatology, 19,* 83–94.

Hamilton, W. D. (1964). The genetical evolution of social behaviour. *Journal of Theoretical Biology, 7,* 1–52.

Harcourt, A. H. (1978). Strategies of emigration and transfer by primates, with particular reference to gorillas. *Zeitschrift für Tierpsychologie, 48,* 401–420.

Harlow, H. K., Harlow, M. K., Dodsworth, R. O., & Arling, G. L (1966). Maternal behavior of rhesus monkeys deprived of mothering and peer association in infancy. *Proceedings of the American Philosophical Society, 110,* 58–66.

Hartup, W. W., Laursen, B., Stewart, M. I., & Eastenson, A. (1988). Conflict and the friendship relations of young children. *Child Development, 59*, 1590–1600.

Hawley, P. H. (1999). The ontogenesis of social dominance: A strategy-based evolutionary perspective. *Developmental Review, 19*, 97–132.

Hawley, P. H. (2002). Social dominance and prosocial and coercive strategies of resource control in preschoolers. *International Journal of Behavioral Development, 26*, 167–176.

Hawley, P. H. (2003). Prosocial and coercive configurations of resource control in early adolescence: A case for the well-adapted Machiavellian. *Merrill-Palmer Quarterly, 49*, 279–309.

Hawley, P. H., & Little, T. D. (1999). Winning some and losing some: A social relations approach to social dominance in toddlers. *Merrill-Palmer Quarterly, 45*, 185–214.

Hawley, P. H., Little, T. D., & Pasupathi, M. (2002). Winning friends and influencing peers: Strategies of peer influence in late childhood. *International Journal of Behavioral Development, 26*, 466–474.

Hawley, P. H., & Vaughn, B. E. (2003). Aggression and adaptive functioning: The bright side to bad behavior. *Merrill-Palmer Quarterly, 49*, 239–246.

Hold, B. (1977). Rank and Behavior: An ethological study of preschool children. *Homo, 28*, 158–188.

Huesmann, L. R., Eron, L. D., Lefkowitz, M. M., & Walder, L. O. (1984). Stability of aggression over time and generations. *Developmental Psychology, 20*, 1120–1134.

James, W. (1890). *The principles of psychology.* New York: Henry Holt.

Juvonen, J., Graham, S., & Schuster, M. A. (2003). Bullying among young adolescents: The strong, the weak, and the troubled. *Pediatrics, 112*, 1231–1237.

Kappeler, P. (1993). Female dominance in primates and other mammals. In P. P. G. Bateson, et al. (Eds.), *Perspectives in ethology, Vol. 10: Behavior and evolution.* New York: Plenum.

Koyama, N. F. (2003). Matrilineal cohesion and social networks in *macaca fuscata. International Journal of Primatology, 24*, 797–811.

Kuester, J. P. A. (1988). Rank relations of juvenile and subadult natal males of Barbary macaques (Macaca sylvanus) at Affenberg Salem. *Folia Primatologica, 5*, 33–44.

LeBlanc, S. (2003). *Constant battles.* New York: St. Martin's Press.

LaFreniere, P., & Charlesworth, W. R. (1983). Dominance, attention, and affiliation in a preschool group: A nine-month longitudinal study. *Ethology and Sociobiology, 4*, 55–67.

LaFreniere, P. J., & Charlesworth, W. R. (1987). Effects of friendship and dominance status on preschooler's resource utilization in a cooperative/competitive paradigm. *International Journal of Behavioral Development, 10*, 345–358.

Lorenz, K. (1966). *On aggression.* New York: Harcourt Brace.

Low, B. S. (2000). *Why sex matters.* Princeton, NJ: Princeton University Press.

Manson, J. H., & Wrangham, R. W. (1991). Intergroup aggression in chimpanzees and humans. *Current Anthropology, 32*, 369–390.

Marx, K., & Engels, F. (1848). *Manifest der Kommunistischen Parte* [the communist manifesto]. London: Burghars.

McGrew, W. C. (1972). *An ethological study of children's behavior*. New York: Academic Press.

Miller, N. E., Sears, R. R., Mowrer, O. H., Doob, L. W., & Dollard, J. I. (1941). The frustration–aggression hypothesis, *Psychological Review, 48*, 337–342.

Missakian, E.A. (1976, June). Aggression and dominance relations in peer groups of six to forty-five months of age. Paper presented at the Annual Meeting of the Animal Behavior Society, Colorado.

Missakian, E. A. (1980). Gender differences in agonistic behavior and dominance relations of Synanon communally reared children. In D. R. Omark, F. F. Strayer, & D. G. Freedman (Eds.), *Dominance relations: An ethological view of human conflict and social interaction* (pp. 397–414). New York: Garland.

Mitani, J., Merriwether, D. A., & Zhang, C. (2000). Male affiliation, cooperation, and kinship in wild chimpanzees. *Animal Behavior, 59, 885–893.*

Mitani, J. C., & Watts, D. P. (2001). Why do chimpanzees hunt and share meat? *Animal Behavior, 61,* 915–924.

Mitani, J. C., Watts, D. P., & Muller, M. N. (2002). Recent developments in the study of wild chimpanzee behavior. *Evolutionary Anthropology, 11,* 9–25.

Moffitt, T. E., Caspi, A., Dickson, N., Silva, P. S., & Stanton, W. (1996). Childhood-onset versus adolescent-onset antisocial conduct problems in males: Natural history from ages 3 to 18 years. *Development and Psychopathology, 8,* 399–424.

Nashida, T. (1983). Alpha status and agonistic alliance in wild chimpanzees (*Pan troglodytes scshweinfurthii*). *Primates, 24,* 318–336.

Nashida, T., Hiraiwa-Hasegawa, M., Hasegawa, T., & Takahata, Y. (1985). Group extinction and female transfer in wild chimpanzees in the Mahale National Park, Tanzania. *Zeitschrift fur Tierpsychologie, 67,* 284–301.

Nashida, T., & Kawanaka, K. (1985). Within-group cannibalism by adult male chimpanzees. *Primates, 26,* 274–285.

Nashida, T., & Hosaka, K. (1996). Coalition strategies among adult male chimpanzees of the Mihale Mountains, Tanzania. In W. McGrew, L. Marchant, & T. Nashida, (Eds.), *Great ape societies* (pp. 114–134). Cambridge: Cambridge University Press.

Oli, M. K. (2003). Hamilton goes empirical: estimation of inclusive fitness from life-history data. *Proceedings of the Royal Society of London, 270,* 307–311.

Parsons, T. (1947). Certain primary sources and patterns of aggression in the social structure of the Western world. *Psychiatry, 10,* 167–181.

Patterson, G. R. (1982). A social learning approach to family intervention: III. *Coercive Family Process.* Eugene, OR: Castalia.

Patterson, G. R., DeBaryshe, B., & Ramsay, E. (1989). A developmental perspective on antisocial behavior. *American Psychology, 44,* 329–335.

Pellegrini, A. D. (1998). Bullies and victims in school: A review and call for research. *Journal of Applied Developmental Psychology, 19,* 165–176.

Pellegrini, A. D. (2003). Perceptions and possible functions of play and real fighting in early adolescence. *Child Development, 74,* 1459–1470.

Pellegrini, A. D., & Bartini, M. (2001). Dominance in early adolescent boys: Affiliative and aggressive dimensions and possible functions. *Merrill-Palmer Quarterly, 47,* 142–163.

Pellegrini, A. D., Bartini, M., & Brooks, F. (1999). School bullies, victims, and aggressive victims: Factors relating to group affiliation and victimization in early adolescence. *Journal of Educational Psychology, 91*, 216–224.

Pellegrini, A. D., & Long, J. D. (2003). A sexual selection theory longitudinal analysis of sexual segregation and integration in early adolescence. *Journal of Experimental Child Psychology, 85*, 257–278.

Pellis, S. M., Pellis, V. C., & Foroud, A. (2005). Play fighting: Aggression, affiliation, and the development of nuanced social skills. In R. E. Tremblay, W. W. Hartup, & J. Archer (Eds.), *Developmental origins of aggression* (pp. 47–62). New York: Guilford.

Pereira, M. E. (1992). The development of dominance relations before puberty in cercopithecine societies. In J. Silverberg & P. Gray, (Eds.), *Aggression and peacefulness in humans and other primates* (pp. 117–149). New York: Oxford University Press.

Pereira, M. E. (1995). Development and social dominance among group-living primates. *American Journal of Primatology, 37*, 143–175.

Pereira, M. E., & Fairbanks, L. A. (2002a). *Juvenile primates: Life history, development, and behavior.* Chicago: University of Chicago Press. (Reprint originally published in 1993)

Pereira, M. E., & Fairbanks, L. A. (2002b). What are juvenile primates all about? In M. E. Pereira & L. A. Fairbanks (Eds.), *Juvenile primates: Life history, development, and behavior.* Chicago: University of Chicago Press. (Reprint originally published by Oxford University Press, 1993)

Prinstein, M. J., & Cillessen, A. H. N. (2003). Forms and functions of adolescent aggression associated with high levels of peer status. *Merrill-Palmer Quarterly, 49*, 310–342.

Pusey, A., Williams, J., & Goodall, J. (1997). The influence of dominance rank on the reproductive success of female chimpanzees. *Science, 277*, 828–831.

Raffaelli, M. (1997). Young adolescents' conflicts with siblings and friends. *Journal of Youth and Adolescence, 26*, 539–558.

Riss, D., & Goodall, J. (1977). The recent rise to the alpha rank in a population of free-living chimpanzees. *Folia Primatologica, 27*, 134–151.

Rodkin, P. C., Farmer, T. W., Pearl, R., & Van Acker, R. (2000). Heterogeneity of popular boys: Antisocial and prosocial configurations. *Developmental Psychology, 36,* 14–24.

Rowell, T. E. (1974). The concept of social dominance. *Behavioral Biology, 11*, 131–154.

Salmivalli, C., & Nieminen, E. (2002). Proactive and reactive aggression among school bullies, victims, and bully-victims. *Aggressive Behavior, 28*, 30–44.

Sannen, A., Heistermann, M., van Elsacker, L., Mohle, U., & Eens, M. (2003). Urinary testosterone metabolite levels in Bonobos: A comparison with Chimpanzees in relation to social system. *Behaviour, 140*, 683–696.

Santos, A. J., & Winegar, L. T. (1999). Child social ethology and peer relations: A developmental review of methodology and findings. *Acta Ethologica, 2*, 1–11.

Sapolsky, R. M. (2004). Social status and health in human and other animals. *Annual Review of Anthropology, 33*, 393–418.

Schjelderup-Ebbe, T. (1922). Beitra"ge zur Sozialpsychologie des Haushuhns (Contributions to the social psychology of domestic chickens). *Zeitschrift für Psychologie, 88,* 225–252.

Sluckin, A., & Smith, P. (1977). Two approaches to the concept of dominance in preschool children. *Child Development*, 48, 917–923.

Smith, P. K., Cowie, H., Olafsson, R. F., & Liefooghe, A. P. D. (2002). Definitions of bullying: A comparison of terms used, and age and gender differences, in a fourteen-country international comparison. *Child Development, 73,* 1119–1133.

Strayer, F. F. (1980a). Current problems in the study of dominance. In D. R. Omark, F. F. Strayer, & D. Freedman (Eds.), Dominance relations: *An ethological view of human conflict and social interaction* (pp. 443–452). New York: Garland STPM Press.

Strayer, F. F. (1980b). Social ecology of the preschool peer group. In W. A. Collins (Ed.), *Minnesota symposium on child development, Vol. 13* (pp. 165–196). Hillsdale, NJ: Lawrence Erlbaum Associates.

Strayer, F. F. (1989). Co-adaptation within the peer group: a psychobiological study of early competence. In B. Schneider, G. Atilia, J. Nadel, & R. Weisman (Eds.), *Social competence in developmental perspective* (pp.145–174). Dordecht, Netherlands: Kluwer.

Strayer, F. F. (1992). The development of agonistic and affiliative structures in preschool play groups. In J. Silverberg & P. Gray (Eds.), *Aggression and peacefulness in humans and other primates* (pp. 150–171). New York: Oxford University Press.

Strayer, F. F., Bovenkert, A., & Koopman, P. F. (1975). Social affiliation and dominance in captive squirrel monkeys (*Saimiri sciureus*). *Journal of Comparative and Physiological Psychology, 89,* 308–318.

Strayer, F. F., Chapeskie, T., & Strayer, J. (1978). The perception of preschool social dominance. *Aggressive Behavior, 4,* 183–192.

Strayer, F. F., & Harris, P. J. (1978). Social cohesion among captive squirrel monkeys (*Saimiri sciureus*). *Behavioral Ecology and Sociobiology, 5,* 93–110.

Strayer, F. F., & Noel, J. M. (1986). The prosocial and antisocial functions of preschool aggression: An ethological study of triadic conflict among young children. In C. Zahn-Waxler (Ed.), *Social and sociobiological origins* (pp. 107–131). New York: Cambridge University Press.

Strayer, F. F., & Strayer, J. (1976). An ethological analysis of social agonism and dominance relations among preschool children. *Child Development, 47,* 980–989.

Strayer, F. F., & Trudel, M. (1984). Developmental changes in the nature and function of social dominance among young children. *Ethology and Sociobiology, 5,* 279–295.

Symons, D. (1978). *Play and aggression: A study of rheseus monkeys.* New York: Columbia University Press.

Tinbergen, N. (1951). *The study of instinct.* New York: Oxford University Press.

Tremblay, R. E. (2000). The development of aggressive behaviour during childhood: What we have learned in the past century. *International Journal of Behavioral Development, 24,* 129–141.

Tremblay, R. E., Nagin, D. S., Seguin, J. R., Zoccolillo, M., Zelazo, P. D., Boivin, M., et al. (2004). Physical aggression in early childhood: Trajectories and predictors. *Pediatrics, 114*, 43–50.

Tremblay, R. E., & Nagin, D. S. (2005). The developmental oritins of physical aggression in humans. In R. E. Tremblay, W. W. Hartup, & J. Archer (Eds.), *Developmental origins of aggression* (pp. 83–106). New York: Guilford.

Trivers, R. L. (1974). Parent–offspring conflict. *American Zoologist, 14*, 249–264.

Vaughn, B. E. (1999). Power is knowledge (and *vice versa*): A commentary on "on winning some and losing some: A social relations approach to social dominance in toddlers". *Merrill-Palmer Quarterly, 45*, 215–225.

Vaughn, B. E., Vollenweider, M., Bost, K. K., Azria-Evans, M. R., & Snider, J. B. (2003). Negative interactions and social competence for preschool children in two samples: Reconsidering the interpretation of aggressive behavior for young children. *Merrill-Palmer Quarterly, 49*, 245–278.

Vaughn, B. E., & Waters, E. (1980). Social organization among preschooler peers: Dominance, attention and sociometric correlates. In D. R. Omark, F. F. Strayer, & D. Freedman (Eds.), *Dominance relations: An ethological view of human conflict and social interaction.* (pp. 359–380). New York: Garland STPM Press.

Vaughn, B. E., & Waters, E. (1981) Attention structure, sociometric status, and dominance: interrelations, behavioral correlates, and relationships to social competence. *Developmental Psychology, 17*(3), 275–288.

Verbeek, P., & de Waal, F. B. M. (2001). Peacemaking among preschool children. *Peace and Conflict: Journal of Peace Psychology, 7*, 5–28.

de Waal, F. (1982). *Chimpanzee politics: Power and sex among apes.* Baltimore: The Johns Hopkins University Press.

de Waal, F. B. M. (1986a). The integration of dominance and social bonding in primates. *Quarterly Review of Biology, 61*, 459–469.

de Waal, F. B. M. (1986b). The brutal elimination of a rival among captive male chimpanzees. *Ethology and Sociobiology, 7*, 237–251.

de Waal, F. B. M. (1989a). *Peacemaking among primates.* Cambridge, MA: Harvard University Press.

De Waal, F. B. M. (1989b). Dominance "style" and primate social organization. In V. Standen & R. A. Foley (Eds.), *Comparative socioecology* (pp. 243–264). Oxford, UK: Blackwell.

De Waal, F. B. M. (1992). Aggression as a well-integrated part of primate social relationships: A critique of the Seville Statement on Violence. In J. Silverberg & P. Gray (Eds.), *Aggression and peacefulness in humans and other primates* (pp. 37–56). New York: Oxford University Press.

de Waal, F. B. (1995). Bonobo sex and society. *Scientific American, 272*, 82–88.

de Waal, F. B. M. (2000). Primates: A natural heritage of conflict resolution. *Science, 289*, 586–590.

De Waal, F. B. M., & Johanowicz, D. L. (1993). Modification of reconciliation behavior through social experience: An experiment with two macaque species. *Child Development, 64*, 897–908.

De Waal, F. B. M., & Yoshihara, D. (1983). Reconciliation and redirected affection in rhesus monkeys. *Behavior, 85*, 224–241.

Watts, D. P. (1989). Infanticide in mountain gorillas: New Cases and a reconsideration of the evidence. *Ethology, 81*, 1–18.

Watts, D. P. (2004). Intracommunity coalitionary killing of an adult male chimpanzee at Ngogo, Kibale National Park, Uganda. *International Journal of Primatology, 25*, 507–521.

Watts, D. P., & Mitani, J. C. (2000). Infanticide and cannibalism by male chimpanzees at Ngogo Kibale National Park, Uganda. *Primates, 41*, 357–365.

Weaver, A., & de Waal, F. B. M. (2003). The mother-offspring relationship as a template in social development: Reconciliation in captive brown Capuchins (*cebus apella*). *Journal of Comparative Psychology, 117*, 101–110.

Weisfeld, G., Omark, D. R., & Cronin, C. L. (1980). A longitudinal and cross-sectional study of dominance in boys. In D. R. Omark, F. F. Strayer, & D. Freedman (Eds.), *Dominance relations: An ethological view of human conflict and social interaction* (pp. 205–216). New York: Garland.

Wilson, E. O. (1975). *Sociobiology.* Cambridge, MA: Belknap.

Wilson, M., Hauser, M., & Wrangham, R. (2001). Does participation in intergroup conflict depend on numerical assessment, range location, or rank for wild chimpanzees? *Animal Behavior, 61*, 1203–1216.

Wilson, M. L., & Wrangham, R. W. (2003). Intergroup relations in chimpanzees. *Annual Review of Anthropology, 32*, 563–592.

Watts, D., & Mitani, J. (2001). Boundary patrols and intergroup encounters among wild chimpanzees. *Behaviour, 138*, 299–327.

Wrangham, R. W. (1999). The evolution of coalitionary killing. *Yearbook of Physical Anthropology, 42*, 1–30.

Wrangham, R., & Peterson, D. (1996) *Demonic males.* New York: Houghton-Mifflin Company.

York, A. D., & Rowell, T. E. (1988). Reconciliation following aggression in patas monkeys, *Erythrocebus patas. Animal Behavior, 36*, 502–509.

Zillman, D. (1979). *Hostility and aggression.* Hillsdale, NJ: Lawrence Erlbaum Associates.

3

WHY HAS AGGRESSION BEEN THOUGHT OF AS MALADAPTIVE?

Peter K. Smith
Goldsmiths College, University of London

This chapter attempts an ideological history of thinking about aggression, especially in children, and especially among developmental psychologists. It does not present new data, but rather explore why the labeling of aggression as maladaptive gained such widespread acceptance over such a considerable period of time.

Aggressive behavior is prevalent throughout nonhuman species, and serves a variety of functions. For interspecific aggression, these include obtaining prey items (food), and defending self or offspring/kin against predators. For intraspecific aggression, these include competition for resources, status, and ultimately reproductive opportunities. Aggressive behavior is also prevalent throughout human societies, and throughout the lifespan in both genders; it is often successful at least at certain levels.

Despite the ubiquity of aggression and its apparent functionality, a strong tradition of work in childhood social development has uncritically characterized aggression as "maladaptive" or "socially incompetent" behavior, and aggressive children as "lacking social skills." Some examples of this tradition of thinking will be given. This view has been challenged recently within child development, with evidence that aggressive behavior can, in some contexts, be associated with popularity, status, social skills and social competence. Some of those putting forward this revised view argue that the traditional view confounds what is socially desirable, with what is socially competent or successful.

But why did the traditional view—of aggression as maladaptive— come to be so influential for so long? I explore the history of this and suggest some reasons. The two main reasons I suggest are (1) the sheltered disciplinary ethos of psychology in much of the 20th century (ignoring both evolutionary explanations, and wider sociological contexts and conflicts of interest between individuals and groups), and (2) the strong "social engineering" or policy-oriented ethos of early child development work (with the objective of raising good healthy children).

DEFINITION, TYPES AND MODES OF AGGRESSION

Aggression is generally taken as referring to an attack on or harm to other(s), that is intentional; it can be seemingly unprovoked (proactive aggression), or in response to aggressive provocation (reactive aggression). Related terms are violence (often defined as only physical forms of aggression, but might involve damage to property as well as persons); bullying (usually defined as repeated aggression where there is an imbalance of power); and delinquent or antisocial behavior (generally defined in more legal terms).

Types of Aggression

Considering the range of types of aggression seen in nonhuman species, as well as humans, there is a broad division between interspecific and intraspecific aggression. Interspecific aggression—from one species to another—would include predation (you certainly harm another being when you eat it!). It would also include defensive aggression (against a predator, for example); and mobbing behavior, as when smaller birds may harass a potential predator to drive it away.

Intraspecific aggression—within members of a species—is generally, and very broadly, over resources. These may be direct fights over, for example, mating opportunities, a breeding or nesting site, food, or possession of a territory that is proxy for access to any of these. Another category of aggression would be dominance conflicts; these may be apparently unprovoked, but in group-living species can be important as a proxy for avoiding prolonged resource conflicts. Described early on in domestic fowl (the "pecking order"), dominance hierarchies are characteristic of many mammalian species including ungulates, canids, and primates (Moore, 1993). The dominance hierarchy provides a way of avoiding lots of damaging fights over resources. Usually, a lower ranking animal gives way to a higher ranking animal over a resource. This is to the benefit of the lower ranking animal, as it avoids a high probability of unnecessary injury. However it does not get the resource; and in the long run, this could be very disadvantageous. Thus at times, challenges to dominance status will occur. Such challenges are especially likely in two situations. One is developmental; a younger animal approaches maturity and fuller strength, and/or an older animal loses power. The other is structural; a new animal joins a social group. Both such dominance challenges are commonly seen in ground-living primates, such as rhesus macaques. Dominance rankings are important for both males and females (though the two rankings are rather separate). Dominance is more fluid in males; as a juvenile male approaches adult status, he will either need to fight for a higher dominance ranking within his own troop, or, as quite often happens, leave his natal troop for another and fight to establish his ranking within that one.

What appears to us as a particularly nasty kind of aggressive behavior, is abuse of infants, and infanticide. These are not rare in animal species. In lions, for example, who are organized on a pride system (a few males and several females and their young), an incoming group of younger males (often related to each other, though not to the pride) may drive away the resident males and take over the mating rights with the females. When this happens, young lion cubs are likely to be attacked and killed by the incoming males (the females try to avoid this, but will not risk a deadly fight with the males). The likely reason is that these cubs are unrelated to the incoming males, and the females will conceive again more quickly (with the incoming males' own offspring) if these cubs are not suckling (Bertram, 1976).

Such phenomena are common in primates too. They may not be such overt attacks and killing as in the case of lions, but maltreatment of infants can occur. This is often in the context of allomothering—females other than the mother, carrying an infant. This is often helpful when the other female is a sister, or related; but sometimes females who are not related, and from a different and maybe more dominant matriline, will "kidnap" an infant and mistreat it physically (Hrdy, 1977).

Examples of aggressive behavior are thus widespread in animals. Indeed I know of no species of animal where there is no repertoire of aggressive behavior. The reason is obvious and is spelled out in evolutionary theory. Animals are competing for limited resources. This does not mean continual fighting and competition (see discussion of games theory, in the following section). Animals often need to cooperate too, especially in group-living species and in kin groups. But an animal that cannot be aggressive at times to defend its interests is unlikely to survive long, and unlikely to have many offspring. In summary, the capacity for aggressive behavior is vital for reproductive success, and has clearly been selected for in every species.

Modes of Aggression in Humans. In animal species, aggressive behavior most obviously takes the form of direct physical attack. In humans, however, we see (or are aware of) a much wider variety of forms, due to our linguistic abilities and complicated social groupings. Physical attacks may also be indirect (e.g., on someone's belongings, or property). Direct verbal attacks (orally, or by letter, text, or e-mail) can be hurtful and damaging. So can indirect verbal attacks (spreading rumors detrimental to someone in a social group). Systematic social exclusion from normal group activities can be considered aggressive. Indeed, social exclusion and rumor spreading are often described as relational aggression (Crick & Grotpeter, 1995).

There are yet more sophisticated ways of damaging someone, in adults especially and in institutional settings. Björkqvist, Österman, and Lagerspetz (1994) have described manipulative practices of institutional aggression, such as setting unrealistic workloads in order that someone will fail, or insinuating without direct accusation.

Sex differences characterize these types of human aggression (Card & Little, this volume). Males relatively commit more physical kinds of attacks; females relatively commit more relational kinds of attacks (Björkqvist, 1994). A likely reason grounded in evolutionary theory is that (given that most aggression is within one sex) each sex chooses forms of aggression that are most damaging: For males, physical strength is a sign of status and a physical attack directly threatens such status. For females, reputation in the social network (rather than physical strength) is a measure of status, and relational aggression is probably more effective.

There are also characteristic age trends. The frequency of aggressive behavior tends to increase with age and then decrease, but is very dependent on type and mode. Physical aggression peaks earlier than verbal, relational, and later still institutional aggression (Björkqvist, Lagerspetz, & Kauklainen, 1992). Such phenomena are of course heavily mediated by culture and practices such as subsistence economy, schooling, and work practices. However a widespread observation is that dominance conflicts peak in adolescence, whether this takes the form of risk-taking behaviors, noncompliance with adult rules, or direct physical violence (Arnett, 1992). Again, this has a basis in evolutionary reasoning, as adolescence signals the beginning of entry into adulthood and the need to challenge for a position or status both vis-à-vis one's peers, and with the adult world.

Finally, in humans especially, aggressive behavior can vary in social complexity in terms of numbers. Much aggression is one-to-one, or by a small group or gang (against one, or against another group or gang). But, in addition, we can witness aggression by larger groups; for example in mob violence, or in village conflicts or tribal warfare (Chagnon, 1968). And, of course, we can see aggression at the state or nation level, or by an alliance of nations, in modern warfare.

Cultural factors greatly influence the expression and frequency of aggression. Some societies are relatively warlike (Chagnon, 1968); others are relatively peaceful, and discourage the overt expression of aggression (Kemp & Fry, 2004). However in no society is aggression absent. In summary, aggressive behavior is ubiquitous in humans, as individuals, groups or societies.

Aggression in Childhood has Often Been Seen as "Maladaptive."   The raison d'être for this book is exactly this—that those of us who have been working in the area of childhood social development in recent decades know that aggression in children has often been labeled as "maladaptive." The precise label varies, but common epithets are "socially incompetent," "showing deficits in social information processing," and "exhibiting maladaptive behavior." In addition, such behavior has often been labeled "deviant," a concept that requires a slightly different analysis.

The view of aggression as maladaptive behavior has been put recently in its strongest form by proponents of the Social Information Processing model (SIPS). For example, Crick and Dodge (1996) wrote that "Skillful processing at each step is hypothesized to lead to competent performance within a situation, whereas biased or deficient processing is hypothesized to lead to deviant social behavior (e.g., aggression)," and "Social maladjustment is related to the formulation of social goals that are likely to be relationship-damaging" (p. 994).

This view of childhood aggression as "maladaptive" is often reproduced and transmitted to students of child development, in textbooks. For example, in *Child Psychology: A Contemporary Viewpoint*, Hetherington and Parke (1993) state that "aggressive children may behave in a hostile and inappropriate fashion because they are not very skilled at solving interpersonal problems" (p. 603). In *Child Development*, Berk (2000) states that "social-cognitive deficits and distortions add to the maintenance of aggressive behavior" (p. 515).

In *How Children Develop* (2003), Siegler, DeLoache, and Eisenberg review work on aggressive behavior and social cognition. They summarize the evidence (p. 559) as showing that aggressive children are more likely to:

- "Attribute hostile motives to others in contexts in which the other person's motives and intentions are unclear"
- Have goals "hostile and inappropriate to the situation"
- "Come up with fewer options ... and these options are more likely to involve aggressive or disruptive behaviors"
- "Evaluate aggressive responses more favorably, and competent, prosocial responses less favorably"

- "Expect aggressive behavior to result in positive outcomes (e.g., getting their own way) and to reduce negative treatment by others"
- "Feel more confident of their ability to perform acts of physical and verbal aggression."

These statements may well provide a reasonably accurate factual summary of a considerable body of literature. However, it hardly seems a basis for labeling aggressive children as incompetent. Admittedly, some studies suggest that they come up with fewer response options, and that could legitimately be argued to be a deficit. On the other hand, expecting aggressive responses to produce positive outcomes and reduce negative treatment by others might well be skillful, competent behavior; further, feeling more confident in their ability to perform acts of aggression must be a sign of competence, not incompetence. Nevertheless the authors label prosocial as distinct to aggressive responses as "competent," and go on to state that "not all aggressive children exhibit the same deficits" (p. 560)—implying that for most aggressive children, these are "deficits."

Questioning Whether Childhood Aggression Is Maladaptive

There are very good reasons to doubt this "received wisdom," as exemplified in a considerable body of child development research, and in child psychology texts. The reasons are both theoretical, and empirical. I take my theoretical arguments from (a) evolutionary theory, (b) developmental theories within psychology, and (c) sociological theory.

Evolutionary Theory.   As we saw earlier, evolutionary theory suggests that aggressive behavior is universal, and multifaceted. It must often be adaptive, or else it would not have been selected. Furthermore, its adaptive nature is obvious, in terms of individual reproductive success.

This does not mean that we should expect an animal to be aggressive frequently, or in every situation. Aggressive behavior is always risky—there is an obvious danger of retaliation and injury. The work of Maynard Smith (1982) and others, who applied game theory analyses to animal behavior, shows this clearly. In a simple model, Maynard Smith imagined a "hawk" strategy (when, in conflict over a resource, always attack), and a "dove" strategy (who always retreat). In a population of "doves," a single "hawk" wins every conflict at zero cost, so obviously "hawks" multiply. But in a population of "hawks," they are always fighting, injuring, and killing each other; a "dove" avoids injury and survives. So the optimal strategy is actually some balance between the two. More sophisticated models build in elements such as assessing the opponent's strength, and responding depending on what the opponent's previous act was (e.g., "tit-for-tat"). In summary, what these analyses show—and consistent with what is observed in actual animal behavior—is that some mixed strategy is most effective. The most successful patterns are a mix of cooperative and competitive strategies. Aggressive behavior is an option, just as is cooperative and even altruistic behavior (Trivers, 1971). The balance will depend on the individual, the circumstances, and the species. But a "competent" or "well-adapted" animal will certainly have aggressive behavior within its repertoire.

Developmental Theories Within Psychology.   In terms of skill development, there are certainly views within psychology that would see conflict situations and even aggressive behaviors, as developing important social and cognitive abilities. These may be ignored if we focus on victims of aggression (as Vaughn, this volume, points out), but are often present for the aggressor(s).

Some of these skills would be intrinsic to aggression itself. Only by engaging in fights or other forms of aggressive behavior will you learn, for example, about your own strengths and weaknesses (physically, verbally, and psychologically) in such situations. You will learn how to be aggressive more effectively—when to attack, which mode of aggression to use, when to stop, and so on. In other words, if aggression is a conditional strategy, we need to learn about these conditions and how to operate within them—don't attack a much stronger opponent (usually); it's best to trust someone first and only attack them if they attack you (usually)—the kinds of knowledge operationalized in the game theory analyses just described.

Such arguments could be accused of being circular. These skills are only needed if aggression is needed. But it is also possible and perhaps likely that other skills can be acquired through aggressive behaviors that have more general application. Certain aggressors (an example is ring-leader bullies; Salmivalli, Lagerspetz, Björkqvist, Osterman, & Kaukianen, 1996) would need skills such as leading a gang, choosing the right place to attack a victim, avoiding detection, choosing the most effective way to hurt a victim. These involve more general skills such as understanding social dynamics and the thoughts and emotions and likely plans of others.

Sociological Theory.   Another set of relevant perspectives comes from writings in the sociological tradition. Sociologists have, more than developmental psychologists, kept apart the interests of the individual and the interests of the social group or the wider society. This is noticeable in writings about delinquent and antisocial behavior, for example in adolescence. Whereas child psychologists have generally taken delinquent and antisocial behavior as a sign of lacking social skills (and hence using social skills training programs; e.g., Bullis, Walker, & Sprague, 2001), sociologists and some social psychologists have taken different perspectives.

One set of arguments would posit that aggressive and antisocial behavior can enhance status in a peer group, especially a delinquent peer group. Reputation enhancement theory suggests that delinquent adolescents and adolescent peer groups have different values concerning antisocial behavior; for nondelinquent groups antisocial behavior might be a reason for exclusion, but for delinquent groups it is a reason for inclusion (Carroll et al., 1999; Emler, Reicher, & Ross, 1987).

Another argument is that aggression can sometimes be seen as a "rational" response when other developmental pathways do not appear to offer much chance or reward. This could be the case for youth in very disadvantaged environments; conventional career prospects are small or nonexistent, and aggressive or antisocial acts may provide an alternative "career path" that offers more promise in terms of money, prestige and opportunity. More broadly, aggression can be seen sometimes as a legitimate response to oppression (Galtung, 1969). This could be at the level of individuals within a repressive institution or society; or at the level of a group, or even a nation state, feeling threatened or repressed by another.

Empirical Evidence.   As much of this book is taken up with empirical evidence counteracting the view that childhood aggression is necessarily maladaptive, it is not necessary to go into details about this here. I just mention a few examples—two very relevant to the evolutionary approach, two to the developmental approach.

Hawley's (2002, 2003) research shows that in resource competition situations, a mixed strategy (sometimes prosocial, sometimes coercive) enhances social dominance with "bistrategic controllers" being most effective. For example, her study with 3- to 5-year-old U.S. preschoolers found that "bistrategic controllers, although aggressive, were morally mature and preferred play partners by their peers" (Hawley, 2003, p. 213). This was not true of those children just using coercive control. Such findings are very compatible with the evolutionary game theory analyses described earlier.

Pellegrini and Long (2003) obtained a range of longitudinal data on 138 U.S. early adolescents aged 12–13 years. Their work suggests the importance of social dominance and aggression at this age, although differently for the two sexes. They found that dating popularity correlated with dominance, for boys. For girls, dating popularity correlated with relational aggression. Again, this emphasis on the role of dominance and ways of obtaining it, fits well with evolutionary thinking.

Two other studies relate more to possible developmental benefits of aggression (of course, evolutionary and developmental arguments are often compatible). Vaughn, Vollenweider, Bost, Azria-Evans, & Snider (2003), in a study of 471 U.S. 3-year-olds in Head Start programs, found a complex pattern of correlations between measures of aggression and measures of social competence, but make a fair summary in stating that "for the most part, aggression and negative behavior measures were positive predictors of social competence," and "we are inclined to see these negative episodes as opportunities for learning and for social-cognitive development." Working with a sample of 206 English 7- to 10-year-olds, Sutton, Smith, and Swettenham (1999a) found that ring-leader bullies (but not other aggressive children) scored higher on measures of social cognition—advanced theory-of-mind tasks, and emotion recognition tasks. They argued that ring-leader bullies especially needed to develop such skills, to be able to lead a gang, choose effective ways of hurting a victim, avoid detection, and generally maintain their reputation.

In summary, these and other studies provide ample evidence that equating aggressive behavior with social incompetence is much too simple, if not plain wrong. At various age levels through childhood, some aggressive behavior (e.g., bistrategic controller, ring-leader bully) is associated positively with social competence and/or popularity, even if other aggressive behavior (e.g., coercive controller, assistant, or follower bully) is not.

AVOIDING CONFUSION

At this point it is important to avoid possible confusion between scientifically appraising the correlates of aggressive behavior, and approving it or taking a moral stance. Of course, aggressive behavior is unpleasant or dangerous to others. Although it should not be labeled as "socially incompetent" or "maladaptive," in any general sense, it might well be labeled as "socially undesirable" (Sutton, Smith, & Swettenham, 1999b). In between these two labels, aggressive behavior is often labeled as "deviant." It may be deviant from social norms (i.e., socially undesirable), but it is not really deviant developmentally (i.e., many children show aggressive behavior, competently). We should not confuse "socially undesirable" with "socially incompetent"; and we should not confuse social interests, with the interests of an individual. I return to further consideration of these labels, and of moral judgment issues, at the end of this chapter.

Why was Childhood Aggression Thought to be Maladaptive?

It appears that we have a tradition of thinking and summarizing about childhood aggression, in research and in textbooks, that is at best one-sided if not basically erroneous. This research has ignored competing viewpoints, and confused social undesirability with social incompetence. Why did this happen? I argue that there are two important causes. One lies in the origins of the discipline of child psychology, and the "social engineering" ethos that pervaded it through much of the 20th century. The other lies in the disciplinary isolation of child psychology, especially from evolutionary theories, and from sociological approaches.

The "Social Engineering" Ethos of Much Child Psychology in the 20th Century

As Fagan (1992) writes, "the late 19th and early 20th centuries marked an era of social reforms, many of which were directed at children" (p. 236). In North America (United States, Canada) and in European countries such as the United Kingdom, the origins of child psychology were bound up with other practical disciplines and hopes of social reform and improvement, including the child study movement. Universal and compulsory schooling was coming to these developing industrialized countries, and the new discipline of child study was intimately involved in both documenting normal patterns of behavior, and in diagnosing and dealing with patterns that proved difficult for schooling, or more generally for behavior in line with social reform aspirations. As Witmer (who founded the first psychological clinic in the United States, in 1896) put it, an important aim of clinic work with "slum children" was to "discover mental and moral defects and to treat the child in such a way that these defects may be overcome or rendered harmless" (Witmer, 1910; cited in Fagan, 1992, p. 238).

According to Fagan (1992) "after 1910, the more scientific fields of child and educational psychology and psychoeducational testing emerged to replace traditional child study" (p. 241). Child psychology, clinical/school psychology, and special education, influenced each other and developed symbiotically in the United States, in the early decades of the 20th century. "All these relationships developed interdependently, and all were prompted by the reform era and associated with broad expressions of a new psychotechnology" (Fagan, 1992, p. 241).

During the 1920s to 1940s, many child development institutes and welfare stations were set up in North America. The Society for Research in Child Development (SRCD) started in 1933. Looking back at 70 years of SRCD and child development research in his 2003 Presidential address, Parke (2004) wrote that these reflected "societal concerns about ways of improving the rearing of children" (p. 2). A striking phrase from Cora Bussey Hillis, "an early supporter of these activities," is: "If research could improve corn and hogs, it could improve children" (Parke, 2004, p. 2; citing Sears, 1975). This phrase epitomizes what can be called a "social engineering ethos"; a wish to "improve children" so that they behave in accordance with the wishes of social reformers. They should behave well in school, and not engage in deviant or anti-social behaviors.

A similar philosophy can be seen at work in England. At the start of the 20th century the mental hygiene movement was concerned with practices of investigation, diagnosis and reformation of maladjusted and delinquent children. According to Rose (1985, p. 197), juvenile courts and child guidance clinics arose through the 1920s and 1930s as part of the mental hygiene movement. "This psychology entered into an alliance with welfare workers, providing the rationale for a new theory and practice of social work"; "the difficult child was gradually re-conceived in terms of maladjustment" (p. 165).

Maladjustment was taken as "disharmony between the individual and the social relations in which he must live." The U.K. Underwood Report of 1955, Report of the Committee on Maladjusted Children, stated that "the surest way to prevent maladjustment from arising in children is to encourage in every possible way their healthy develop-ment, particularly on the emotional side" (cited in Rose, 1990, p. 172). Much of the intervention work inspired by this movement was directed against aggression and delinquency in children.

Of course, a great deal of this thought and effort can be seen as jus-tifiable, especially taking as one's premise the efficient working of soci-ety and of socially approved institutions (such as schools). However it does take the society as a given "good" and it does conflate what might be in an individual's interests with what is in society's interests. As Rose (1985) puts it, "This problem is exacerbated further when what counts as abnormality is set by a norm of adaptation to the conventions of a socioeconomic order" (p. 231). This is by now a not unfamiliar cri-tique of psychological thinking from a sociological perspective. But why has it taken so long to have an impact?

DISCIPLINARY ISOLATION OF CHILD PSYCHOLOGY

Child study followed by child psychology developed in an ideological context of social reform, mental hygiene, and social engineering. Although laudable in principle, these aims ran the risk of routinely conflating individual benefit with social benefit, and of taking as a given a particular kind of society or socioeconomic order. Insights from evolutionary thinking, from sociological thinking, and even different areas of thinking in developmental psychology, might have helped produce a broader and more reflective perspective on this ideological context. It did not happen. The cause seems to have been an unthinking disciplinary isolation, possibly rooted in a concern to establish child psychology as a scientific discipline in its own right. As Parke (2004) wrote about the 70 years of SRCD, reviewing the decades 1943 to 1963, "In terms of the twin themes of application and interdisciplinarity, this historical period was not a cause for celebration. In our eagerness to achieve respectability as a science, we developed a disciplinarity that reduced the flow of ideas and influence across disciplinary boundaries" (p. 4).

Isolation From Evolutionary Theories

Although biological/evolutionary theories were influential at the start of the 20th century, for example in the work of Hall (1904), on the whole the reaction against "social Darwinism" seems to have negated this. Throughout much of the last century, debate on biological influences on development in child psychology was largely limited to the heredity/environment issue and their relative influence (often treated dichotomously). The evolutionary approach was not seriously considered in child development research until the 1970s. It then began to appear through the child ethology movement (Blurton Jones, 1972). Even then, child ethology remained a minority concern, and also was mainly involved in advocating more naturalistic, observational studies, rather than strongly pushing an evolutionary perspective in terms of adaptation. The advent of sociobiology (Wilson, 1975) gradually changed this, together with the development of evolutionary psychology. However only in very recent years has a true evolutionary developmental psychology begun to have some influence in mainstream thinking (Bjorklund & Pellegrini, 2000, 2002; Bjorklund & Smith, 2003; Geary & Bjorklund, 2000; Hawley, 2003).

Isolation From Sociological Approaches

There has been a consistent area of research in the sociology of childhood, in topics such as peer relationships (Corsaro, 1997) and delinquency (Sumner, 1994). A distinctive program for a sociological approach to childhood has, however, only been fully articulated in the last 20 years (James & Prout, 1990; Jenks, 1982), perhaps more strongly in Europe than in North America. Related to this have been radical critiques of developmental psychology (e.g., Burman, 1994). The program presented by James and Prout (1990, pp. 8–9) and in associated critiques, would certainly lead to a rethink of the "aggression equals maladjustment" assumption, because they stress the strong influence of social ideology on the kind of developmental psychology that is encouraged or pursued.

However, although not ignored, these perspectives have seldom interacted in any substantial way with mainstream research by psychologists on social development. This is perhaps because the broad brush critique often presented by such sociological thinkers, not only attacks many other targets (e.g., quantitative methodology, the positivistic viewpoint), but also can be seen as insensitive to what have been broader interests and developments in mainstream developmental psychology in recent decades. In any event, the insights of this kind of perspective, for example into career paths in antisocial behavior and delinquency, and the distinction between individual needs and wider societal needs, have had little impact into research as published in flagship child psychology journals such as *Child Development* and *Developmental Psychology*.

Insights from either evolutionary thinking, or from sociological thinking, could have served as antidotes to the social engineering ethos of mainstream child psychology (especially regarding social development) in the 20th century. In fact, for various reasons (that deserve much fuller exploration than sketched out here), these perspectives only began to have an impact in the 1980s, and only started to impact significantly on mainstream thinking in very recent years.

SUMMARY ON AGGRESSION AS MALADAPTIVE

To summarize so far, aggression in children has often been labeled as "maladaptive" or "socially incompetent" by developmental psychologists. This is not a tenable position, either empirically or theoretically. Aggressive behavior is a universally available part of the behavioral repertoire of all species, including humans. Social competence means being able to use aggressive behavior in suitable ways, at suitable times, in suitable contexts. This will, of course, depend on the social context, and some societies and historical periods, more than others, have tried to moderate or decrease aggressive behavior.

The prevalent misconception just discussed may have arisen through a combination of a social engineering ethos that motivated and guided much of child study and child psychology through the 20th century. Further, a disciplinary isolation during this period from other perspectives, notably from evolutionary psychology on the one hand, or sociological thinking on the other, might have inoculated against such short-sightedness. As it is, many developmental psychologists have confused "socially incompetent" with "socially undesirable."

Of course, individual episodes of aggressive behavior may be socially incompetent, and some individuals may be more aggressive than is good for them. But just because too much aggression or the wrong kind of aggression can sometimes be bad for an individual, does not justify labeling all aggressive behavior as "incompetent." After all, some individuals eat too much than is good for them, or eat the wrong foods, but we do not say that eating per se is "incompetent"! To my mind, the argument that aggression is socially incompetent, as a generality, is a nonstarter. But some of the other labels are more challenging. Often childhood aggression is labeled as "deviant social behavior" (Crick & Dodge, 1996, p. 994). And is aggression necessarily "socially undesirable"?

IS AGGRESSION "DEVIANT"?

Deviant is described as "different from the norm or from accepted standards" (*Encarta World English Dictionary,* 1999). Again, there is confusion between what happens, and what is socially desirable. Highly aggressive children would certainly be different from the norm, and would certainly offend against accepted standards in modern Western society. However aggressive behavior generally is not different from the norm; it would be a hard task to find a child who has never been aggressive—indeed, and especially including relational aggression, to find a child who has not been aggressive on many occasions. Thus, using "socially deviant behavior" as a general label for aggression in children (rather than just for unusually highly aggressive children) can only be referring to the "accepted standards" part of the definition; in other words, saying that aggressive behavior is socially undesirable.

IS AGGRESSION ALWAYS SOCIALLY UNDESIRABLE?

Many societies have actually encouraged childhood aggression, especially physical fighting in boys and young men. For individuals, fighting prowess was a mark of manhood and a route to status and reproductive success. And for the tribe, skilled fighters were essential for intertribal conflicts over resources. This does not mean that nomadic and tribal peoples were necessarily very aggressive. This was very variable. Conflicts could often be resolved by ritualized aggression rather than serious fights. Indeed, individuals who could not control very high aggression were often seen as dangerous. As Fry (2005) summarizes,

"For humans, the practice of fighting skills may be a more complex task than in some other species. Humans may have to practice not only fighting maneuvers but also restraint within a social world that includes rules for fighting and dispute resolution. It is interesting to contemplate how much aggression among humans is restrained, curtailed, or limited through social conventions, enforced by the participants themselves and by other members of the group" (p. 79).

In modern societies, aggressive behavior less often involves direct physical fighting, especially in warfare. There has arguably been a historical trend to put more constraints on violence and warfare (Ruff, 2001), even if success is obviously very partial and patchy. This goes with a socialization rhetoric that puts a negative value on aggressive behavior, and especially physical aggression. This rhetoric is especially strong in the "socially reforming" professions, such as teachers and social workers.

It is clear that aggression harms others, and that it is justifiable for society to negatively sanction much aggressive behavior, and for parents to socialize their children into not being unduly aggressive (Tremblay, 2003). Nevertheless, there is scope for further honest debate concerning when we permit aggression and when we sanction it. It is arguable that the rhetoric against aggression, against never fighting back, the exhortation to "turn the other cheek," are examples of what Campbell (1975) called "social preaching." Following Campbell's line of reasoning in this respect, the general optimum for society is for less aggression than might be in an individual's own interest. Individuals may thus be somewhat recalcitrant to social preaching, so that the social preaching needs to be for even less aggression than might be socially optimal, in order that the actual balance reached is near the societal optimum. This could explain why some of these exhortations not to fight back do not always ring true with parents of children. We may want a fairer society, but we do not want our child to be bottom of the pile (and of course not all parents share the same ideals of a fairer society).

For most of us, clearly excessive aggression is undesirable. Also, bullying—repeated aggression against a weaker target—seems morally and socially contemptible. Whatever benefits there may be to an individual persistent aggressor or bully, there are large social costs. Given the kind of society we are in, and the kind of social contract that most of us feel we belong to, then efforts to reduce excessive violence, chronic physical aggression, and bullying, are a very important and worthwhile goal (Smith, Pepler, & Rigby, 2004; Tremblay, 2003). But how far do we go? Should we really try to stop all playground fights?

Discourage defensive aggression? "Turning the other cheek" is an ideal that is very seldom lived up to in practice.

The fiction that childhood aggression is socially incompetent needs to be left behind us. Our ability for, and tendency toward, aggressive behavior needs to be faced honestly. Rather than condemn all aggressive behavior, we should discuss acceptable limits, ways of preventing aggression going too far, ways of resolving conflicts without too much damage. The real debate is about social desirability. It is a debate that should bring developmental psychologists into a broader interdisciplinary arena. It is a debate that will not be definitively resolved, but will be part of our ongoing process of trying to manage our social relationships and our societies, and of trying to change them so that we can deal with interpersonal conflicts effectively; this is one of the major issues that threaten our survival as a species.

CONCLUSIONS

This chapter has attempted to give some reasons as to why aggression has come to be thought of as maladaptive by many developmental psychologists. Following some discussion of the definitions, types, and modes of aggression, a case is first made that aggressive behavior has adaptive functions in nonhuman species and in humans. The adaptiveness of aggression is conditional and depends on context. Nevertheless, in children, aggressive behavior has been widely considered as maladaptive or socially incompetent, with aggressive children lacking social skills. Some examples of this tradition of thinking were discussed, together with some recent emotional challenges to this. The chapter argues that the traditional view confounds what is socially desirable, with what is socially competent or successful. The chapter then explores why the traditional view may have come about. Two main reasons are suggested. One is the sheltered disciplinary ethos of psychology in much of the 20th century, in which psychology in general and developmental psychology in particular ignored both evolutionary explanations, and wider sociological contexts and conflicts of interest between individuals and groups). The second is the strong "social engineering" or policy-oriented ethos of early child development work, which had the objective of raising good healthy children for society. It is finally argued that a more clear-sighted view of the individual benefits that may accrue from aggression will enable a better societal debate on the extent to which aggressive behaviors should be discouraged, and how this should be done.

REFERENCES

Arnett, J. (1992). Reckless behavior in adolescence: A developmental perspective. *Developmental Review, 12*, 339–373.

Berk, L. (2000). *Child development* (5th ed.). Boston: Allyn & Bacon.

Bertram, B. C. R. (1976). Kin selection in lions and in evolution. In P. P. G. Bateson & R. A. Hinde (Eds.), *Growing points in ethology* (pp. 281–301). Cambridge, UK: Cambridge University Press.

Bjorklund, D. F., & Pellegrini, A. D. (2000). Child development and evolutionary psychology. *Child Development, 71*, 1687–1798.

Bjorklund, D. F., & Pellegrini, A. D. (2002). *The origins of human nature: Evolutionary developmental psychology.* Washington, DC: APA Press.

Bjorklund, D. F., & Smith, P. K. (2003). Evolutionary developmental psychology: Introduction to the special issue. *Journal of Experimental Child Psychology, 85*, 195–198.

Björkqvist, K. (1994). Sex differences in physical, verbal, and indirect aggression: A review of recent research. *Sex Roles, 30*, 177–188.

Björkqvist, K, Lagerspetz, K, & Kaukiainen, A. (1992). Do girls manipulate and boys fight? Developmental trends in regard to direct and indirect aggression. *Aggressive Behavior, 18*, 117–127.

Björkqvist, K, Österman, K., & Lagerspetz, K. M. J. (1994). Sex differences in covert aggression in adults. *Aggressive Behavior, 20*, 27–33.

Blurton Jones, N. (Ed.). (1972). *Ethological studies of child behaviour.* Cambridge, UK: Cambridge University Press.

Bullis, M., Walker, H. M., & Sprague, J. R. (2001). A promise unfulfilled: Social skills training with at-risk and antisocial children and youth. *Exceptionality, 9*, 67–90.

Burman, E. (1994). *Deconstructing developmental psychology.* London: Routledge.

Campbell, D. T. (1975). On the conflicts between biological and social evolution and between psychology and moral tradition. *American Psychologist, 30*, 1103–1126.

Carroll, A., Houghton, S., Hattie, J., & Durkin, K. (1999). Adolescent reputation enhancement: Differentiating delinquent, nondelinquent, and at-risk youths. *Journal of Child Psychology & Psychiatry, 40*, 593–606.

Chagnon, N. (1968). *Yanamamo: The fierce people.* New York: Holt, Rinehart & Winston.

Corsaro, W. (1997). *The sociology of childhood.* Thousand Oaks, CA: Pine Forge Press

Crick, N. R., & Dodge, K. A. (1996). Social information-processing mechanisms in reactive and proactive aggression. *Child Development, 67*, 993–1002.

Crick, N. R., & Grotpeter, J. K. (1995). Relational aggression, gender, and social-psychological adjustment. *Child Development, 66*, 710–722.

Emler, N., Reicher, S., & Ross, A. (1987). The social context of delinquent conduct. *Journal of Child Psychology & Psychiatry, 28*, 99–109.

Encarta World English Dictionary. (1999). London: Bloomsbury Publishing.

Fagan, T. K. (1992). Compulsory schooling, child study, clinical psychology, and special education. *American Psychologist*, 47, 236–243.

Fry, D. P. (2005). Rough-and-tumble social play in children. In A. D. Pellegrini & P. K. Smith (Eds.), *Play in humans and great apes* (pp. 54–85). New York: Guilford.

Galtung, J. (1969). Violence, peace, and peace research. *Journal of Peace Research*, 6, 167–191.

Geary, D. C., & Bjorklund, D. F. (2000). Evolutionary developmental psychology. *Child Development*, 71, 57–65.

Hall, G. S. (1904). *Adolescence: Its psychology and its relation to physiology, anthropology, sociology, sex, crime, religion, and education (Vols. 1-2)*. New York: Appleton.

Hawley, P. H. (2002). Social dominance and prosocial and coercive strategies of resource control in preschoolers. *International Journal of Behavioral Development*, 26, 167–176.

Hawley, P. H. (2003). Strategies of control, aggression and morality in preschoolers: An evolutionary perspective. *Journal of Experimental Child Psychology*, 85, 213–235.

Hetherington, E. M. & Parke, R. D. (1993). *Child psychology: A contemporary viewpoint* (4th ed.). New York: McGraw-Hill.

Hrdy, S. B. (1977). Infanticide as a primate reproductive strategy. *American Scientist*, 65, 40–49

James, A., & Prout, A. (1990). *Constructing and reconstructing childhood*. Basingstoke: Falmer.

Jenks, C. (1982). *The sociology of childhood*. London: Batsford.

Kemp, G., & Fry, D. P. (Eds.). (2004). *Keeping the peace: Conflict resolution and peaceful societies around the world*. New York: Routledge.

Maynard Smith, J. (1982). *Evolution and the theory of games*. Cambridge, UK: Cambridge University Press.

Moore, A. (1993). Towards an evolutionary view of social dominance. *Animal Behaviour*, 46, 594–596.

Parke, R. D. (2004). The Society for Research in Child Development at 70: Progress and promise. *Child Development*, 75, 1–24.

Pellegrini, A. D., & Long, J. D. (2003). A sexual selection theory longitudinal analysis of sexual segregation and integration in early adolescence. *Journal of Experimental Child Psychology*, 85, 257–278.

Rose, N. (1985). *Governing the soul: The shaping of the private self*. London: Routledge.

Rose, N. (1990). *The psychological complex: Psychology, politics and society in England 1869–1939*. London: Routledge & Kegan Paul.

Ruff, J. R. (2001). *Violence in early modern Europe 1500–1800*. Cambridge, UK: Cambridge University Press.

Salmivalli, C., Lagerspetz, K. M. J., Björkqvist, K., Osterman, K., & Kaukiainen, A. (1996). Bullying as a group process: Participant roles and their relations to social status within the group. *Aggressive Behavior*, 22, 1–15.

Sears, R. R. (1975). Your ancients revisited: A history of child development. In E. M. Hetherington (Ed.), *Personality and the Behavior Disorders*, Vol.1. (pp. 306–322). New York: Ronald Press.

Siegler, R., DeLoache, J., & Eisenberg, N. (2003). *How children develop.* New York: Worth.

Smith, P. K., Pepler, D. K., & Rigby, K. (Eds.). (2004). *Bullying in schools: How successful can interventions be?* Cambridge, UK: Cambridge University Press.

Sumner, C. (1994). *The sociology of deviance: An obituary.* Buckingham: Open University Press.

Sutton, J., Smith, P. K., & Swettenham, J. (1999a). Social cognition and bullying: Social inadequacy or skilled manipulation? *British Journal of Developmental Psychology, 17,* 435–450.

Sutton, J., Smith, P. K., & Swettenham, J. (1999b). Socially undesirable need not be incompetent: A response to Crick and Dodge. *Social Development, 8,* 132–134.

Tremblay, R. E. (2003). Why socialization fails: The case of chronic physical aggression. In B. B. Lahey, T. E. Moffitt, & A. Caspi (Eds.), *Causes of conduct disorder and juvenile delinquency* (pp. 182–224). New York: Guilford Press.

Trivers, R. L. (1971). The evolution of reciprocal altruism. *Quarterly Review of Biology, 46,* 35–57.

Vaughn, B. E., Vollenweider, M., Bost, K. K., Azria-Evans, M. R., & Snider, J. B. (2003). Negative interactions and social competence for preschool children in two samples: Reconsidering the interpretation of aggressive behavior for young children. *Merrill-Palmer Quarterly, 49,* 245–278.

Wilson, E. O. (1975). *Sociobiology: The new synthesis.* Cambridge, MA: Belknap Press.

4

IS AGGRESSION ADAPTATIVE? YES: SOME KINDS ARE AND IN SOME WAYS

Anthony D. Pellegrini
University of Minnesota, Twin Cities Campus

In a 2003 panel discussion at the peer pre-conference of the Society for Research in Child Development entitled, "Is Aggression Maladaptive?" most of the participants took a measured approach and answered the question, correctly I think: It depends. It depends on what you mean by aggression and what you mean by adaptive. In the course of the paper presentations and discussion, the issue of the different types of aggression was explicitly and thoroughly addressed whereas discussion of the meaning of "adaptation" was strikingly absent. The use of aggression to defend one's self (i.e., protective aggression) was almost universally endorsed as beneficial.

The two positions that aggression may or may not be adaptive may reflect two traditions in the study of aggression. In the social and behavioral sciences, generally, aggression is often studied in response to larger societal concerns and with the problems associated with aggression. Concomitantly, social scientists studying aggression have been concerned with individuals embedded in groups, such as societies, cultures, and schools. In the United States, at least, the study of aggression is often supported by the private foundations and the federal government as part of an effort to control it. From this view, much research on aggression has had some concerns with reducing its frequency and intensity, and for good reason. In the 20th century, arguably the most aggressive and violent period in recent human history (Hobsbawm, 1996), governments have tried to use science to engineer a better society. Toward this end, the National Institute of Health supports research in aggression from the point of view of it being problematic to public health. This has lead to the general view that aggression may not have a function, or at least a positive one, and thus it may be considered "maladaptive."

A second tradition in the study of aggression is represented by the biological sciences, most thoroughly in the fields associated with behavioral ecology (e.g., Archer, 1988), ethology (e.g., Hinde, 1980), and sociobiology (Wilson, 1975). A motivation for the biological study of aggression may have been in response to the ubiquity of aggression in the animal kingdom, from invertebrates, such as sea coral, Scolymia lacera (Lang, 1971, cited in Archer, 1988) to the great apes (such as chimpanzees, Pan troglodytes, Wrangham, 1999).

In this chapter I show how different types of aggression are adaptive, in the biological sense, for males and females. Toward this end, I present a model suggesting that sex differences in aggression are based, ultimately, on different mating strategies. More proximally, I show how sexual dimorphism in physical size relates to differences in physical activity and aggressive and competitive behaviors where males, in sexually segregated groups, are more competitive and physically aggressive, relative to girls.

The study of animal behavior, including aggression, is often rooted in Darwin's theory of evolution by natural selection. One view of this theory holds that if a behavior, like aggression, is frequently observed in nature, it probably has a function and was probably selected for. That is, a frequently observed class of behavior (both within and across species) probably was naturally selected because the benefits associated with the behavior probably outweigh the costs; if it did not have a function it would not have been selected. From this view, aggression may have costs, but it also has benefits that outweigh the cost, thus aggression is naturally selected for. For natural selection to occur, there must be variation in reproductive success within a population (Silk, 1986). The ability to reproduce is labeled "fitness" (or "ultimate function) and fitness is a result of "adaptations." For biologists, adaptations are traits or behaviors that confer reproductive advantage on individuals possessing them (Silk, 1986). Consequently, adaptation relates to reproductive fitness. If aggression increases reproductive fitness, it is adaptive. That is, it should relate to an individual's fitness, or the number of reproducing offspring. Unlike many social science models, individuals (indeed the gene; Dawkins, 1976), not groups (though see Boyd & Richerson, 1985, for an alternative view), are the units of natural selection. From this view, it is perhaps more understandable to consider the advantages associated with aggression.

The idea that individuals, not groups, are considered the appropriate unit of analysis has implications for the way in which adaptation is defined.

Not surprisingly, explication of what it is we mean by adaptation is as important as the ways in which we define aggression (Hartup, 1974). As just noted, the issue of what adaptive means was not addressed explicitly in that SRCD panel discussion. Instead it was implicitly defined in terms of "beneficial consequences" (Hinde, 1980) of a behavior. So, for example, a beneficial consequence, or function, of aggression might be that it, in some samples of adolescent males, positively and significantly correlated with subsequent measures of social status, such as popularity with peers (e.g., Pellegrini & Long, 2003; Rodkin et al., 2000). Clearly this is different than function in the biological sense of adaptation; thus it is important to specify how function is being used.

In this chapter, I discuss one form of aggression, "competitive aggression" (Archer, 1988), and suggest how it may relate to function of a different sort- adaptations associated with "ultimate function." Ultimate function is concerned with the degree to which individuals reproduce and maximize the survival of their offspring.

IS AGGRESSION ADAPTIVE? IT DEPENDS ON WHAT IS MEANT BY AGGRESSION AND WHAT IS MEANT BY ADAPTIVE

Two Types of Aggression

Aggression can be defined from a number of perspectives and as serving a variety of functions. For example, it has been defined in terms of function (e.g., to do harm) and in terms of the structural characteristics (e.g., hitting, kicking, biting, destroying property). Consistent with the theme of this volume I (following Hartup [1974] and Archer [1988]) take a functional perspective on defining aggression. I consider aggression as one of many ways in which individuals can solve problems and there are at least two specific problems for which aggression may be useful: To protect one's self or kin and as a way in which to compete for resources (e.g., food and mates in the animal kingdom, toys in preschool children).

Protective aggression is defensive and it is used to remove different types of threats and danger (Archer, 1988). It also includes the use of aggression in retaliation to a threat to one's self or one's offspring (i.e., parental aggression). Protective aggression also tends to be more serious and consequently, more costly to both the perpetrator and the target (in terms of risks associated with injury and death) than competitive aggression (Archer, 1988) because individuals' safety is clearly at risk. The lack of sex differences in protective aggression in much of the animal kingdom probably reflects the importance of aggression in solving the different problems faced by males (e.g., defense against attacks) and females (to protect offspring) alike. Consequently, the answer to the question, Is protective aggression adaptive, we can answer: Yes.

Competitive aggression is different from protective aggression. Primarily, it is used as one of many competitive strategies to secure resources and is a strategy associated with content competitions for resources. By contrast, scramble competition for resources does not rely on aggression. The choice governing the use of competitive aggression is typically guided by two levels of decisions (usually implicitly): Is the resource scarce and worth fighting for? Is it worth fighting this/these particular opponent(s) for this resource? Answering these questions usually involves estimating the value of the resource and the strength of the opponent. A highly valuable resource (e.g., where there is a shortage of available and high-quality mates) typically corresponds to willingness to use (and costly in terms of risks associated with injury, death, punishment, caloric expenditure, etc) aggression. Implementation of costly aggression strategies, is however, typically preceded by other, less costly, strategies, such as using threats and dominance displays (Clutton-Brock & Albon, 1979). If these fail to secure the contested resources, aggression is a default.

The cost of using an aggressive strategy is also influenced by the specific opponent against whom one is competing. Higher costs are associated with certain opponents, thus adjusting the value of the resource in the cost:benefit ratio. So, it would be more costly to aggress against a bigger and stronger opponent, relative to a weaker and smaller one. Correspondingly, using aggression against a specific opponent may have different costs depending on the context in which it is embedded. For example, fighting in a school with strict and consistent rules is more expensive (high likelihood of severe enforcements) than in a more tolerant school. In cases where it is too costly to compete for resources or when resources are readily available, individuals may use a "scramble" strategy, where they try to access resources without challenging another, though to my knowledge this hypothesis has not been tested.

Unlike protective aggression, sex differences are observed in competitive aggression among many human and nonhuman primates, where males, more than females, use direct and physical aggression to compete for resources. This sex difference in aggression is part of the more general sex difference where males are more competitive than females (Pellegrini & Archer, 2005). As I specify in the following discussion, this difference is consistent with sexual selection theory whereby males (of many primate species) are more competitive and physically active than females. This difference is reflected in the social dominance organization of male groups where there is more competition and use of direct aggression, as well as other agonistic and competitive strategies, in their quest to dominate same sex peers (see Pellegrini & Archer, 2005, and Pellegrini, Kato, Blatchford, & Baines, 2003, for fuller discussions). These dominance hierarchies, in turn, relate to access to resources. It should be noted, though, dominance organization in group is fluid, and status changes as members, resources, and the more general ecologies change.

All of this is not to say that females (at least adolescents and adults) do not use aggressive strategies to compete for resources. The form of aggression they use is less direct and less physically vigorous than the sort used by males. Instead, they more frequently than males tend to use indirect, social forms of aggression to access resources (Björkqvist, Lagerspetz, & Kaukiainen, 1992; Campbell, 1999; 2002; Crick & Grotpeter, 1995; Galen & Underwood, 1997). Although different forms of aggression, including direct and indirect aggression (Hartup, 1974; Little, Henrich, Jones, & Hawley, 2003), are often correlated both in the sense that the same target has relatively lower and higher frequencies/ rates and in the sense that both can be seen in a single episode or exchange between individuals, they also have unique dimensions. Sex differences in the use of direct aggressive strategies are also consistent with sexual selection theory to the extent that females are physically smaller (by 10%–15%) and less vigorous than males (Pellegrini, 2004; Pellegrini, Long, & Mizerak, 2005). Further females' use of indirect, less confrontational aggressive strategies is consistent with their role as the more investing in the reproductive role of the two sexes (Campbell, 1999; Trivers, 1972). That is, females may use indirect aggression more frequently than males because it is safer than the more direct types— enabling them to "stay alive" to protect and provision their offspring (Campbell, 1999). This view leads to the prediction that males should use dominance/physical aggressive strategies to access resources and females should use indirect aggressive strategies.

A MODEL FOR SEX DIFFERENCES IN THE FUNCTIONS OF AGGRESSION

Darwin (1871) and later Trivers (1972) recognized explicit differences between males' and females' aggression. For example, Darwin observed that males of many (but not all) species tend to be bigger, more physically active, and more physically aggressive than females. Darwin also pointed out that differences in size, aggression, and levels of vigorous behavior seemed to be related to differences in mating strategies. Specifically, in polygnous species (where males have many mates), relative to monogamous species (where males and females form stable pair bonds), males are larger, more physically vigorous, and also more competitive and physically aggressive.

Consistent with this theory, the converse also seems to be true, as in cases of where reproductive roles are reversed (i.e., where males take on most of the care of offspring, relative to females). The best examples of these cases come from polyandrous (females take many mates) shore birds, such as the spotted sand piper, Actitis macularia (Erckmann 1983) and the American Jacana, Jacana spinosa (Jenni,1974). In these species, predictions hold: Females are larger than males, there is sexual segregation, and there is intrasexual female competition where females are more aggressive than males.

In the case of humans (as well as great apes; Pellegrini, 2004), competition and direct aggression are especially evident when there is a shortage of females and in both polygynous and promiscuous mating systems. In the case of polygyny, there is greater variation in males', relative to females', reproductive success: One male copulates with a number of females. This results in males competing with each other for the chance to mate, probably causing males to be more competitive and aggressive (direct) than females.

Darwin also suggested that females had an active role in securing mates; they were not passive pawns in the male reproductive game (See also Campbell, 2002; Smuts, 1987; 1995; Trivers, 1985). Females' reproductive strategies relate to their actively choosing the best mates and this often involves manipulating intrasexual social relationships, such as alliances, to access mates and to protect themselves and their offspring. Females' use of indirect/relational aggression is consistent with this view (Campbell, 1999).

Darwin could not, however, determine why males were competitive and females choosy, and not vice versa. Based on the earlier work of Bateman (1948), Trivers (1972) suggested that differences in parental investment are responsible for a number of sex differences, including levels of types of aggression, in different species. The basic consideration that sex is inexpensive for males (i.e., one-off mating efforts) and expensive for females (mating efforts, gestation, and provisioning and care of infants/juveniles) leads to the general rule that female investment leads to female choosiness and concerns with maximizing investment in offspring. Females are therefore less likely than males to risk harm or danger because it would compromise their ability to provision and protect their offspring. Females, in other words, are more concerned with "staying alive" (Campbell, 1999, 2002).

Behaviorally, this means that they use more indirect and safer strategies to access and protect resources. Males, on the other hand, are much less choosy in mating. This view is also supported by Buss's (1989)

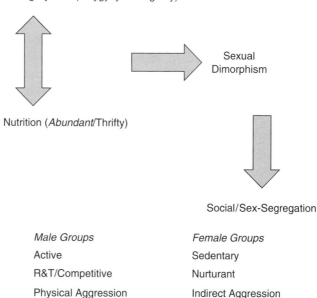

Mating System (*Polygyny*/Monogamy)

Sexual
Dimorphism

Nutrition (*Abundant*/Thrifty)

Social/Sex-Segregation

Male Groups	Female Groups
Active	Sedentary
R&T/Competitive	Nurturant
Physical Aggression	Indirect Aggression

FIGURE 4.1   Mating system (polygyny/monogamy).

findings on human males' tendency toward promiscuity. The strategy of frequent mating and lack of paternal investment results in intrasexual competition for mates, sexual dimorphism, and differences in aggression. The patterns related to mating strategies, competitiveness, and uses of different forms of aggression, however, are related to the environment in which individuals develop.

To conclude this section, sex differences in aggression, where males use direct strategies more than females and females use more indirect strategies than males, seem to derive, ultimately, from reproductive roles. These roles and associated sex differences in aggression and competitive behavior, however, are moderated by contextual factors.

Contextual Moderation

Although I have argued that evolutionary history has an impact on human development, I must further clarify the moderating role of context in understanding human development. My position is that genes and environments, and indeed behavior (Stamps, 2003), are dynamically interdependent (Archer & Lloyd, 2002; Bateson, 2005; Bjorklund & Pellegrini, 2000; Gottlieb, 1998). My model is presented in Figure 4.1.

Genetic history interacts with other layers of social complexity. Specifically, the environment in which an individual develops, starting with conception, influences the ways in which evolutionary history is expressed. Bateson and Martin (1999) use a jukebox metaphor to describe this process. Individuals within each species have a genetic endowment that can be realized through a wide variety of options (similar to the collection of records in a jukebox) but the specific developmental pathway taken (similar to the specific record selected) by an individual is influenced by the perinatal environment (i.e., from conception through infancy) of the developing organism. Thus, a number of developmental pathways are possible, but which one is selected is determined by the environment in which the organism develops (Archer, 1992; Caro & Bateson, 1986).

For the purposes of this chapter, perhaps the most relevant aspect of the environment is nutrition, as it affects the sexual dimorphism in size, which, in turn, affects sex segregation of juvenile peer groups and direct competitive aggression where the physically larger sex is the more physically active and more physically aggressive (Pellegrini, 2004). Specifically, the nutritional history of the human mother impacts the physical size of the offspring, and more specifically that of males (Bateson & Martin, 1999). Further, ecological conditions and the availability of resources seem to affect human mating systems and sexual dimorphism. Alexander and colleagues (Alexander, Hoogland, Howard, Noonan, & Sherman, 1979) used the Human Relations Area File to partition human societies as ecologically imposed monogamy (e.g., Lapps of Norway, Cooper and Labrador Eskimo), polygynous (e.g., Bedouin Arabs and Khmer) and culturally-monogamous (most Western societies). They found that the ecological-imposed groups, that is, groups whose monogamous mating system was determined by their environments rather than by legal systems, were significantly less dimorphic than the other two but there were no differences between the polygynous and culturally imposed monogamy groups. They argued that in ecologically imposed monogamous cultures efforts of both parents are needed to protect and make provisions for the offspring. From this view, sexual dimorphism in physical size results from the confluence of ecological and mating systems. Dimorphism is, in turn, hypothesized to be an antecedent condition for different energetic and physical activity demands of males and females as well as an antecedent to both sex segregation and sex differences in aggression (Pellegrini et al., 2005; Ruckstuhl & Neuhaus, 2005).

Differences in body size are associated with differences in physical activity and associated with competitiveness and aggressiveness such that males and females view themselves differently very early in development and then segregate (see Pellegrini, 2004, for a fuller discussion). Later, these differences are translated into different social roles and differences in agonistic behaviors associated with different energetic demands.

To conclude this section, I have argued that although sex differences in aggression are derived from evolutionary history, the expression of these differences is moderated by the ecology in which individuals develop. This view of the role of evolution in human development and behavior is consistent with current conceptions of gene–environment transactions (e.g., Bateson, 2005; Stamps, 2003).

Sexually Segregated Groups as Socialization Contexts for Differences in Aggression

I suggest that males' early bias toward physically active behavior (Eaton & Enns, 1986) is an antecedent to rough and physically aggressive behaviors that are learned and practiced in sexually segregated peer groups. These behaviors are probably functional in terms of learning motor skills associated with male reproductive roles. Females avoid these active behaviors and interact with each other because they find vigorous behavior, especially in the presence of males, to be aversive and possibly dangerous (Pellegrini, 2004). In these segregated groups, males and females learn and practice, possibly through observational learning and reinforcement, (Boyd & Richerson, 1985) the social roles associated with being an adult male or female.

First, it is important to note that there are varying degrees of social segregation (Conradt, 1998). In "no segregation" cases, juveniles meet randomly. With "complete segregation," males and females are found in separate groups whereas in "partial segregation," a proportion of the group segregates and the remaining proportion do not. Degree of segregation is often assayed by the proportion of males or females in a group (e.g., Pellegrini & Long, 2003). For example, in a study of early adolescents observed in a variety of unstructured venues (e.g., hallways, cafeteria, dances) the proportion of males: males + females in focal males' groups ranged from .92 to .77 across 2 years of observation (Pellegrini & Long, 2003). In a study of primary school children's playground behavior, segregation was measured as presence in "mostly" segregated (where 60% or more were of the same sex) or "mixed" (where .40 or less were of the same sex) groups (Blatchford, Baines, & Pellegrini, 2003); both boys and girls were observed in the "mostly" segregated groups in 80% of the observations. Some scholars have defined and measured segregation more absolutely—whether the group was same or mixed-sex—and found that .39 and .40 of male and female groups (in this case of preschoolers), respectively, were segregated, or same-sex (Fabes, Martin, Hanish, Anders, & Madden-Derdich, 2003).

Different levels of physical activity are an important antecedent for sexually segregated peer groups and different forms of aggression during childhood. Males and male groups, from the preschool through early adolescent years, are more physically more vigorous and competitive than female groups (Pellegrini, 2004; Pellegrini et al., 2002), and it is in these groups that different uses of competitive aggression are learned and develop. This difference continues at both the individual and group levels through the juvenile period, despite sex differences in maturation (Eaton & Yu, 1989; Pellegrini, 2004).

That males are more active than females is probably due to their larger size and corresponding need to develop skeletal, muscle, and neural systems as well as differences in hormonal systems (Pellegrini & Smith, 1998). For example, young girls with abnormally high levels of male hormones, relative to controls, are more likely to interact with male peers and toys (Berenbaum & Snyder, 1995). These vigorous behaviors, in turn, relate to males' social roles as adults. Specifically, the vigorous activity characteristic of juvenile males' groups is related to the development of neural (cerebellar) and muscle systems used in behaviors associated with fighting and predation (Byers & Walker, 1995). Consequently, males use segregated groups not only to engage in vigorous physical exercise (Pellegrini, Horvat, & Huberty, 1998) and competitive games (Pellegrini et al., 2002) but also to practice behaviors and roles related to physical aggression and social dominance relationships during childhood and adolescence (Pellegrini, 2003).

Social dominance can be defined as a social relationship where individuals are hierarchically ordered for access to some resource (Dunbar, 1988; Gottman & Ringland, 1981; Hawley, 1999; Pellegrini & Long, 2003; Strayer, 1980). Dominance relationships are typically established by a combination of agonisitic (e.g., threats, winning fights) and cooperative strategies (e.g., reconciling defeated peers; deWaal, 1986; Pellegrini & Bartini, 2001; Strayer, 1980)—depending on the type of competition. Male groups, more so than female groups, are characterized by dominance hierarchies predicated on the use of aversive strategies.

When individuals are forming new social groups, especially during adolescence and when they enter a new school, dominance relationships are being established. Consequently, aggression is high as dominance relationships are established. With the passage of time, aggression decreases as dominance relationships are established and recognized (Pellegrini & Bartini, 2001). Consequently, dominance hierarchies minimize aggression as individuals recognize their place in the group.

TESTING HYPOTHESES DERIVED FROM
THE PROPOSED MODEL

In this section, I present data relevant to hypotheses derived from my model. The data were collected as part of a larger project addressing the role of aggression and peer relations during early adolescence. The project was a multimethod, longitudinal study conducted in a rural county in north Georgia. Fuller details of the procedures relevant to the analyses presented here can be found in Pellegrini and Long (2003) and Pellegrini (2003). The first set of hypotheses relates to sex segregation and differential uses of aggression in these groups.

Research has found that females find high levels of activity and the possibility of encountering rough play and physical aggression aversive and typically avoid males groups (Maccoby, 1998). Further, female groups are smaller, more nurturant, and, correspondingly, the social roles enacted are related to adult reproductive roles. For example, females' pretend play is usually characterized by the enactment domestic roles (Garvey, 1990). In keeping with the relative importance of close relationships in female groups, they more frequently use indirect and social, relational forms of aggression to access resources.

Using social, relational aggression (for example, spreading rumors; Björkqvist, 1994; Crick & Grotpeter, 1995; Galen & Underwood, 1997) does not involve direct confrontation between peers. In order to secure a resource, such as a date and especially in adolescence, females may try to damage social reputations of their rivals and form alliances and coalitions against them.

The same biological and socialization forces that maintained sexual segregation during childhood conspire to bring the two sexes together with the onset of puberty and adolescence (Maccoby, 1998). Hormonal changes during adolescence as well as societal stress on heterosexual relationships (Collins & Sroufe, 1999) result in boys and girls showing increased interest in one another. This interest is realized by an increase in cross-sex contact as well as increased interest in dating (Dunphy, 1963).

One way to understand the beginnings of heterosexual relationships is to study youngsters as they first make the transition into middle school and follow them longitudinally. In this way the natural history of relationships with opposite sex peers can be studied from the point when youngsters first encounter each other in an institution designed for young adolescents.

Sexual selection theory and dominance theory are useful in understanding the ways in which boys' and girls' groups become integrated during early adolescence. Sexual selection theory posits separate strategies for males and females: Males compete directly with each other for mates and females choose mates; where they compete, it should be indirect rather than direct. Thus, males should compete with each other, in the form of intrasexual aggression, for dominance status. Male–male aggression should be more frequent than male–female aggression. Secondly, males' dominance status should covary with the degree to which their peer groups are sexually segregated to predicted heterosexual interaction. As boys' dominance increases their peer groups should become correspondingly less segregated, reflecting the interrelation among dominance, sexual segregation, and heterosexual relationships. More specifically, during early adolescence heterosexual relationships are important resources and competition for these resources is reflected in dominance relationships. Dominance status, in turn, should predict the extent to which boys interact in sexually integrated groups and in boys' heterosexual activity. In our work, we have defined heterosexual activity as the degree to which males are nominated by female peers for hypothetical dates. Although this measure has obvious limitations (e.g., it is not a direct measure of either dating or of reproductive success), it is a starting point for testing relations between male dominance and reproductive fitness.

In adolescence and with the onset of puberty, heterosexual relationships, in the form of dating, become a very important resource for both males and females (Collins & Sroufe, 1999; Pellegrini & Bartini, 2001). Dominant males should have access to females and females should find these males attractive and nominate them for hypothetical dates (Bukowski, Sippola, & Newcomb, 2000; Pellegrini & Bartini, 2001; Pellegrini & Long, 2003). Dominant boys are also leaders of their peer groups and, consequently, girls often want to associate with high-status boys. The importance of a high-status "date" is consistent with the notion that early dating is a group-oriented phenomenon and by choosing to "go out" with high-status boys, girls enhance their status with both same and opposite sex peers.

Girls, however, are not as reliant on direct physical aggression and dominance-related strategies as boys. As just noted, girls tend to use indirect, or relational, aggression as a way in which to manipulate their female peers, and enhance their reputation in the wider peer group (Björkqvist, 1994; Campbell, 1999; Crick & Grotpeter, 1995; Galen & Underwood, 1997). Relational aggression is where individuals enhance themselves by damaging reputations and social relations of rivals through the use of gossip, rumor, and threats.

Our data support these claims (Pellegrini & Long, 2003). As displayed in Table 4.1, male–male aggression is more frequent than cross-sex aggression, consistent with meta-analyses of sex differences in aggression (Pellegrini & Archer, 2005).

TABLE 4.1

Descriptive Statistics for Frequency/Observation of R&T and Aggression by Time by Sex of Initiator and Sex of Target

	Boy to Girl		Boy to Boy		Girl to Boy		Girl to Girl	
	M	SD	M	SD	M	SD	M	SD
6th/Fall								
R&T	.25	.57	1.03	1.50	.42	.76	.47	.72
Aggression	.03	.18	.13	.41	.07	.26	.01	.20
6th/Spring								
R&T	.45	.83	1.93	2.45	.48	.69	.85	1.33
Aggression	.03	.12	.31	.65	.16	.43	.12	.06

Further, and as displayed in Tables 4.2 and 4.3, the differential functions of dominance/direct aggression and indirect/relational aggression for boys and girls in relation to segregated peer groups and dating was partially supported. Table 4.2 displays the bivariate correlations, by sex, for these relations and Table 4.3 shows tests of the hypothetical models, using general linear modeling. Results indicate that for boys, increases in dominance and decreases in segregation lead to dating popularity. That is, dominant boys are aggressive first, then rise in dominance, then are chosen for hypothetical dates. Relational aggression was not important for boys. For girls, on the other hand and counter to the hypothesis, increases in relational aggression predicted increases in segregation and lead to increases in dating popularity.

That there was an increase, not decrease, in girls' segregation, along with an increase in relational aggression to predicting dating was counter to the hypothesis. It may be that as girls' dating activity increased, along with their use of relational aggression. A very speculative interpretation is that girls may have retreated into same-sex groups in order to self-disclose their feelings on dating and to damage their female rivals' reputations.

Although there are socialization and biological pressures to initiate heterosexual relationships during adolescence, we must also recognize that cross-sex interaction is very difficult for youngsters of this age. Initial cross-sex contact is quite risky to initiate to the extent that it breaks well-established patterns of sex segregation entrenched since early childhood (Maccoby, 1998; Pellegrini, 2004; Serbin et al., 1977). Further, there is a real risk that overtures to opposite sex peers will be publicly rejected, resulting in public embarrassment for the initiator. One way in which youngsters can minimize these risks is to use overtures that are playful and ambiguous in their intent. Specifically, youngsters of

TABLE 4.2
Correlations Predicting Dating Popularity by Sex
Correlations (N) between Dating Popularity as the Criterion Measure
and Segregation, Dominance, Relational Aggression

Males	6th Fall	6th Spring	7th Fall	7th Spring
Segregation	−0.15(54)	−0.30* (43)	−0.11(69)	−0.24(37)
Dominance	0.07(46)	0.34** (59)	0.42** (64)	0.46** (64)
Relational Aggression	−0.04(42)	−0.05(27)	0.11(61)	0.05(63)
Females				
Segregation	0.10 (44)	−0.11(43)	0.06(51)	0.17(28)
Dominance	−0.21 (27)	0.16(53)	0.06(50)	−0.03(51)
Relational Aggression	0.15 (40)	0.37* (30)	0.07(49)	0.15(54)

Note. The criterion variable is dating popularity; $*p < .05$, $**p < .01$

this age sometimes resort to "poke and push" courtship behaviors, a construct that bares close resemblance to rough- and- tumble play (R&T), for example, playfully hitting, pushing, grabbing, and teasing an opposite sex peer (Maccoby, 1998; Pellegrini, 2003; Schofield, 1981). These behaviors can be interpreted as affiliative overtures by the recipient and reciprocated. Alternatively, they can be rejected. When the overture is reciprocated, cross-sex contact has been successfully initiated. When the overture is rejected, the initiator saves face because the bout can be dismissed as playful and not serious. R&T between males, on the other, hand, should relate to aggression and dominance.

The second set of predictions posits that male–male R&T initially serves dominance and aggressive functions during adolescence but, with time, male–female R&T is a nascent form of heterosexual interaction, or poke and push courtship.

Data for these analyses were derived from the same source as those just reported and a more thorough description of procedures can be found in Pellegrini (2003). Briefly, I directly observed adolescent boys' R&T and physical aggression across the first full year of middle school and made the following predictions. First, males' R&T, dominance, and aggression should be intercorrelated. This is based on the proposition that adolescent male–male R&T is used to establish and maintain dominance. Second, if boys are using R&T for dominance, they should target other boys more than they target girls. However, the targets of boys' R&T bouts should change with time. In the second half of the year, after dominance is

TABLE 4.3
Dynamic Covariate Analysis

		Segregation		Dominance	
		Main Effect	*Sex Interaction*	*Main Effect*	*Sex Interaction*
Model[a]	χ^2	$\hat{\gamma}_0(SE)$	$\hat{\gamma}_1\ (SE)$	$\hat{\gamma}_2\ (SE)$	$\hat{\gamma}_3\ (SE)$
1	18.33***	−1.34*** (.22)	1.63*** (.41)	.83*** (.11)	−.84*** (.21)
2	20.52***	−.33*** (.22)	164*** (.41)	.85*** (.11)	−.87*** (.21)

Note. The criterion variable is dating popularity; ***$p < .001$; [a]Model 2 is identical to Model 1 with the exception that γ_4 is set to zero; omnibus χ^2 $df = 3$; fixed effects t-tests $df = 111$.

established, boys should target girls more than in the first part of the year, perhaps as a playful strategy to initiate heterosexual contact.

First, males' R&T was significantly intercorrelated with observed aggression, $r = .31$, $p < .01$, and with dominance (as assessed by peer ratings), $r = .25$, $p < .05$. Dominance and aggression were also interrelated, but only marginally, $r = .21$, $p < .06$. These analyses support the hypothesis that males' R&T during early adolescence is related to dominance and aggression. The relation between R&T and dominance and aggression is consistent with earlier work (Humphreys & Smith, 1987; Neill, 1976; Pellegrini, 1995). This pattern, different from that in childhood, is probably related to the increasing importance of peer status, rapid changes in body size during, and the transition into a new school. These forces may have converged to exacerbate dominance-related conflicts.

Second, I tested the hypothesis that targets for males' R&T should change with time: If it is used to establish dominance it should be intrasexual more than intersexual at the start of the year. With the passage of time, and the stabilization of dominance relationships, males should use R&T intersexually more frequently as a way in which to explore heterosexual relationships. Descriptive statistics for these analyses are displayed in Table 4.1.

For R&T, significant main effects were observed for sex of the target, F (1,259) = 22.51, $p <. 001$, where more R&T was aimed at boys than girls, and for time, F (1,259) = 19.29, $p <. 001$, where more R&T was observed in the second half of the year compared to the first half. There was also a significant time by sex of focal youngster by sex of target, F (1,259) = 13.29, $p < .001$, interaction. Consistent with the hypothesis, boys targeted girls for R&T more during the second half of sixth grade than during the first half of sixth grade. The finding that boys also targeted other boys more than girls in the second half of the year may suggest that girls may be more receptive to boys' advances in Spring and may encourage this push–poke activity. (I acknowledge Pat Hawley for this interpretation.)

These results can best be explained as boys using both R&T and aggression with other boys across the whole first year of middle school to sort out their status. Boys were aggressive with each other but not aggressive with girls, consistent with the finding that their R&T was related to aggression and dominance. I suggest that male–female R&T in the second half of the year was more playful than aggressive and may be a form of poke-and-push courtship.

Schofield (1981) described a similar phenomenon where young adolescents used rough and playful overtures to initiate contact with members of the opposite sex. Consistent with this argument, the observational data just presented showed that males and females are not aggressive with each other. Further, the increase with time of intersexual R&T fits with other findings showing that cross-sex interaction and interests in heterosexual relationships dynamically influence each other across early adolescence. That is, the extent to which adolescent males and females interact with each other is affected by their interest in dating and conversely, heterosexual interaction influences interest in dating (Pellegrini & Long, 2003).

CONCLUSIONS

I have argued that one way in which aggression can be understood is in terms of sexual selection theory. From this view, aggression takes different forms for males and females. Males' aggression is physical and used in the service of dominance, albeit at a marginally significant level. Dominance, especially in adolescence and adulthood, is associated with accessing heterosexual relationships. Our data support this process model.

Females, on the other hand, use less direct and physical forms of aggression. Further, female groups, do not seem to be organized according to dominance relationships in the same way as male groups. Specifically, indirect aggression is not related to agonism-based dominance but it is related to females' heterosexual relationships. Thus, females used aggression to access heterosexual relationships, but we do not know the processes by which this is done. One possibility is that girls' use of indirect, or relational, aggression is moderated by their physical attractiveness. The less attractive the girls, the more likely they are to be aggressive.

Another, related, hypothesis derived from research by feminist evolutionary psychologists (Campbell, 2002) and primatologists (Smuts,

1987; 1995) is that females use indirect aggression to form coalitions and alliances. Specifically, females may use indirect aggression to damage the reputations of their more attractive peers who are also rivals for heterosexual relationships.

In short, boys and girls use aggression in different ways, but in each case it is related to their being nominated for dates with opposite sex peers. Adolescent males use physical aggression, dominance, and R&T to serve dominance exhibition and maintenance functions (Pellegrini & Smith, 1998). These strategies, in turn, relate to hypothetical dating popularity (Pellegrini & Long, 2003). Females use other strategies, such as alliances with other females (Smuts, 1995) and manipulation of relationships (Björkqvist et al., 1992; Campbell, 1999; Crick & Grotpeter, 1995; Galen & Underwood, 1997), to gain and maintain status in their groups.

REFERENCES

Alexander, R. D., Hoogland, J. L., Howard, R. D., Noonan, K. M., & Sherman, P. W. (1979). Sexual dimorphisms and breeding systems in pinnipeds, ungulates, primates, and humans. In N. A. Chagnon & W. Irons (Eds.), *Evolutionary biology and human social behavior* (pp. 402–435). North Scituate, MA: Duxbury Press.

Altringham, J., & Senior, P. (2005), Sexual segregation in bats. In K. Ruckstuhl & P. Neuhaus (Eds.), *Sexual segregation in vertebrates* (pp. 280–302). Cambridge, UK: Cambridge University Press.

Archer, J. (1988). *The behavioural biology of aggression.* Cambridge, UK: Cambridge University Press.

Archer, J., & Lloyd, B. (2002). *Sex and gender (2nd ed.).* London: Cambridge University Press.

Bateman, A. J. (1948). Intrasexual selection in *Drosophilia. Heredity, 2,* 349–368.

Bateson, P. P. G. (2005). Play and its role in the development of great apes and humans. In A. D. Pellegrini & P. K. Smith (Eds.), *The nature of play: Great apes and humans* (pp. 13–26). New York: Guilford.

Bateson, P. P. G., & Martin, P. (1999). *Design for a life: How behaviour develops.* London: Jonathan Cape.

Berenbaum, S. A., & Snyder, E. (1995). Early hormonal influences on childhood sex-typed activity and playmate preferences: Implications for the development of sexual orientation. *Developmental Psychology, 31,* 31–42.

Bjorklund, D. F., & Pellegrini, A. D. (2000). *Evolutionary developmental psychology.* Washington, DC: American Psychological Association.

Björkqvist, K. (1994). Sex differences in physical, verbal, and indirect aggression: A review of recent research. *Sex Roles, 30,* 177–188.

Björkqvist, K., Lagerspetz, K. M. J., & Kaukiainen, A. (1992). Do girls manipulate and boys fight? Developmental trends in regard to direct and indirect aggression. *Aggressive Behavior 18,* 117–127.

Blatchford, P., Baines, & Pellegrini, A. D. (2003). The social context of school playground games: Sex and ethnic differences and changes over time after entry into junior school. *British Journal of Developmental Psychology, 21,* 481–505.

Boyd, R., & Richerson, P. J. (1985). *Culture and the evolutionary process.* Chicago: The University of Chicago Press.

Bronfenbrenner, U., & Ceci, S. J. (1994). Nature–nurture reconceptualized in developmental perspective: A bioecological model. *Psychological Review, 101,* 568–586.

Brown, B. S., Eicher, S. A., & Petrie, S. (1986). The importance of peer group ("crowd") affiliation in adolescence. *Journal of Adolescence, 9,* 73–96.

Bukowski, W. M., Sippola, L. A., & Newcomb, A. F. (2000). Variations in patterns of attraction to same- and other-sex peers during early adolescence. *Developmental Psychology, 36,* 147–154.

Buss, D. M. (1989). Sex differences in human mate preferences: Evolutionary hypotheses tested in 37 cultures. *Behavioral and Brain Sciences, 12,* 1–49.

Byers, J. A., & Walker, C. (1995). Refining the motor training hypothesis for the evolution of play. *American Naturalist, 146,* 25–40.

Campbell, A. (1999). Staying alive: Evolution, culture, and women's intrasexual aggression. *Behavioral and Brain Sciences, 22,* 203–252.

Campbell, A. (2002). *A mind of her own: The evolutionary psychology of women.* Oxford, UK: Oxford University Press.

Caro, T. M., & Bateson, P. (1986). Ontogeny and organization of alternative tactics. *Animal Behaviour, 34,* 1483–1499.

Clutton-Brock, T. H., & Albon, S. D. (1979). The roaring of red deer and the evolution of honest advertisement. *Behaviour, 69,* 145–170.

Coie, J. D., & Dodge, K. A. (1998). Aggression and antisocial behavior. In N. Eisenberg (Ed.), *Manual of child psychology, Vol. 3, Social, emotional, and personality development* (pp. 779–862). New York: Wiley.

Collins, W. A., & Sroufe, L. A. (1999). Capacity for intimate relationships: A developmental construction. In W. Furman, B. B. Brown, & C. Feiring (Eds.), *The development of romantic relationships in adolescence* (pp. 125–147). New York: Cambridge University Press.

Conradt, L. (1998). Measuring the degree of sexual segregation in group-living animals. *Journal of Animal Ecology, 67,* 217–226.

Crick, N. R., & Grotpeter, J. K. (1995). Relational aggression, gender, and social-psychological adjustment. *Child Development, 66,* 710–722.

Darwin, C. (1871). *The descent of man, and selection in relation to sex.* London: John Murray

deWaal, F. B. M. (1986). The integration of dominance and social bonding in primates. *Journal of Theoretical Biology, 61,* 459–479.

Dawkins, R. (1976). *The selfish gene.* New York: Oxford University Press.

Dunbar, R. I. M. (1988). *Primate social systems.* Ithaca, NY: Cornell.

Dunphy, D. C. (1963). The structure of urban adolescent peer groups. *Sociometry, 26,* 230–246.

Eaton, W. O., & Enns, L. (1986). Sex differences in human motor activity level. *Psychological Bulletin, 100,* 19–28.

Eaton, W. C., & Yu, A. (1989). Are sex differences in child motor activity level a function of sex differences in maturational status? *Child Development, 60*, 1005–1011.

Erckmann, W. W. (1983). The evolution of polyandry in shorebirds: An evaluation of hypotheses. In S. K. Wasser (Ed.), *Social behavior of female vertebrates* (pp. 113–168). New York: Academic Press.

Fabes, R. A., Martin, C. L., Hanish, L. D., Anders, M. C., & Madden-Derdich, D. A. (2003). Early school competence: The roles of sex-segregated play and effort control. *Developmental Psychology, 39*, 848–858.

Galen, B. R., & Underwood, M. K. (1997). A developmental investigation of social aggression among children. *Developmental Psychology, 33*, 589–600.

Garvey, C. (1990). *Play* (2nd. ed.). Cambridge, MA: Harvard University Press.

Gottlieb, G. (1998). Normally occurring environmental and behavioral influences on gene activity: From central dogma to probabilistic epigenesis. *Psychological Review, 105*, 792–802.

Gottman, J. M., & Ringland, J. T. (1981). The analysis of dominance and bidirectionality in social development. *Child Development, 52*, 393–412.

Hartup, W. (1974). Aggression in childhood: Developmental perspectives. *American Psychologist, 29*, 336–341.

Hawley, P. H. (1999). The ontogenesis of social dominance: A strategy-based evolutionary perspective. *Developmental Review, 19*, 97–132.

Hinde, R. (1980). *Ethology*. London: Fontana.

Hobsbawm, E. J. (1996). *The age of extremes: A history of the world, 1914–1991*. New York: Vintage Books.

Humphreys, A., & Smith, P. K. (1987). Rough-and-tumble play, friendship and dominance in school children: Evidence for continuity and change with age. *Child Development, 58*, 201–212.

Jenni, D. A. (1974). Evolution of polyandry in birds. *American Naturalist, 14*, 129–144.

Little, T. D., Henrich, C. C., Jones, S. M., & Hawley, P. H. (2003). Disentangling the "whys" from the "whats" of aggressive behaviour. *International Journal of Behavioral Development, 27*, 122–133.

Maccoby, E. E. (1998). *The two sexes: Growing up apart, coming together*. Cambridge, MA: Harvard University Press.

Neill, S. (1976). Aggressive and non-aggressive fighting in twelve- to-thirteen year old pre-adolescent boys. *Journal of Child Psychology and psychiatry, 17*, 213–220.

Pellegrini, A. D. (1995). A longitudinal study of boys' rough and tumble play and dominance during early adolescence. *Journal of Applied Developmental Psychology, 16*, 77–93.

Pellegrini, A. D. (2003). Perceptions and possible functions of play and real fighting in early adolescence. *Child Development, 74*, 1459–1470.

Pellegrini, A. D. (2004). Sexual segregation in childhood: A review of evidence for two hypotheses. *Animal Behaviour, 68*, 435–443.

Pellegrini, A. D., & Archer, J. (2005). Sex differences in competitive and aggressive behavior: A view from sexual selection theory. In B. J. Ellis & D. J. Bjorklund (Eds.), *Origins of the social mind: Evolutionary psychology and child development* (pp. 219–244). New York: Guilford.

Pellegrini, A. D., & Bartini, M. (2001). Dominance in early adolescent boys: Affiliative and aggressive dimensions and possible functions. *Merrill-Palmer Quarterly, 47,* 142–163.

Pellegrini, A. D., Bartini, M., & Brooks, F. (1999). School bullies, victims, and aggressive victims: Factors relating to group affiliation and victimization in early adolescence. *Journal of Educational Psychology, 91,* 216–224.

Pellegrini, A. D., Horvat, M., & Huberty, P. D. (1998). The relative cost of children=s physical activity play. *Animal Behaviour, 55,* 1053–106.

Pellegrini, A. D., Kato, K., Blatchford, P., & Baines, E. (2002).A short-term longitudinal study of children's playground games across the first year of school: Implications for social competence and adjustment to school. *American Educational Research Journal, 39,* 991–1015.

Pellegrini, A. D., & Long, J. D. (2003). A sexual selection theory longitudinal analysis of sexual segregation and integration in early adolescence. *Journal of Experimental Child Psychology, 85,* 257–278.

Pellegrini, A. D., Long, J., & Mizerak, E. (2005). Sexual segregation in humans.In K. Ruckstuhl & P. Neuhaus (Eds.), *Sexual segregation in vertebrates* (pp. 200–217). Cambridge, UK: Cambridge University Press.

Pellegrini, A. D., & Smith, P. K. (1998). Physical activity play: The nature and function of a neglected aspect of play. *Child Development, 69,* 577–598.

Ralls, K. (1977). Sexual dimorphism in mammals: Avian models and unanswered questions. *The American Naturalist, 11,* 917–938.

Rodkin, P. C., Farmer, T. W., Pearl, R., & Van Acker, R. (2000). Heterogeneity of popular boys: Antisocial and prosocial configurations. *Developmental Psychology, 36,* 14–24.

Ruckstuhl, K., & Neuhaus, P. (2005). (Eds.) *Sexual segregation in vertebrates.* Cambridge, UK: Cambridge University Press.

Schofield, J. W. (1981). Complementary and conflicting identities: Images and interactions in an interracial school. In S. R. Asher & J. M. Gottman (Eds.), *The development of children's friendships* (pp. 53–90). New York: Cambridge University Press.

Serbin, L. A., Tonick, I. J., & Sternglanz, S. H. (1977). Shaping cooperative cross-sex play. *Child Development, 48,* 924–929.

Silk, J. B. (1986). Social behavior in evolutionary perspective. In B. B. Smuts, D. C. Cheyney, R. M. Seyforth, R. W. Wrangham, & T. Struhsaker (Eds.), *Primate societies* (pp. 318–329). Chicago: University of Chicago Press

Smuts, B. B. (1987). Gender, aggression, and influence. In B. B. Smuts, D. C. Cheyney, R. M. Seyforth, R. W. Wrangham, & T. Struhsaker (Eds.), *Primate societies* (pp. 400–412). Chicago: University of Chicago Press.

Smuts, B. B. (1995). The evolutionary origins of patriarchy. *Human Nature, 6,* 1–32.

Stamps. J. (2003). Behavioural processes affecting development: Tinbergen's fourth question comes to age. *Animal Behaviour, 66,* 1–13.

Strayer, F. F. (1980). Social ecology of the preschool peer group. In W. A. Collins Ed.), *Minnesota symposium on child development, Vol. 13* (pp. 165–196). Hillsdale, NJ: Lawrence Erlbaum Associates.

Trivers, R. (1972). Parental investment and sexual selection. In B. Campbell (Ed.), *Sexual selection and the descent of man* (pp. 136–179). Chicago: Aldine.

Trivers, R. L. (1985). *Social evolution*. Menlo Park, CA: The Benjamin Cummings
   Publishing Co.
Wilson, E. O. (1975). *Sociobiology: The new synthesis*. Cambridge, MA: Harvard
   University Press.
Wrangham, R. W. (1999). Evolution of coalitionary killing. *Yearbook of Physical
   Anthropology, 42*, 1–30.

5

DIFFERENTIAL RELATIONS OF INSTRUMENTAL AND REACTIVE AGGRESSION WITH MALADJUSTMENT: DOES ADAPTIVITY DEPEND ON FUNCTION?

Noel A. Card
University of Arizona

Todd D. Little
University of Kansas

In order to examine questions of whether and to what degree aggression is adaptive or maladaptive, an important consideration is why the aggression is enacted. As we describe in more detail in the following section, researchers have described various forms of aggression (i.e., the act itself) as well as their functions (i.e., why it was enacted). The most common function-related distinction is that between instrumental and reactive aggression. Instrumental aggression generally refers to agonistic acts that are planful and goal-oriented. Reactive aggression generally refers to agonistic acts that are enacted in response to perceived threats and is characterized by a degree of emotional dysregulation.

In this chapter, we focus on the distinction between the instrumental and reactive functions of aggression. We begin with a review of the extant literature regarding the theoretical and empirical distinctions between these two functions of aggression and examine the adjustment correlates of each. In the review, we note problematic limitations of this work, including issues related to both theory and measurement. Addressing the measurement issues, we describe a measurement and analysis approach that can be used to disentangle the forms (i.e., overt, social) and functions (i.e., instrumental, reactive) of aggression and present findings from this approach that elucidate the distinct adjustment correlates between the instrumental and reactive functions of aggression. Finally, we discuss theoretical rationales for why reactive aggression would be associated with maladaption whereas instrumental aggression would not. Limitations and suggestions for future research are also elaborated.

DISTINGUISHING INSTRUMENTAL AND REACTIVE AGGRESSION

Aggressive behavior has long been distinguished in terms of its two general functions (i.e., the motives of the aggressor; see e.g., Dodge & Coie, 1987; Hartup, 1974; Lorenz, 1966). Although various terms have been used to describe this distinction, we prefer the terms instrumental and reactive aggression. As we see, precise definitions of this distinction are lacking. Broadly speaking, then, instrumental aggression (cf. proactive, offensive, or "cold-blooded" aggression) generally refers to aggression that is deliberately enacted and directed toward obtaining desired goals. Reactive aggression (cf. defensive or "hot-blooded" aggression) generally refers to aggression that is an angry, often emotionally dysregulated, response to perceived offenses or frustrations. Consistent with Bushman and Anderson's (2001) arguments, any given act of aggressive behavior can consist of a mixture of instrumental and reactive function; thus whether an aggressive act is instrumental or reactive is not the question. On the other hand, the functions of aggression are distinct dimensions that, when measured independently, can be used to understand individuals' tendencies to aggress more or less instrumentally, more or less reactively, or both (see Little, Brauner, Jones, Noch, & Hawley, 2003).

Aggression has been distinguished in other ways, most notably by form. Broadly speaking, the most common distinction is that between overt and social-relational aggression. Overt aggression generally refers to (a) physical acts such as pinching, pushing, kicking, and hitting; (b) verbal acts such as name calling, threatening, harmful sarcasm, and harassment; (c) nonverbal acts such as "eye-daggers" and offensive gestures; and sometimes (d) material acts such as defacing, damaging, or destroying a target's personal property. Social-relational aggression generally refers to interpersonal acts of reputational or emotional harm such as talking about others behind their back, intentionally excluding from the group, spreading rumors, gossiping, and hurtful manipulation of relationships (see Table 5.1 for an alternative schematic overview of the different forms of aggression, and for detailed discussions of them see e.g., Björkqvist, Lagerspetz, & Kaukiainen, 1992; Cairns, Cairns, Neckerman, Ferguson, & Gariépy, 1989; Crick & Grotpeter, 1995; Galen & Underwood, 1997; Lagerspetz, Björkqvist, & Peltonen, 1988; Parke & Slaby, 1983; Xie, Cairns, & Cairns, 2005).

For the most part, the various forms of aggression have pronounced associations with various maladjustment outcomes (Card, Stucky, Sawalani, & Little, 2006). Importantly, however, this literature often does not account for the functions that the aggressive acts serve. Our focus, therefore, is on the distinction between instrumental versus reactive functions that children's aggression serves, because we view these two functional dimensions as key to considering the potential adaptivity of agonistic behavior. We believe that this distinction is especially critical given that (a) different social-cognitive processes are believed to underlie the enactment of each function of aggression; and, as is reviewed shortly, (b) these functions might be expected to differentially relate to psychosocial adjustment.

Instrumental and reactive functions of aggression derive from distinct theoretical perspectives. These perspectives posit that different social-cognitive processes are responsible for enacting aggressive behavior (see Fig. 5.1 and Crick & Dodge, 1994, 1996; Dodge & Coie, 1987; Gifford-Smith & Rabiner, 2004). Instrumental aggression is related to Bandura's (1973, 1986) social-cognitive learning theory, which describes aggressive behavior as a product of high self-efficacy for aggression, outcome values for aggression, and valuation of these outcomes obtained through aggressive means. Each of these social-cognitive processes has been shown to independently predict instrumental aggression among children (Boldizar, Perry, & Perry, 1989; Crick & Dodge, 1996; Egan, Monson, & Perry, 1998; Perry, Perry, & Rasmussen, 1986; Schwartz et al., 1998; Slaby & Guerra, 1988; Smithmyer, Hubbard, & Simmons, 2000). As shown in Figure 5.1, these social cognitions are incorporated most directly in Steps 4 (response access or construction) and 5 (response decision) of Dodge's social information-processing model of aggression (1986; see Crick & Dodge, 1994; Gifford-Smith & Rabiner, 2004). Reactive aggression, on the other hand, is related to the frustration-aggression model (Dollard, Doob, Miller, Mowrer, & Sears, 1939; see Berkowitz, 1993) and is incorporated as Steps 1 (encoding of cues) and 2 (interpretation of cues) in Dodge's social-information processing

TABLE 5.1

Schematic Overview of the Different Forms of Aggression and Example Acts.

	Physical Acts	Verbal Acts	Non-Verbal Acts	Interpersonal Acts	Passive Acts
Direct (confrontational)	Hitting, kicking, punching, pushing, etc. the target (overt)	Berating; calling the target names; sarcasm; threats (overt)	"eye-daggers" directed at the target; gestures (overt)	Enlisting others to gang up against the target (social)	Ignoring or refusing to acknowledge the target's presence
Indirect (Non-confrontational)	Destroying or defacing the target's property (overt)	Gossiping; spreading rumors about the target (social)	"eye-rolling"; gesturing about the target (social)	Keeping a target from joining a clique or group; hurtful manipulation of target's relationships (social)	Not sharing secrets; withholding information or materials that would benefit the target

Note. Passive acts are not commonly assessed in measures of aggression.

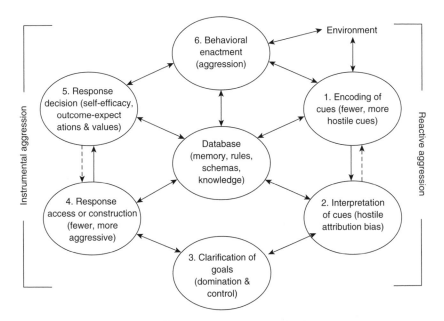

FIGURE 5.1   Social Information Processing model of aggressive behavior (adapted from Crick & Dodge, 1994).

model. Evidence suggests that reactively aggressive youths have biases and deficits in these social information-processing components, such as hostile-attribution biases, which are consistent with this model (e.g., Crick & Dodge, 1996; Dodge & Coie, 1987; Dodge, Coie, Pettit, & Price, 1990; Schwartz et al., 1998).

CORRELATES OF INSTRUMENTAL AND REACTIVE AGGRESSION

Guided by the theoretical distinctions between the functions of aggression, numerous researchers have sought to explore the differential correlates of instrumental and reactive aggression. In this section, we review the psychosocial correlates of each function of aggression that have been elucidated in prior work using traditional measurement strategies (in contrast to the newer approach described in the following discussion). Specifically, we report results of a meta-analytic review of the correlates of instrumental and reactive aggression to internalizing problems, prosocial behavior, dysregulation and hyperactivity, delinquency, academic performance, peer rejection, and peer victimization (for a full report, see Card & Little, in press). These correlates were selected because they together represent a broad range of psychosocial adjustment.

Works were included in this review if they utilized normative samples (i.e., psychiatric and juvenile justice samples were excluded) and reported sufficient information to compute an effect size of instrumental and reactive aggression with any of the seven correlates of interest. The effect size (r) of the association of instrumental and reactive aggression with each of these correlates was coded using procedures described by Rosenthal (1991), and were combined using sample-size-weighted fixed-effects procedures (see Hedges & Olkin, 1985; Hedges & Vevea, 1998). In order to compare the associations of instrumental versus reactive aggression to these correlates, t scores representing the differences between the dependent correlation coefficients were computed for each study (see pp. 56–57 of Cohen & Cohen, 1983), which were, in turn, transformed to d scores in order to be combined across studies (using sample-size-weighted fixed effects; see Card & Little, 2005, for more details).

Table 5.2 summarizes these effect sizes from prior literature and shows the meta-analytically combined relations of instrumental and reactive aggression with seven indices of psychosocial adjustment. From these combined relations, we see that both instrumental and reactive functions of aggression generally exhibited reliable correlations of small to moderate magnitude with personal and interpersonal maladjustment correlates. Specifically, both exhibited moderately strong associations with low prosocial behavior and with peer rejection or low social preference, both had small to moderate relations with dysregulation and hyperactivity, delinquency, and peer victimization, and both had little relation to internalizing problems or academic performance.

In contrast to these generalities, there was mixed evidence to suggest that these functions of aggression are differentially related to maladjustment. Although there was no evidence to suggest that either function of aggression is more strongly related than the other to delinquency, and there was insufficient evidence to draw conclusions regarding academic achievement, other results are more conclusive. Specifically, internalizing problems, low prosocial behavior, dysregulation and hyperactivity, peer rejection and low social preference, and peer victimization were all more strongly associated with reactive than instrumental aggression. These findings shed new light on the differential relations of instrumental and reactive aggression to psychosocial maladjustment, suggesting

TABLE 5.2

Correlates of Instrumental and Reactive Aggression.

Correlate	Study	N	Age (years)	Instrumental (r)	Reactive (r)	Difference (d)
Internalizing Problems						
	Day et al. (1992)	88	8.6	-.25	.14	-.76**
	Dodge & Coie (1987)	158	7.0	-.09	-.12	.09
	Dodge et al. (1997)	502	8.0	.31	.36	-.13
	Orobio de Castro et al. (2005)	84	10.1	.10	-.04	.37
	Pulkkinen (1996)	369	8.7	-.04	-.07	.05
	Salmivalli et al. (2005)	589	12.0	-.17	-.14	-.10
	Schippell et al. (2003)	90	12.9	-.01	.07	-.17
	Vitaro et al. (2002)	1203	10.5	.03	.07	-.10
	Weighted fixed effects means:			.02	.05**	-.08*
Prosocial Behavior						
	Day et al. (1992)	88	8.6	-.20	-.29	.16
	Dodge & Coie (1987)	158	7.0	.01	.01	.01
	Hegland & Rix (1990)	64	6.2	-.16	-.10	-.12
	Marcus & Kramer (2001)	107	5.3	-.57	-.59	.06
	Price & Dodge (1989)	70	6.0	.07	-.17	.51*
	Salmivalli et al. (2005)	589	12.0	-.28	-.35	.25*
	Vorbach (2000)	112	13.1	-.24	-.30	.08
	Weighted fixed effects means:			-.24**	-.30**	.17**
Dysregulation / Hyperactivity						
	Day et al. (1992)	88	8.6	.16	.20	-.08
	Farver (1996)	64	4.3	.31	.48	-.46
	Hubbard et al. (2002)	272	8.0	.01	.04	-.08
	Orobio de Castro et al. (2005)	84	10.1	.30	.37	-.21
	Price & Dodge (1989)	70	6.0	.14	.37	-.52*

TABLE 5.2 (CONTINUED)

Correlate	Study	N	Age (years)	Instrumental (r)	Reactive (r)	Difference (d)
	Pulkkinen (1996)	369	8.7	.14	.02	.16
	Ramsden (2001)	120	9.0	.35	.62	-.21
	Schippell et al. (2003)	90	12.9	.35	.62	-.72**
	Vorbach (2002)	112	13.1	.16	.25	-.14
	Washburn et al. (2004)	211	12.5	.15	.18	-.08
	Weighted fixed effects means:			.16*	.19**	-.12**
Delinquency						
	Atkins et al. (2002)	157	10.4	.23	.34	-.26*
	Brown et al. (1996)	186	9.0	.42	.49	-.21
	Frick et al. (2003)	98	12.4	.35	.28	.19
	Pulkkinen (1996)	369	8.7	.14	.00	.18
	Schippell (2001)	96	13.0	.55	.57	-.07
	Vitaro et al. (2002)	1203	10.5	.09	.07	.06
	Weighted fixed effects means:			.18**	.16*	.03
Academic Performance						
	Day et al. (1992)	88	8.6	.05	-.22	.51*
	Pulkkinen (1996)	369	8.7	-.02	.02	-.05
	Weighted fixed effects means:			-.01	-.03	.06
Peer Rejection / Low Social Preference						
	Brown et al. (1996)	186	9.0	.26	.26	.00
	Coie et al. (1991)	131	7.0	.22	.10	.24
	Day et al. (1992)	88	8.6	-.17	.18	-.68**
	Dodge et al. (1990)	129	7.0	.26	.10	.39*
	Dodge et al. (1997)	422	8.0	.25	.35	-.25*
	Poulin & Boivin (1999)	149	10.5	.32	.41	-.28

TABLE 5.2 (CONTINUED)

Correlate	Study	N	Age (years)	Instrumental (r)	Reactive (r)	Difference (d)
	Price & Dodge (1989)	70	6.0	.06	.32	-.57*
	Prinstein & Cillessen (2003)	235	16.3	-.14	.02	-.26
	Ramsden (2001)	120	9.0	.26	.28	-.05
	Smithmyer (2001)	76	8.0	.42	.56	-.44
	Volling et al. (1993)	896	7.6	.13	.20	-.16*
	Vorbach	112	13.1	.22	.29	-.10
	Waschbusch et al. (1998)	405	7.5	.73	.78	-.22*
Weighted fixed effects means:				.26**	.34**	-.17**
Peer Victimization						
	Camodeca et al. (2002)	242	8.8	-.17	.25	-2.96**
	Lento (2001)	3884	11.5	.10	.20	-.24**
	Roland & Idsøe (2001)	3884	11.5	.10	.20	-.24**
	Salmivalli & Nieminen (2002)	1062	12.0	.16	.29	-.27**
	Schwartz (1994)	442	12.0	.18	.28	-.35**
	Schwartz et al. (1998)	66	8.0	-.07	.48	-1.33**
Weighted fixed effects means:				.10**	.23**	-.22**

Note. Tests of significance were performed on the differences in correlations within each study, the sample-size-weighted average correlations of each type aggression with the correlate, and of the sample-size-weighted differences across studies: $* p < .05$, $** p < .01$.

that, where differences can be detected, reactive aggression is generally more strongly related to maladjustment than instrumental aggression.[1]

DIFFICULTIES IN DIFFERENTIALLY ASSESSING INSTRUMENTAL AND REACTIVE AGGRESSION

Instrumental and reactive aggression should be quite distinct from one another because the concepts emanate from quite distinct theoretical conceptualizations and they have different underlying social cognitive functions. However, traditional work has been hampered by the inability to assess these two functions of aggression in an empirically unique manner. As a result, traditional measures of instrumental and reactive aggression are often very highly correlated. This high degree of correlation has led some to conclude that youths who are highly instrumentally aggressive are also highly reactively aggressive (Coie & Dodge, 1998). This high degree of correlation (i.e., lack of empirical distinctiveness) may also explain the mixed findings regarding their differential associations with maladjustment.

To determine the magnitude of this intercorrelation, we meta-analytically combined correlations between instrumental and reactive aggression for 36 studies (consisting of 17,360 youths), that report this intercorrelation. As is shown in Table 5.3, the sample-size-weighted average correlation was $r = .68$ ($Z = 108.8$, $p < .001$, 95% C. I. = .671 to .687). When one corrects for measurement error (using internal consistencies reported in studies, with the mean $\alpha = .88$ for both instrumental and reactive aggression used for studies not reporting this value), the mean estimate of disattenuated correlation is .78 ($Z = 122.0$, $p < .001$, 95% C. I. = .773 to .786).

---

[1]It is worth noting that the differential relations, as indexed by the d-statistic that were detected through this meta-analysis were not consistently found within the individual studies included. This fact both supports the importance of this meta-analytic work and indicates the difficulty of detecting these differential correlates in single studies. Some individual studies have made similar conclusions based on multiple regression weights or partial/semipartial correlations of each function of aggression predicting maladjustment after controlling for the other function. These independent relations indicate the associations of maladjustment with the portion of each function of aggression that does not overlap with the other function (e.g., the part of reactive aggression that does not overlap with instrumental aggression). These independent relations are conceptually distinct from the differential relations examined here (indexed with the d-statistic), which capture the magnitude to which one function of aggression is more or less strongly related to maladjustment than is the other function.

TABLE 5.3
Correlations Between Instrumental and Reactive Aggression.

Study	N	Age	Reporter	r	α inst.	α react.	rcorrect
Arsenio et al. (2004)	100	15.9	teacher	.68	nr	nr	.77
Atkins et al. (2002)	238	10.4	teacher	.62	.83	.92	.71
Brendgen et al. (2001)	516	13.0	teacher	.68	.86	.86	.79
Brown et al. (1996)	186	9.0	teacher	.70	.94	.92	.75
Camodeca et al. (2002)	242	8.8	teacher	.87	.95	.93	.93
Crain (2002)	134	10.2	peer	.95	.95	.96	.99
Crick & Dodge (1996)	624	11.0	teacher	.68	.90	.90	.76
Day et al. (1992)	88	8.6	teacher	.41	.84	.73	.52
Dodge & Coie (1987) – study 1	259	10.0	teacher	.76	.91	.90	.84
Dodge & Coie (1987) – study 2	339	7.0	teacher	.76	.87	.88	.87
Dodge et al. (1997)	504	8.0	teacher	.64	.93	.95	.68
Frick et al. (2003)	98	12.4	self + parent	.70	.81	.85	.84
Hegland & Rix (1990)	32	6.2	observ.	.06	nr	nr	.07
Marcus & Kramer (2001)	107	5.3	mother	.62	.85	.70	.80
Orobio de Castro et al. (2005)	84	10.1	teacher	.71	.90	.87	.80
Phillips & Lochman (2003)	50	11.0	teacher	.78	.93	.95	.83
Poulin & Boivin (2000)	167	11.0	teacher	.73	.91	.91	.80
Poulin et al. (1997)	66	8.0	observ.	.47	nr	nr	.53
Price & Dodge (1989)	70	6.0	observ.	.04	.96	.84	.04
	70	6.0	teacher	.83	.94	.95	.88
Prinstein & Cillessen (2003)	235	16.3	peer	.23	nr	nr	.26
Pulkkinen (1996)	369	8.7	peer	-.27	.87	.83	-.31
	369	8.7	teacher	-.32	.84	.77	-.40

TABLE 5.3 (CONTINUED)

Study	N	Age	Reporter	r	α inst.	α react.	rcorrect
Ramsden (2001) / Ramsden & Hubbard (2002)	348	10.0	teacher	.82	.91	.93	.89
Roland & Idsøe (2001)	3884	11.5	self	.66	1.00	1.00	.66
Salmivalli & Nieminen (2002)	1062	12.0	peer	.67	.87	.89	.76
Salmivalli & Nieminen (2002)	1062	12.0	teacher	.32	.55	.70	.52
Salmivalli et al. (2005)	589	12.0	peer	.82	.90	.90	.91
Schippell et al. (2003)	90	12.9	teacher	.55	.80	.84	.67
Schwartz (1994)	442	12.0	peer	.89	.96	.90	.96
Schwartz (1994)	334	12.0	teacher	.73	.93	.95	.78
Schwartz et al. (1998)	66	8.0	observ.	.48	nr	nr	.55
Smithmeyer (2002) / Hubbard et al. (2002)	556	8.0	teacher	.78	.90	.95	.84
Strassberg et al. (1994)	273	5.0	observ.	.18	nr	nr	.21
Van Manen et al. (2001)	115	9.4	teacher	.43	.85	.90	.49
Vazzana (2001)	222	9.3	teacher	.79	.92	.93	.85
Vitaro et al. (2002)	3825	11.0	teacher	.72	.82	.83	.87
Vitaro et al. (1998)	742	12.0	teacher	.71	.84	.86	.84
Waschbusch et al. (1998)	405	7.5	teacher	.68	.92	.97	.72
Washburn et al. (2004)	116	12.5	teacher	.76	.89	.85	.87
	233	12.5	self	.69	.86	.69	.90
Weighted fixed effects mean				.68	.88	.88	.78
Median				.68			.78

Note. nr = not reported

These correlations are clearly different from one (i.e., the confidence intervals do not include 1.0), supporting the distinction between instrumental and reactive aggression found in factor analytic studies (i.e., Day, Bream, & Pal, 1992; Poulin & Boivin, 2000). Nevertheless, this extremely high correlation does draw into question the extent to which traditional measurement approaches can distinctly assess instrumental and reactive aggression. At best, this extremely high overlap obscures the potential differential correlates of instrumental and reactive aggression and may explain the inconsistencies evident in prior work in detecting differential relations to maladjustment.

TOWARD A NEW APPROACH TO ASSESSING INSTRUMENTAL AND REACTIVE AGGRESSION

We believe that the high overlap between instrumental and reactive aggression may be an artifact of traditional methods of assessment, rather than representing the true relation between the constructs of instrumental and reactive aggression. Traditional methods of assessing the two functions of aggression have typically used items that include overlapping forms of aggression (e.g., instrumental and reactive items that both imply acts of overt aggression, such as "hits or pushes others to get what they want" and "hits or pushes other when angry"); thus, part of this overlap is due to the variance shared in the form of aggression (see Little, Jones, Henrich, & Hawley, 2003). Furthermore, the associations of instrumental and reactive aggression with adjustment (see the previous discussion) raise significant uncertainty regarding the extent to which the associations are due to the specific function of aggression or the form of aggression inherent in the traditional assessment instruments. In other words, the associations cannot be interpreted because of the fundamental confound of form and function in the tradition measures of instrumental and reactive aggression.

In response to these problems with traditional measures of instrumental and reactive aggression, a methodological and analytic approach was developed to assess the functional components of aggression in an unconfounded manner (Little, Jones, et al., 2003). This approach utilized a questionnaire that was specifically designed to assess six subscales of aggressive behavior (see Fig. 5.2): two assess the pure overt and social aggression in which no function is implied (e.g., pure overt aggression: "I'm the type of person who hits, kicks, or punches others," pure social aggression: "I'm the kind of person who gossips or spreads rumors"). The other four scales assess the four possible combinations of the two forms (overt, social) and two functions (instrumental, reactive) of aggression: overt-instrumental (e.g., "I often start fights to get what I want"), overt-reactive (e.g., "If others have angered me, I often hit, kick, or punch them"), social-instrumental (e.g., "To get what I want, I often gossip or spread rumors about others"), and social-reactive (e.g., "If other have hurt me, I often try to keep them from being in my group of friends").

As shown in Figure 5.2, this measurement system allows for the decomposition of variability on the four form-function scales into that due to form (i.e. the two pure latent variables with indicators) and that due to function. In Figure 5.2, this information is captured by the two latent variables that encompass the information from the four form-function scales after controlling for form. Utilizing a sample of 1,723 students in Grades 5 through 10 (ages 11 to 16) in Berlin, Germany, this unique methodology and analytic strategy revealed that instrumental and reactive aggression—after removing the effects of the overt and social forms of aggression—were essentially unrelated (disattenuated r = −.10; see Little, Jones, et al., 2003). Ongoing research with a sample of 6th- through 8th-grade students in the United States yields similarly low correlations between instrumental and reactive aggression using a similar methodology (disattenuated r = .23; Card & Little, 2006)

Using these measures of instrumental and reactive aggression that are freed of common form variance, it is also possible to more clearly study the distinct correlates of these functions of aggression. Little, Jones, et al. (2003) found that reactive aggression exhibited moderate positive associations with hostility, frustration intolerance, and peer-reported antisocial behavior, whereas instrumental aggression was unrelated (or had a small negative relation) to these constructs. On the other hand, instrumental aggression was strongly related to self-reports (but not peer-reports) of coercively influencing others, whereas reactive aggression had a small positive relations to self- and peer-reported coercive influence.

Because instrumental and reactive functions of aggression were essentially orthogonal using this new methodology, Little, Brauner et al. (2003), using the same data from the German sample as Little, Jones, et al. (2003), distinguished five meaningful configurations of youths along the dimensions of instrumental and reactive aggression (see Fig. 5.3): an "instrumental" group (high on instrumental aggression only), a "reactive" group (high on reactive aggression only), a "both" group (high on both functions of aggression), a "typical" group (near average on both functions), and a "neither" group (low on both functions). These groups were found to differ in meaningful ways: the "reactive" and "both" groups displayed higher levels of hostility and frustration

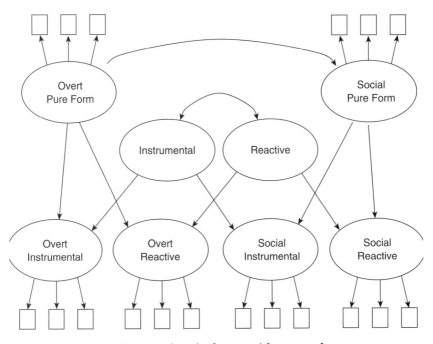

FIGURE 5.2   Disentangling the forms and functions of aggression.

intolerance (as measured by self-, peer-, and best-friend-reports, with the exception of self-reported hostility), as well as lower academic ability and school performance, than did the "instrumental" group. In fact, the "instrumental" group generally did not differ from the "typical" group on these variables, and the "instrumental" group actually had lower frustration intolerance than the "typical" group. The "neither" group, although not displaying elevated levels of emotional dysregulation, were maladjusted on several other indicators (e.g., hostility and self-concept).

Although it has seen limited usage to date, it is clear that this method of disentangling form from function of aggressive behavior yields measures of instrumental and reactive aggression that avoid the problems of high intercorrelations inherent in traditional approaches. Given this purer assessment of the functions of aggression, we expect that future research using this approach will be better able to identify the distinct adjustment correlates of instrumental and reactive aggression. Preliminary results (i.e., Little, Brauner, et al., 2003; Little, Jones, et al., 2003) are promising, but more work is clearly needed.

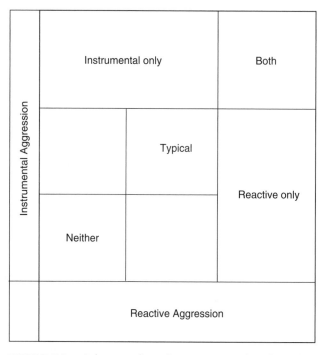

FIGURE 5.3   Subgroups based on instrumental and reactive
functions of aggression.

IS ONLY REACTIVE AGGRESSION
PREDICTIVE OF MALADJUSTMENT?

There are three perspectives that might offer explanation for greater
maladjustment for reactive than for instrumental aggressors. These
include evolutionary theory, action-control theory, and consideration
of the dyadic nature of aggression.

Evolutionary Theory

As numerous contributors to this volume have attested (see chapters
by Hawley, Pellegrini, Smith, and Vaughn, this volume), there is ample
theoretical basis from an evolutionary perspective to expect that
aggressive behavior would be implemented in the social context and
that the maladaptive consequences of the action would not be universal. Because these perspectives are covered thoroughly throughout
this volume, we do not discuss them here. Our position is simply that

other perspectives, particularly the action-control perspective, are in harmony with evolutionary perspectives (see Hawley & Little, 2002; Little, Hawley, Henrich, & Marsland, 2002)

Action-Control Theory. Similar to self-efficacy theory, action-control theory provides an elaborated view of human self-regulation that focuses on goal-directed behavior and the personal beliefs that one develops about the various means that are available to the individual for obtaining a desired outcome. From this perspective, aggression is one possible means to obtain a given outcome. Through various personal- and social-learning mechanisms, individuals develop a sense of how effective different forms of aggression (i.e., as a means) can be for obtaining a goal (ends) and they develop a personal sense of how effective they are in implementing the means (e.g., a particular aggressive act; see Table 5.1). From this perspective then, the instrumental use of aggression as a means to obtain a goal would be both common and, if effective, it would be wielded in various contexts. Action-control theory also focuses on the interface between context and behavioral regulation. In this regard, the instrumental use of aggression would be wielded primarily in contexts that support such use. The classroom, for example, presumably monitored by teachers and aides, would not support the overt use of aggression but may allow more covert forms of aggression (e.g., passing disparaging notes about a classmate). Outside the classroom and perhaps off of the school property, the context would more likely support overt forms of aggression but not the more covert forms.

Youths who are highly effective in the social arena might be expected to have various forms of aggression at their disposal, and many might willingly use them. Action-control theory would also posit that the amount and degree of aggression would be tempered to the context. In this regard, the agentic use of aggression would not only be goal directed, it would also be measured in both the form chosen and the degree needed to attain the goal. Agentic use of aggression implies the skills and awareness to determine the right nature and severity of the aggressive act (e.g., name calling vs. a verbal berating vs. a pushing match vs. a fisticuffs) that would be sufficient to attain the desired end. For example, enacting a defensive response to a clear threat with an aggressive behavior that is of appropriate severity (i.e., knowing when a push or shove will be sufficient to quell the threat as opposed to responding immediately with fists and feet) would be agentic and adaptive. Depending on the context, the amount of aggression exhibited by instrumental youths that is needed to be effective may only be minimal or it may be routine.

On the other hand, reactive aggression lacks the measured, planful, and goal-directed qualities that make the instrumental use of aggression effective. Reactively aggressive youth have deficits such as hostile dispositions and hostile information-processing biases (Crick & Dodge, 1996) as well as problems with emotional regulation (e.g., ease of frustration; see Little, Jones, et al., 2003 as well as the results of the meta-analysis just discussed). Compared to instrumentally aggressive youth, those who are reactively aggressive are likely to aggress more indiscriminately and more severely than needed. Such a pattern implies a lack of awareness and skills needed to be effective. As a result, the intensity and frequency of aggressive acts would begin to alienate the peer world and generally would lead to various maladaptive consequences.

The Dyadic Nature of Aggression

Recent conceptualizations of aggression as a dyadic phenomenon (e.g., Pierce & Cohen, 1995) may also provide explanations as to why reactive aggression is more strongly related to social maladjustment. Perry, Perry, and Kennedy (1992) described two types of aggressors: "effectual aggressors," who "apply force swiftly and unemotionally to gain what they want" versus "ineffectual aggressors," who "perform aggression primarily in the context of extended and emotionally heated conflicts" (p. 310; Perry et al., 1992). These descriptions are similar to the functions of instrumental and reactive aggression. Perry et al. (1992) suggested that effectual aggressors would be aggressive but not victimized in the peer group (aggressive nonvictims), whereas ineffectual aggressors would be both aggressive and victimized (aggressive victims).

In an extension of this conceptualization to dyadic aggressor-victim relationships within the school setting (in contrast to studies of artificial playgroups; see Coie et al., 1999; Hubbard, Dodge, Cillessen, Coie, & Schwartz, 2001), Card and colleagues (Card, 2001; Card, Isaacs, & Hodges, 2000) found that aggressive nonvictims (i.e., those that Perry and colleagues described as effectual aggressors) aggress primarily against peers who are viewed as victims by the larger peer group, whereas aggressive victims (i.e., ineffectual aggressors) target a variety of peers. These findings point to one possible explanation for the greater maladaptivity of reactive aggression. Youths who use aggression in an unplanned, emotionally dysregulated manner may attempt aggression against peers whom they either can not successfully dominate or who are well established in the peer group, and therefore bring social censure for aggression toward themselves. Youths who use aggression in a planned manner, on the other hand, may select peers who are easily dominated, will give up resources, and who are in poor standing in the peer group, and hence these aggressors will successfully obtain rewards and not suffer negative social ramifications for their aggression. Although studies explicitly testing these ideas have not yet been performed, this consideration of the dyadic nature of aggression (aggressive behaviors occurring between specific aggressors and victims) offers a potentially fruitful explanation of the greater adaptivity of instrumental than reactive aggression.

Remaining Questions

In the heading of this section we posed the question "Is only reactive aggression predictive of maladjustment?" Although we have provided rationales from three theoretical perspectives of why reactively aggressive might be more strongly associated with maladjustment than instrumental aggression, more work is certainly needed before a conclusive answer can be provided to this question. We have reviewed the extant empirical literature and some findings from a recent methodological advancement that allows for the disentangled assessment of instrumental and reactive functions of aggression. These findings converge to suggest that reactive aggression is associated with several indices of social and emotional maladjustment. In contrast, instrumental aggression is generally not associated with these indices, and in some cases is related in a direction that suggests improved adjustment of instrumentally aggressive youths. However, three unexplored issues must be considered before one can conclude that instrumental aggression is not related to maladjustment or may in fact forecast healthy adjustment.

First, the relatively recent advances in methodology to disentangle instrumental and reactive aggression have allowed for only one study to assess the adaptivity of these functions of aggression. The reports from this study (Little, Brauner, et al., 2003; Little, Jones, et al., 2003) have examined only a small portion of potential maladjustment correlates, and have been limited in terms of the culture (i.e., German) and age range studied. Current research is underway that uses this procedure in a sample of youth from the United States (Card & Little, 2006), which will allow evaluation of the generalizability of these findings. Future research will need to broaden the range of adjustment correlates considered, the cultural contexts in which this methodology is used, and (especially) the range of ages sampled.

Second, no prior studies have used this methodology and examined longitudinal relations. In fact, any longitudinal studies of instrumental and reactive aggression are rare. In our review of the extant empirical literature, we found no studies that evaluated adjustment correlates as both antecedents (i.e., predicting change in instrumental and reactive aggression over time) and consequences (i.e., change in adjustment over time being predicted by instrumental and reactive aggression). Future longitudinal research using the disentangling methodology is clearly needed to establish that adjustment indices serve as antecedents, which serve as consequences, and which serve as both antecedents and consequences of instrumental and reactive aggression. Moreover, it will be necessary to consider the results of long-term longitudinal studies before any definitive conclusions regarding the degree of adaptivity or maladaptivity of instrumental and reactive aggression can be made.

Finally, the concept of "adaptive" must be considered in light of who is impacted by the aggression. Even if it is found that the individuals enacting instrumental aggression do not suffer maladjustment for their aggression, this does not account for potential negative adjustment suffered by the victims and observers of this aggression. Ample evidence indicates that the victims of aggression are negatively impacted (e.g., Hodges & Perry, 1999; see Card, 2003). Although there is no evidence to suggest that this impact differs depending on the function the aggression serves for the aggressor, it is an unstudied topic that warrants future work. Similarly, youths who are not directly involved in aggression, but who witness aggressive acts, may feel unsafe and experience anxiety and other consequences similar to the victims themselves. Whether this differs depending on whether the aggression is instrumental or reactive in nature is unknown, but it seems likely that this function at most weakly moderates the impact on observers (e.g., observers are generally poor judges of the motives of the aggressor).

CONCLUSIONS

In summary then, prior literature examining instrumental and reactive aggression has provided, when combined using meta-analytic techniques, evidence that reactive aggression is related to maladjustment, whereas instrumental aggression is generally unrelated or, in some cases, is related to positive adjustment. Much of this literature is limited, however, by the confounded measurement of these functions of aggression. The methods of assessing instrumental and reactive aggression developed by Little and colleagues (Little Brauner, et al., 2003; Little, Jones, et al., 2003) represents a promising direction for better assessing these functions, and ongoing research (e.g., Card & Little, 2006) will likely provided further answers of the distinct relations of instrumental and reactive aggression to adjustment. However, we believe that future research is needed in at least four generally overlapping directions.

First, as just mentioned, future research should consider the broad range of constructs that may have distinct relations with instrumental and reactive aggression. Aside from measures of adjustment, general social orientations, motivations, and self-regulatory styles would enlighten our understanding of what it means to be instrumentally aggressive versus reactively aggressive. The action-control model of self-regulation (see e.g., Little, Hawley, et al., 2002), for example, could be readily adapted to study the belief profiles and means-ends understandings about various aggression acts as well as prosocial acts directed for the same ends. Understanding the belief and motivational profile of instrumentally aggressive youth would provide a way to develop tailored aggression-reduction programs that would be suited to the particular belief profile of sub-groups of aggressive youth (see e.g., Little, Brauner, et al., 2003).

Second, it should be recognized that the instrumental versus reactive dichotomy is somewhat imprecise, and further refinement of the functions that aggression serve will likely improve our understanding of the adaptivity of aggressive behavior. Although the measurement and analysis approach developed by Little and colleagues (Little, Jones et al., 2002; Little, Brauner et al., 2002) is a step in the right direction, it is also not without its limitations. For example, a responsive act of aggression can be planful and goal-directed—it may appear as a reactive outburst, but it is enacted with the full intent of gaining a desired outcome. The Little system currently does not adequately capture this distinction between reactive aggression that is truly reactionary in the sense of an undercontrolled anger or hostile misattribution. Moreover, the Little system does not adequately capture the intensity of the reactive response nor the severity of the behavior enacted. Both intensity and severity are likely to have distinct correlates with socioemotional status and adjustment. High-intensity reactive aggression would likely be less easily regulated than low-intensity reactive aggression, and it would likely be linked with greater maladaptation than low-intensity reactive aggression. Moreover, the severity of a given aggressive act is not considered. A direction for future work would be the development of a severity index for aggressive acts.

A third limitation is the general lack of information about the context of the aggression behavior: Developing measures of the context and how it might support aggressive behavior would be advantageous. For example, Vernberg and colleagues (Vernberg, Jacobs, & Hershberger, 1999) have developed a violence audit that includes some contextual factors such as the degree to which peers encourage and incite aggressive encounters (i.e., aggressive by-standing) and the degree to which adults monitor and intercede during aggression episodes. Such measures should be further elaborated and refined to identify the characteristics of the contexts that support or inhibit the expression of aggressive behavior and the conditions under which instrumental aggression is effective and reactive aggression is particularly ineffective.

A fourth direction for future work is to focus much greater attention to the targets and their relationship to the aggressor. A critical distinction among these aggressor–victim relationships might be whether they involve instrumental, effectual aggressive interactions or reactive, and perhaps non-effectual, aggression (see Perry et al., 1992). It is also expectable that the study of these relationships will partially overlap with our understanding of other peer relationships; for example, antipathetic relationships (i.e., relationships based on mutual dislike) have been shown to more often have aggressive interactions than other relationships (e.g., friendships or neutral acquaintanceships; see Card, in press; Card & Hodges, in press). Thus, understanding the relationship contexts in which aggression occurs is a promising direction for research, especially in combination with considering the instrumental or reactive motives of this aggression.

Therefore, we do not feel that it is "time to pull the plug" (Bushman & Anderson, 2001) on the instrumental versus reactive aggression distinction. The key argument against the distinction outlined in Bushman and Anderson is the futility of classifying any given act of aggression as hostile or instrumental. As we have just outlined, this distinction is fruitful if one focuses on assessing function as unique dimensions that individuals can vary along. In this regard, the body of research that we have reviewed demonstrates the distinct adaptivity versus maladaptivity of instrumental versus reactive aggression. Moreover, the recent conceptual and methodological advances described here highlight this distinction as a promising direction for future research (Little, Brauner et al., 2003; Little, Jones et al., 2003).

ACKNOWLEDGMENTS

This work was supported in part by grants from the NIH to the University of Kansas through the Mental Retardation and Developmental Disabilities Research Center (5 P30 HD002528), the Center for Biobehavioral Neurosciences in Communication Disorders (5 P30 DC005803), an NRSA fellowship to the first author while at the University of Kansas (1 F32 MH072005), and a new faculty grant to the second author from the University of Kansas (NFGRF 2301779). Its contents are solely the responsibility of the authors and do not necessarily represent the official views of these funding agencies.

REFERENCES

References marked with an asterisk indicate studies included in the meta-analyses.

*Arsenio, W. F., Gold, J., & Adams, E. (2004). Adolescents' emotion expectancies regarding aggressive and nonaggressive events: Connections with behavior problems. *Journal of Experimental Child Psychology, 89*, 338–355.

*Atkins, M. S., McKay, M. M., Frazier, S. L., Jakobsons, L. J., Arvanitis, P., Cunningham, T., Brown, C., & Lambrecht, L. (2002). Suspensions and detentions in an urban, low-income school: Punishment or reward? *Journal of Abnormal Child Psychology, 30*, 361–371.

Bandura, A. (1973). *Aggression: A social learning analysis.* Englewood Cliffs, NJ: Prentice Hall.

Bandura, A. (1986). *Social foundations of thought and action.* Englewood Cliffs, NJ: Prentice Hall.

Berkowitz, L. (1993). *Aggression: Its causes, consequences, and control.* Philadelphia, PA: Temple University Press.

Björkqvist, K., Lagerspetz, K. M. J., & Kaukiainen, A. (1992). Do girls manipulate and boys fight? Developmental trends in regard to direct and indirect aggression. *Aggressive Behavior, 18*, 117–127.

Boldizar, J. P., Perry, D. G., & Perry, L. C. (1989). Outcome values and aggression. *Child Development, 60*, 571–579.

*Brendgen, M., Vitaro, F., Tremblay, R. E., & Lavoie, F. (2001). Reactive and proactive aggression: Predictions to physical violence in different contexts and moderating effects of parental monitoring and caregiving behavior. *Journal of Abnormal Child Psychology, 29*, 293–304.

*Brown, K., Atkins, M. S., Osborne, M. L., & Milnamow, M. (1996). A revised teacher rating scale for reactive and proactive aggression. *Journal of Abnormal Child Psychology, 24*, 473–480.

Bushman, B. J., & Anderson, C. A. (2001). Is it time to pull the plug on hostile versus instrumental aggression dichotomy? *Psychological Review, 108*, 273–279.

Cairns, R. B., Cairns, B. D., Neckerman, H. J., Ferguson, L. L., & Gariépy, J. L. (1989). Growth and aggression: I. Childhood to early adolescence. *Developmental Psychology, 25*, 320–330.

*Camodeca, M., Goossens, F. A., Terwogt, M. M., & Schuengel, C. (2002). Bullying and victimization among school-age children: Stability and links to instrumental and reactive aggression. *Social Development, 11*, 332–345.

*Camodeca, M., & Goossens, F. A. (2005). Aggression, social cognitions, anger and sadness in bullies and victims. *Journal of Child Psychology and Psychiatry, 46*, 186–197.

Card, N. A. (2001). *Who aggresses against whom?: An examination of aggressors and victims in a school setting.* Unpublished Master's research project, St. John's University.

Card, N. A. (2003, April). Victims of peer aggression: A meta-analytic review. In N. A. Card & A. Nishina (Chairs), *Whipping boys and other victims of peer aggression: 25 years of research, now where do we go?* Poster symposium presented at the biennial meeting of the Society for Research in Child Development, Tampa, FL.

Card, N. A. (in press). "I hated her guts!": Emerging adults' recollections of the formation, maintenance, and termination of antipathetic relationships during high school. *Journal of Adolescent Research.*

Card, N. A., & Hodges, E. V. E. (in press). Victimization within mutually antipathetic peer relationships. *Social Development.*

Card, N. A., Isaacs, J., & Hodges, E. V. E. (2000, March). Dynamics of interpersonal aggression in the school context: Who aggresses against whom? In J. Juvonen & A. Nishina (Chairs), *Harassment across diverse contexts.* Poster symposium presented at the 8th biennial meeting of the Society for Research on Adolescence, Chicago, IL.

Card, N. A., & Little, T. D. (in press). Proactive and reactive aggression in childhood and adolescence: A meta-analysis of differential relations with psychosocial adjustment. *International journal of Behavioral Development.*

Card, N. A., & Little, T. D. (2006). *Disentangling form from functions of Aggression: Longitudinal interrelations among instrumental and reactive aggression and psychosocial adjustment.* Manuscript in preparation.

Card, N. A., Stucky, B. D., Sawalani, G., & Little, T. D. (2006). *Overt and social forms of aggression: A meta-analytic review of intercorrelations, gender differences, and relations to maladjustment.* Manuscript in preparation.

Cohen, J., & Cohen, P. (1983). *Applied multiple regression / correlation analysis for the behavioral sciences* (2nd ed.). Hillsdale, NJ: Lawrence Erlbaum Associates.

Coie, J. D., Cillessen, A. H. N., Dodge, K. A., Hubbard, J. A., Schwartz, D., Lemerise, E. A., et al. (1999). It takes two to fight: A test of relational factors and a method for assessing aggressive dyads. *Developmental Psychology, 35,* 1179–1188.

Coie, J. D., & Dodge, K. A. (1998). Aggression and antisocial behavior. In W. Damon (Series Ed.) & N. Eisenberg (Volume Ed.), *Handbook of child psychology* (5th ed., Vol. 3, pp. 779–862). New York: Wiley.

* Coie, J. D., Dodge, K. A., Terry, R., & Wright, V. (1991). The role of aggression in peer relations: An analysis of aggressive episodes in boys' play groups. *Child Development, 62,* 812–826.

* Crain, M. M. (2002). *The relationship of intent attributions, goals and outcome expectancies to relationally aggressive behavior in pre-adolescent girls.* Unpublished doctoral dissertation, California School of Professional Psychology, Alliant International University.

Crick, N. R., & Dodge, K. A. (1994). A review and reformulation of social information-processing mechanisms in children's social adjustment. *Psychological Bulletin, 115,* 74–101.

* Crick, N. R., & Dodge, K. A. (1996). Social information-processing mechanisms in reactive and instrumental aggression. *Child Development, 67,* 993–1002.

Crick, N. R., & Grotpeter, J. K. (1995). Relational aggression, gender, and social-psychological adjustment. *Child Development, 66,* 710–722.

* Day, D. M., Bream, L. A., & Pal, A. (1992). Instrumental and reactive aggression: An analysis of subtypes based on teacher perceptions. *Journal of Clinical Child Psychology, 21,* 210–217.

Dodge, K. A. (1986). A social information processing model of social competence in children. In M. Perlmutter (Ed.), *Minnesota Symposium on Child Psychology* (Vol. 18, pp. 77–125). Hillsdale, NJ: Lawrence Erlbaum Associates.

* Dodge, K. A., & Coie, J. D. (1987). Social information-processing factors in reactive and instrumental aggression in children's playgroups. *Journal of Personality and Social Psychology, 53*, 1146–1158.

* Dodge, K. A., Coie, J. D., Pettit, G. S., & Price, J. M. (1990). Peer status and aggression in boys' groups: Developmental and contextual analyses. *Child Development, 61*, 1289–1309.

* Dodge, K. A., Lochman, J. E., Harnish, J. D., Bates, J. E., & Pettit, G. S., (1997). Reactive and instrumental aggression in school children and psychiatrically impaired chronically assaultive youth. *Journal of Abnormal Psychology, 106*, 37–51.

Dodge, K. A., Price, J. M., Bachorowski, J. A., & Newman, J. P. (1990). Hostile attributional biases in severely aggressive adolescents. *Journal of Abnormal Psychology, 99*, 385–392.

Dollard, J., Doob, L. W., Miller, N. E., Mowrer, O. H., & Sears, R. R. (1939). *Frustration and aggression.* New Haven, CT: Yale University Press.

Egan, S. K., Monson, T. C., & Perry, D. G. (1998). Social-cognitive influences on change in aggression over time. *Developmental Psychology, 34*, 299–309.

* Farver, J. M. (1996). Aggressive behavior in preschoolers' social networks: Do birds of a feather flock together? *Early Childhood Research Quarterly, 11*, 333–350.

* Frick, P. J., Cornell. A. H., Barry, C. T., Bodin, S. D., & Dane, H. E. (2003). Callous-unemotional traits and conduct problems in the prediction of conduct problem severity, aggression, and self-report of delinquency. *Journal of Abnormal Child Psychology, 31*, 457–470.

Galen, B. R., & Underwood, M. K. (1997). A developmental investigation of social aggression among children. *Developmental Psychology, 33*, 589–600.

Gifford-Smith, M. E., & Rabiner, D. L. (2004). Social information processing and children's social adjustment. In K. A. Dodge & J. B. Kupersmidt (Eds.), *Children's peer relations: From development to intervention* (pp. 61–79). Washington, DC: American Psychological Association.

* Hartup, W. W. (1974). Aggression in childhood: Developmental perspectives. *American Psychologist, 29*, 336–341.

Hawley, P. H., & Little, T. D. (2002) Evolutionary and developmental perspectives on the agentic self. In D. Cervone & W. Mischel (Eds.), *Advances in personality science* (pp. 177–195). New York: Guilford.

Hedges, L. V., & Olkin, I. (1985). *Statistical methods for meta-analysis.* Orlando, FL: Academic Press.

Hedges, L. V., & Vevea, J. L. (1998). Fixed- and random-effects models in meta-analysis. *Psychological Methods, 3*, 486–504.

* Hegland, S. M., & Rix, M. K. (1990). Aggression and assertiveness in kindergarten children differing in day care experiences. *Early Childhood Research Quarterly, 5*, 105–116.

Hodges, E. V. E., & Perry, D. G. (1999). Personal and interpersonal antecedents and consequences of victimization by peers. *Journal of Personality and Social Psychology, 76*, 677–685.

Hubbard, J. A., Dodge, K. A., Cillessen, A. H. N., Coie, J. D., & Schwartz, D. (2001). The dyadic nature of social information processing in boys' reactive and proactive aggression. *Journal of Personality and Social Psychology, 80,* 68–280.

* Hubbard, J. A., Smithmyer, C. M., Ramsden, S. R., Parker, E. H., Flanagan, K. D., Dearing, K. F., et al. (2002). Observational, physiological, and self-report measures of children's anger: Relations to reactive versus instrumental aggression. *Child Development, 73,* 1101–1118.

Lagerspetz, K. M. J., Björkqvist, K., & Peltonen, T. (1988). Is indirect aggression typical of females? Gender differences in aggressiveness in 11- to 12-year-old children. *Aggressive Behavior, 14,* 403–414.

* Lento, J. (2001). *The role of child maltreatment and peer victimization in the prediction of playground social behaviors in early elementary school.* Unpublished doctoral dissertation, University of California, San Diego.

Little, T. D., Brauner, J., Jones, S. M., Nock, M. K., & Hawley, P. H. (2003). Rethinking aggression: A typological examination of the functions of aggression. *Merrill-Palmer Quarterly, 49,* 343–369.

Little, T. D., Hawley, P. H., Henrich, C. C., & Marsland, K. (2002). Three views of the agentic self: A developmental synthesis. In E. L. Deci & R. M. Ryan (Eds.), *Handbook of self-determination research* (pp. 389–404). Rochester, NY: University of Rochester Press.

Little, T. D., Jones, S. M., Henrich, C. C., & Hawley, P. H. (2003). Disentangling the "whys" from the "whats" of aggressive behaviour. *International Journal of Behavioral Development, 27,* 122–133.

Lorenz, K. (1966). *On aggression.* New York: Harcourt.

* Marcus, R. F., & Kramer, C. (2001). Reactive and proactive aggression: Attachment and social competence predictors. *The Journal of Genetic Psychology, 162,* 260–275.

* Orobio de Castro, B., Merk, W., Koops, W., Veerman, J. W., & Bosch, J. D. (2005). Emotions in social information processing and their relations with reactive and proactive aggression in referred aggressive boys. *Journal of Clinical Child and Adolescent Psychology, 34,* 105–116.

Parke, R. D., & Slaby, R. G. (1983). The development of aggression. In P. Mussen & M. Hetherington (Eds.), *Handbook of child psychology: Socialization, personality, and social development, Vol. 3* (4th ed., pp. 547–641). New York: Wiley.

Perry, D. G., Perry, L. C., & Kennedy, E. (1992). Conflict and the development of antisocial behavior. In C. U. Shantz & W. W. Hartup (Eds.), *Conflict in child and adolescent development* (pp. 301–329). New York: Cambridge University Press.

Perry, D. G., Perry, L. C., & Rasmussen, P. (1986). Cognitive social learning mediators of aggression. *Child Development, 57,* 700–711.

* Phillips, N. C., & Lochman, J. E. (2003). Experimentally manipulated change in children's proactive and reactive aggressive behavior. *Aggressive Behavior, 29,* 215–227.

Pierce, K. A., & Cohen, R. (1995). Aggressors and their victims: Toward a contextual framework for understanding aggressor-victim relationships. *Developmental Review, 15,* 292–310.

* Poulin, F., & Boivin, M. (1999). Proactive and reactive aggression and boys' friendship quality in mainstream classrooms. *Journal of Emotional and Behavioral Disorders, 7,* 168–177.

* Poulin, F., & Boivin, M. (2000). Reactive and instrumental aggression: Evidence of a two-factor model. *Psychological Assessment, 12*, 115–122.
* Poulin, F., Cillessen, A. H. N., Hubbard, J. A., Coie, J. D., Dodge, K. A., & Schwartz, D. (1997). Children's friends and behavioral similarity in two social contexts. *Social Development, 6*, 224–236.
* Price, J. M., & Dodge, K. A. (1989). Reactive and proactive aggression in childhood: Relations to peer status and social context dimensions. *Journal of Abnormal Child Psychology, 17*, 455–471.
* Prinstein, M. J., & Cillessen, A. H. N. (2003). Forms and functions of adolescent peer aggression associated with high levels of peer status. *Merrill-Palmer Quarterly, 49*, 310–342.
* Pulkkinen, L. (1996). Proactive and reactive aggression in early adolescence as precursors to anti- and prosocial behavior in young adults. *Aggressive Behavior, 22*, 241–257.
* Ramsden, S. R. (2001). *Family expressiveness and parental emotion coaching: Their roles in emotion regulation, social status, and childhood aggression.* Unpublished doctoral dissertation, University of Delaware.
* Ramsden, S. R., & Hubbard, J. A. (2002). Family expressiveness and parental emotion coaching: Their role in children's emotion regulation and aggression. *Journal of Abnormal Child Psychology, 30*, 657–667.
* Roland, E., & Idsøe, T. (2001). Aggression and bullying. *Aggressive Behavior, 27*, 446–462.
Rosenthal, R. (1991). *Meta-analytic procedures for social research.* Newbury Park, CA: Sage.
* Salmivalli, C., & Nieminen, E. (2002). Proactive and reactive aggression among school bullies, victims, and bully-victims. *Aggressive Behavior, 28*, 30–44.
* Salmivalli, C., Ojanen, T., Haanpää, J., & Peets, K. (2005). "I'm OK but you're not" and other peer-relational schemas: Explaining individual differences in children's social goals. *Developmental Psychology, 41*, 363–375.
* Schippell, P. L. (2001). *The role of narcissism, self-esteem and attentional biases in childhood reactive and proactive aggression.* Unpublished doctoral dissertation, Ohio State University.
* Schippell, P. L., Vasey, M. W., Cravens-Brown, L. M., & Bretveld, R. A. (2003). Suppressed attention to rejection, ridicule, and failure cues: A unique correlate of reactive but not proactive aggression in youth. *Journal of Clinical Child and Adolescent Psychology, 32*, 40–55.
* Schwartz, D. (1994). *The social behavior of bullied children.* Unpublished doctoral dissertation, Vanderbilt University.
* Schwartz, D., Dodge, K. A., Coie, J. D., Hubbard, J. A., Cillessen, A. H. N., Lemerise, E. A., & Bateman, H. (1998). Social-cognitive and behavioral correlates of aggression and victimization in boys' play groups. *Journal of Abnormal Child Psychology, 26*, 431–440.
Slaby, R. G., & Guerra, N. G. (1988). Cognitive mediators of aggression in adolescent offenders: I. Assessment. *Developmental Psychology, 24*, 580–588.
* Smithmyer, C. M. (2001). *Reactive aggression and low social preference versus proactive aggression: Differential autonomic reactivity to an anger-inducing social situation.* Unpublished doctoral dissertation, University of Delaware.

Smithmyer, C. M., Hubbard, J. A., & Simons, R. F. (2000). Instrumental and reactive aggression in delinquent adolescents: Relations to aggression outcome expectancies. *Journal of Clinical Child Psychology, 29,* 86–93.

* van Manen, T. G., Prins, P. J. M., & Emmelkamp, P. M. G. (2001). Assessing social cognitive skills in aggressive children from a developmental perspective: The social cognitive skills test. *Clinical Psychology and Psychotherapy, 8,* 341–351.

* Vazzana, A. D. (2001). *Outcome expectations and outcome values of proactive, reactive, and nonaggressive boys.* Unpublished doctoral dissertation, Northern Illinois University.

Vernberg, E. M., Jacobs, A. K., & Hershberger, S. L. (1999). Peer victimization and attitudes about violence during early adolescence. *Journal of Clinical Child Psychology, 28,* 386–395.

* Vitaro, F., Brendgen, M., & Tremblay, R. E. (2002). Reactively and instrumentally aggressive children: Antecedent and subsequent characteristics. *Journal of Child Psychology and Psychiatry, 43,* 495–505.

* Vitaro, F., Gendreau, P. L., Tremblay, R. E., & Oligny, P. (1998). Reactive and proactive aggression differentially predict later conduct problems. *Journal of Child Psychology and Psychiatry, 39,* 377–385.

* Volling, B. L., MacKinnon-Lewis, C., Rabiner, D., & Baradaran, L. P. (1993). Children's social competence and sociometric status: Further exploration of aggression, social withdrawal, and peer rejection. *Development and Psychopathology, 5,* 459–483.

* Vorbach, A. M. (2002). *The relationship between emotional competence and social competence among early adolescents.* Unpublished doctoral dissertation, Alliant International University.

* Waschbusch, D. A., Willoughby, M. T., & Pelham, W. E., Jr. (1998). Criterion validity and the utility of reactive and proactive aggression: Comparisons to attention deficit hyperactivity disorder, oppositional defiant disorder, conduct disorder, and other measures of functioning. *Journal of Clinical Child Psychology, 27,* 396–405.

* Washburn, J. J., McMahon, S. D., King, C. A., Reinecke, M. A., & Silver, C. (2004). Narcissistic features in young adolescents: Relations to aggression and internalizing symptoms. *Journal of Youth and Adolescence, 33,* 247–260.

Xie, H., Cairns, B. D., & Cairns, R. B. (2005). The development of aggressive behaviors among girls: Measurement issues, social functions, and differential trajectories. In D. J. Pepler, K. C. Madsen, C. Webster, & K. S. Levene (Eds.), *The development and treatment of girlhood aggression* (pp. 105–136). Mahwah, NJ: Lawrence Erlbaum Associates.

6

VARIATIONS IN THE ASSOCIATION BETWEEN AGGRESSION AND SOCIAL STATUS: THEORETICAL AND EMPIRICAL PERSPECTIVES

Antonius H. N. Cillessen
University of Connecticut

Lara Mayeux
University of Oklahoma

Classic sociometry-based peer relations research of the 1980s yielded consistent and robust associations between aggression and low peer status, such as being classified as peer-rejected (Coie & Dodge, 1998). This association went unchallenged for more than a decade in part because it is so intuitive: It makes sense to think of children or adolescents who are aggressive, hostile, and disruptive as not likely to be accepted by their peers because of the aversiveness of their behavior. Further, the aggression–rejection link (and the companion link between prosocial behavior and acceptance) might have seemed like perfect parsimony to researchers accustomed to untangling complicated and interacting determinants of behavior.

More recent research in the field of peer relations, as well as in related fields such as the sociology of education, has challenged the long-held assumption that aggression and peer rejection go hand-in-hand. New perspectives have arisen due to innovations in how peer status is defined and measured, recent advances in conceptualizing different forms of aggression, and the use of more complex analytical techniques that allow for the identification of moderators of the status–behavior link. Wider theoretical perspectives on the development, forms, and functions of aggression have also informed our understanding of the potential bright side to aggression (see the chapters by Hawley, Pellegrini, and Vaughn, this volume).

Beyond these advances, the peer relations literature has enjoyed a huge growth since the classic papers of the 1980s. That initially small but consistent body of work linking social behavior and peer status primarily for boys and during the specific period of middle childhood has expanded to include research focusing on both genders and a variety of age groups ranging from preschool to adolescence. As a field, we now know much more about the relationship between multiple forms of aggression and multiple status types, differentially for boys and girls at various ages, and in a variety of social contexts.

This chapter is written by researchers who have their background in developmental and social psychology and have used sociometric and observational methods based on a view that gives primacy to the role of social context in understanding peer relations and social behavior. Our discussion of theoretical perspectives and empirical findings reflects this emphasis on the role of social context. In this chapter, we aim to illustrate that the link between aggression and peer status is more complex than the original studies suggested. We begin by presenting three theoretical perspectives that may explain the link between aggression and high status in the peer group. We then review empirical findings that illustrate the variability in the association between measures of aggression and measures of peer status. In this review, we highlight studies illustrating the conditions under which aggression is positively correlated with measures of high status. Thus, our focus is on aggression as a means of attaining or maintaining very specific social benefits—prominence in the peer group and the perks it affords. Viewed in this light, we argue that aggression in the peer system can function as an adaptive behavior that allows youth to achieve important social goals. We conclude this chapter with directions for future research.

THEORETICAL PERSPECTIVES

The association between aggression and measures of high status represents a change in focus for the sociometric field, which traditionally has been centered on the association between aggression and peer rejection or ostracism (see, e.g., Bierman, 2004, for a review). However, when viewed in the context of several theoretical perspectives, this association is not surprising. Cairns (1979) indicated that from the very beginning, theoretical perspectives on aggression have emphasized that aggression is intimately linked to interpersonal and societal control (p. 161). Aggression can be used to control others, and hence, has advantages for the aggressor. The aggressor may not be liked as a result, but still gain benefits from the control over others in direct or indirect ways.

We address the theoretical underpinnings of the aggression–high status link by framing it in three different theoretical perspectives: social learning theory, group dynamics, and dynamic systems theory. We focus on one theoretical perspective (social learning theory) that has been frequently used by peer relations researchers to explain the associations between aggression and high status. We also discuss two theoretical perspectives (group dynamics and dynamic systems theories) that have been applied less often but offer much promise. We do not intend this to be a comprehensive review of all possible theoretical perspectives that exist to explain aggression. Such reviews exist in other chapters in this volume, and elsewhere (see, e.g., Coie & Dodge, 1998). Our focus here is on social contextual perspectives that have specific implications for understanding aggression and its relationship to sociometric status.

Social Learning Theory

Social learning theory explains individual differences in aggression by acknowledging that much of the development of aggression is due to learning in the context of social groups. Social learning theory states that individuals behave in ways that are reinforced by their social environment, in our case, the peer group. Consequently, some forms of aggression in some contexts are strongly reinforced in the peer culture by the increased social attention, higher status, social power, and other benefits they afford. By this account, many instances of aggression can be viewed as entirely functional and reinforced.

A basic principle of social learning theory (see, e.g., Bandura, 1986, 1997) regards the role of cognitive processes. Adults and children alike form cognitions about the associations between behavior and its consequences, and base their own actions on these cognitions. A second principle is that information about the consequences of behavior does not require direct experience but can be obtained via observing these consequences in others. This theoretical framework emphasizes that observational learning requires attention to the behavior of the model, encoding it, and storing it in the cognitive system so that it can be retrieved and used later. Observing the consequences of behavior in others is considered sufficient to make decisions regarding one's own future behavior. The power of this deferred imitation can be expected to increase with age—as the cognitive system matures, encoding and remembering behavior–response contingencies is expected to become easier.

How might these principles apply to the relationship between aggression and status in the peer group? Two different but related social cognitive processes may play a role. First, children and adolescents observe some of their aggressive peers attaining high social standing in the peer group. As a result, according to this theory, they may form positive expectations about the outcomes of physically or relationally aggressive behavior. Second, whether or not they emulate this behavior will depend on their own social goals. If visibility and dominance are social goals that are valued by a given child or adolescent, the decision to engage in these kinds of aggression may be a relatively easy one.

An example of these principles is found in the classic study by Patterson, Littman, and Bricker (1967). These researchers found that submissive preschoolers who were aggressed against by peers learned to retaliate by imitating the behaviors directed to them. As a result, these children became less submissive over time. In contrast, submissive children who were not victimized remained submissive. Moreover, the initially submissive children who had learned to be aggressive generalized their behavior by initiating aggression against peers who had not been aggressive to them in the first place.

Although the formation of expectations about the outcomes of behavior might be a relatively constant process over developmental time, goals may clearly change. For example, LaFontana (2005) found a curvilinear relationship between age and concern for popularity, with popularity as a social goal peaking in middle school. This suggests that children may be most likely to emulate behaviors they perceive as leading to popularity during the middle school years—and, thus, may be particularly interested in pursuing aggression during this time given the association between aggression and peer popularity in adolescence (discussed in detail in the following discussion). This trend would also explain the high salience of clique formation and social exclusion (especially among girls) during the middle school years (Adler & Adler, 1995; Merten, 1997). This finding is also consistent with Moffitt's (1993) adolescence-limited trajectory of aggression peaking in adolescence in response to contextual cues prevalent during this period.

Group Dynamics

A second view that can be used to explain aggression in the peer group is the group dynamics perspective. Group dynamic principles are often present in peer relations research but not often mentioned explicitly. This view highlights the influence of group dynamic factors on the behavior of individuals, dyads, and groups within the larger social network (e.g., Forsyth, 1990; Lewin, Lippit, & White, 1939). Lewin and his colleagues argued that small manipulations of a social situation can produce large changes in the behaviors of persons in a social field. Specifically, differences in the way group members relate to each other as a whole can create differences in the behaviors of individuals in that group.

An example of the group dynamics perspective can be found in Lewin et al.'s (1939) classic study. These researchers manipulated the social climate of experimentally contrived clubs, creating groups that were dominated by either an authoritarian leadership style or a democratic style. They found that particular styles of interaction (such as scapegoating and hostility) among the members could be heightened or lessened simply by manipulating the style of leadership within the groups.

In a recent example, DeRosier, Cillessen, Coie, and Dodge (1994) demonstrated the effect of group dynamic factors on the occurrence of aggression. In experimental play groups of 7- and 9-year-old boys, group variables affected both the likelihood of occurrence of aggression and the type of reaction that aggression received by the rest of the group (DeRosier et al., 1994). Groups characterized by higher levels of physical activity, overall aversive behavior, and competition experienced more aggression among its members. The group was more likely to notice aggression or become physically or verbally involved if the boys involved in an aggressive act had played well together before the aggression occurred. Furthermore, if the group as a whole was characterized by playful competition, the aggression was discouraged; for groups in which aversive behavior was frequent, the aggression was actually encouraged. Although DeRosier et al. did not measure sociometric status, its implications for the role of context in the status–behavior link are important. These findings suggest that among groups of boys who discourage antisocial behavior, aggressive boys may be less accepted because of their deviance from the group norm. Among highly aggressive groups, boys who are not willing to display aggressive behavior may face similar problems.

Group dynamic factors and processes not only impact aggression, but also the outcomes associated with it. For example, Green, Cillessen, Berthelsen, Irving, and Catherwood (2003) demonstrated that the degree to which 6-year-old boys and girls gain access to a desirable resource in a limited resource situation depends on the gender context of the group. These researchers compared three types of groups consisting of four children: all boys, all girls, and mixed sex (two boys and two girls). The findings indicated that when girls interacted with other girls, everybody won (defined as gaining access to the desired resource). When boys interacted with other boys, everybody lost, due to increased competitiveness and aggression of the group interactions. In mixed-sex groups, boys gained more access than in all-boy groups and girls gained less access than in all-girl groups, suggesting that the boys took control at the expense of the girls. The most verbal threats and competitive behaviors occurred when boys interacted with boys. These interactions between gender of the target person and gender of interaction partners illustrate further how group level factors can influences the dynamical interplay of aggression, dominance, and resource control.

The occurrence of aggression, then, can depend on specific aspects of the immediate social situation in which the aggression occurs. By this view, aggression does not occur as the result of a history of social learning that has taken place over some time, but rather as an immediate response to situational cues. Three further illustrations of this view are the effects of group norms on behavior, the phenomenon of ingroup–outgroup bias, and the effect of threats to the self on aggression.

First, aggression is more likely to occur in groups in which it is normative or accepted. In such groups, aggressive children are less likely to be disliked by others (Wright, Giammarino, & Parad, 1986) than in groups in which aggression is not the norm. This is true in part because these children, despite their use of potentially harmful behaviors, maintained a high degree of fit between their own behavior and that of other group members. Apparently, the positive effects of maintaining individual–group fit override the negative effects of individual aggressive acts.

From a peer relations perspective, group norms can vary by clique or subgroup in the peer culture. Research by Cairns and colleagues, for example, has identified the occurrence of highly aggressive cliques in the classroom or grade (Cairns, Cairns, Neckerman, Gest, & Gariepy, 1988). Once a child or adolescent becomes a member of an aggressive clique, using aggression is simply part of the normative, everyday behaviors of that group, despite the negative consequences associated with the aggression. The strong correlation between physical and relational aggression and perceived popularity suggests that aggression may be quite normative within these high-status cliques, particularly in groups of relationally aggressive adolescent girls (Cillessen & Mayeux, 2004b; Rose, Swenson, & Waller, 2004). Identifying social networks and examining their role in these associations is an important goal for future research.

Second, research by Sherif and Sherif (1970) has demonstrated the role of perceived group membership in the occurrence of aggression. Children who perceived peers as members of an outgroup were more likely to aggress against them then towards other peers. Research with adults has shown that simply dividing individuals randomly into artificial groups can produce enough of an ingroup bias to generate preference for ingroup members over outgroup members (Tajfel, 1982). If these effects occur with randomly assigned groups, it is easy to imagine similar outcomes occurring with existing groups that are not random but that have a history of interaction, such as the cliques that adolescents form in middle and high school. The perception of a peer as a member of another clique may be an additional group dynamic factor in the occurrence of aggression against that peer.

Third, threats to the self are related to aggression in groups in multiple ways. If a child is in a position of high status and a peer threatens that status in some way, the child can be expected to aggress against the competitor. This effect may be exacerbated if status is a central component of the individual's self-concept. Felson (1982) has shown that men whose toughness has been challenged often respond with verbal and physical aggression. Dodge and Somberg (1987) found that threats to the self lead to an increase in hostile attributions in aggressive boys. Similarly, high-status youth may respond to a challenge to their status with behavior that re-emphasizes or re-asserts their status. This might explain why some perceived popular youth use aggression: It may be a means of continually reaffirming their dominant status in the peer group. The empirical finding that perceived popularity leads to increased aggression (Cillessen & Mayeux, 2004b), especially across school transitions when adolescents move into new peer contexts, may be partially mediated by threats to the self.

Dynamic Systems Theory

Dynamic systems theories have been widely used to explain developmental phenomena (see, e.g., Thelen & Smith, 1998), in particular motor development and the association between perception and action. Recently, researchers have begun to apply the principles of dynamical systems to social behavior (Granic & Dishion, 2003; Granic, Hollenstein, Dishion, & Patterson, 2003). These approaches emphasize several factors of importance for research on aggression, including examining aggressive behavior as it unfolds over time, either short-term (microgenetic) or long-term (longitudinal); examining how seemingly small events can influence long-term trajectories; and focusing on the self-perpetuating and self-reinforcing behavioral (attractor) states that influence short- and long-term outcomes.

For example, Granic and Dishion (2003) have conceptualized the amount of deviant talk between peers during a conversation as an attractor state that predicts subsequent problem behaviors. Adolescents who were easily sucked into deviant talk with a peer and who seemed to find it difficult to disengage from deviant talk were more likely to have behavior problems three years later. This finding suggested, among other things, that there are physiological or psychological underpinnings to being influenced by a deviant peer. Similar processes may apply to the association between high status and aggression in the peer group. Certain adolescents who become perceived popular may be more likely to be influenced than others by the aggressive behavior of some of their popular peers. Whereas one adolescent girl who observes her peers engaging in gossip about another girl may be able to listen to the gossip and walk away, another may become embroiled in the discussion, and find it hard not to engage in it. This hypothetical situation again emphasizes the need to study these developmental processes as they unfold over time, with time referring to anything from several minutes to several years.

EMPIRICAL FINDINGS

Although a robust association between aggression and peer rejection has been found in many studies, there is mounting evidence that the association of aggression with measures of peer status is more complex. Several studies have identified children who are aggressive but not peer-rejected (e.g., Bagwell, Coie, Terry, & Lochman, 2000; Bierman, Smoot, & Aumiller, 1993). In their meta-analytic review of the association between sociometric status and social behavior, Newcomb, Bukowski, and Pattee (1993) actually found a larger effect size for the association between a broad-band category of aggression and controversial sociometric status than they did for rejected status, a significant finding that has often been overlooked in the literature because of the relatively small size of the controversial group in sociometric research. This finding is significant, however, because the controversial group consists of peers who are disliked by some, but liked by others. Consistent with the potential association between aggression and the acceptance dimension of peer status, many contemporary researchers are finding that aggression is sometimes associated with high status among peers (e.g., Cillessen & Mayeux, 2004b; Hawley, 2003a; Rodkin, Farmer, Pearl, & Van Acker, 2000; Rose et al., 2004). This association link is quickly gaining academic interest and empirical support (see Cillessen & Rose, 2005).

   In one of the first empirical papers to establish this positive association, a substantial number of aggressive third- through sixth-grade boys were shown to be well-connected socially, compared to other peers (Farmer & Rodkin, 1996). In a similar study with younger children, aggressive first-graders were identified and classified as either at-risk or socially competent and well-connected; approximately equal numbers of children fell into each category (Estell, Cairns, Farmer, & Cairns, 2002). Rodkin and colleagues (2000) identified two subgroups of popular boys in early adolescence: tough boys who were described by peers and teachers as athletic, cool, and antisocial, and model boys, who were also described as athletic and cool but as cooperative instead of antisocial. A number of other studies have also found strong relationships between both physical/overt and relational/indirect forms of aggression and perceived popularity (discussed in detail in the following discussion; see Cillessen & Mayeux, 2004b; LaFontana & Cillessen, 2002; Parkhurst & Hopmeyer, 1998; Prinstein & Cillessen, 2003; Rose et al., 2004).

Collectively, these studies indicate that aggressive behavior is robustly associated with high peer status as well as rejection. An important question is how these contradictory findings can be integrated. The answers lie in a number of variables that have been identified as moderators of the relationship between aggression and social status. In this chapter, we focus on four moderating variables (gender, age, form of aggression, and type of peer status) that have a significant impact on how aggression affects children's or adolescents' position in the peer group. For example, the relationship between aggression and status is not developmentally invariant, but instead varies across age groups (see the following discussion). Adolescents using aggressive behaviors are less likely to be disliked by their peers than children in elementary school (see Cillessen & Mayeux, 2004a, for a review). Although the developmental invariance of the association between social status and behavior may seems obvious at this time, peer relations researchers have typically operated under the assumption that the associations between sociometric status and its correlates are the same across various age groups. The current chapter illustrates, for the case of aggression, that this is not necessarily true—a finding that can be extended to other domains of peer relations research.

Moderators of the Aggression-Status Link

Type of High Status. One of the strongest moderators of the aggression–status link, and one of the most important conceptually, is social status itself. Until recently, most research on the aggression–status relationship focused on sociometric popularity, or being well-accepted by the peer group. Children high on sociometric popularity are nominated by many peers as "someone I like the most" and receive few or no nominations as "someone I like the least" (Coie, Dodge, & Coppotelli, 1982). That is, these children enjoy a high level of liking among the peer group and typically have a number of reciprocated friendships. Sociometric popularity is associated with prosocial behaviors such as cooperation, leadership ability, trustworthiness, and kindness in both childhood and adolescence (Newcomb et al., 1993; Parkhurst & Hopmeyer, 1998).

A second form of popularity has also been identified that is associated with quite different behaviors in youth. Unlike sociometric popularity, which is an index of liking among the peer group, perceived popularity is more an index of social impact, visibility, and reputation. Youth who are perceived popular are nominated by peers as the "most popular" members of the classroom or grade, and are typically very highly socially connected, enjoying high levels of status and influence among their peers (Cillessen & Mayeux, 2004b; Rodkin et al., 2000). Perceived popular youth are often described as athletic, cool, and as good leaders, but not as particularly kind or trustworthy (Parkhurst & Hopmeyer, 1998; Rodkin et al., 2000). Furthermore, the behavioral profile of some perceived popular children and adolescents has a significant antisocial component. This antisocial side is probably one key reason why, although perceived popular youth enjoy high levels of social connectedness and influence, they are not necessarily well-liked, especially in adolescence (Cillessen & Mayeux, 2004b; LaFontana & Cillessen, 2002; Rose et al., 2004). Thus, a key distinction between sociometric and perceived popularity is that sociometric popularity is a marker for liking, whereas perceived popularity may be best conceptualized as a marker for social power.

How does aggression fit into this distinction? As it turns out, aggression appears to be one of the driving forces behind it. Aggression is typically not a characteristic of well-liked children. In a large-scale meta-analysis of the behaviors associated with sociometric status types, sociometrically popular children were among the least aggressive. Aggression was instead strongly associated with peer rejection, or sociometric unpopularity (Newcomb et al., 1993).

A different picture emerges when we consider youth who are socially powerful rather than well-liked. In the first empirical paper to identify and define perceived popularity, Parkhurst and Hopmeyer (1998) found that perceived popular youth were described in prosocial terms if they were also sociometrically popular, indicating that some children and adolescents successfully balance being liked and being powerful. However, perceived popular youth who were not well-liked were also described as arrogant and physically aggressive, unlike sociometrically popular youth who were not described in these negative ways. These findings have since been replicated and extended in a number of important studies. Using different methodologies, each confirmed that there are two distinct forms of high status with different behavioral profiles.

Two studies have investigated the perceptions youth have of perceived popular peers and the construct of popularity in general. LaFontana and Cillessen (1998) found that fourth- and fifth-grade children attributed more hostile intent to hypothetical perceived popular peers than they did to hypothetical peers of unknown status (the control group about whom they were given no popularity information). They also made more stable attributions about perceived popular peers' negative behaviors. In a second study, perceived popular children were described as aggressive and as able to use their social power to get what they want, even if it meant being aggressive or antisocial (LaFontana & Cillessen, 2002). The link between aggression and perceived popularity is not limited to descriptions of hypothetical peers. In a large study of children and adolescents, a significant proportion of highly aggressive youth were nominated as perceived popular by peers (Rose et al., 2004). We found similar patterns in our own data. In fifth through ninth grade, aggression was positively related to perceived popularity, but negatively related to sociometric popularity. Furthermore, causal modeling indicated that high perceived popularity in one school year lead to increases in aggressive behaviors during the next school year (Cillessen & Mayeux, 2004b).

Other researchers have established a link between aggression and high status using a different conceptualization of popularity. Social network centrality refers to social connectedness and can also be considered a measure of social visibility and impact. Youth who are high on social centrality have many friends and are part of large, prominent social cliques (e.g., Cairns et al., 1988). Several studies in this tradition have found significant numbers of aggressive children and adolescents to be well-known, well-connected members of these large social networks (Farmer & Rodkin, 1996; Rodkin et al., 2000; Xie, Swift, Cairns, & Cairns, 2002).

In summary, the question of how aggression relates to social status among youth is not a simple one. Some children and adolescents are apparently able to synthesize antisocial behavior with high peer status quite effectively, as long as our definition of high status is a power-oriented one instead of one based on liking. According to the studies just discussed that measure these dimensions of status separately, youth do not necessarily like their aggressive peers, yet they ascribe a significant amount of social power to them (however, see Hawley, 2003b).

Type of Aggression.   The link between aggression and peer status also varies depending on the type of aggression being considered.

Researchers typically distinguish two major categories of aggression: overt/physical and indirect/relational. Overt/physical aggression includes behaviors such as verbal and physical assault and is stereotypically associated with boys rather than girls. Indirect/relational aggression includes behaviors that are more covert and are usually aimed at harming another person's social status, friendships, or reputation (e.g., Crick, 1996). Some behaviors classified as indirect or relational include malicious gossip, exclusion from activities and groups, and giving someone "the silent treatment."

Both physical and relational forms of aggression are associated with low peer status when traditional sociometric definitions of status are used; physical aggression is one of the strongest predictors of peer rejection in the literature (Bierman, 2004; Coie & Dodge, 1998; Newcomb et al., 1993; Underwood, 2002). In studies assessing concurrent correlates and longer term outcomes of aggression, physical aggression is related to a variety of troubling behaviors, such as having a hostile attribution bias (the feeling that "everyone is out to get me," Dodge & Somberg, 1987), anger expression (Fabes & Eisenberg, 1992), and adjustment difficulties such as school dropout (Parker & Asher, 1987).

Relational aggression has also been found to be associated with negative adjustment outcomes, including loneliness, social isolation, and depression, in addition to its association with peer rejection (Crick & Grotpeter, 1995). However, a strong distinction must be made between relational aggression's link to sociometric rejection and its association with perceived popularity and other measures of social power. Although relationally aggressive youth are typically not well-liked by their peers, they are often some of the most socially powerful and influential members of their grade and enjoy high levels of social centrality (Cillessen & Mayeux, 2004b; Prinstein & Cillessen, 2003; Rodkin et al., 2000; Xie et al., 2002).

Why is relational aggression so consistently and so strongly linked to perceived popularity? Many researchers have hypothesized that these kinds of subtle social manipulation lie at the core of what it means to be popular. Rose and colleagues (2004) suggest that relationally aggressive acts such as threatening to cut friendship ties and excluding certain peers from groups and activities allow the perpetrator to covertly rearrange the social structure of the peer group in such a way that will enhance their own status and visibility. Recent popular books and films on the topic of social meanness and manipulation confirm this hypothesis from an anecdotal standpoint—for example, the movie *Mean Girls,* and the book *Queen Bees and Wannabees*, on which it was based (Wiseman, 2002). There is also empirical support for this suggestion. Perceived popularity in tenth grade was associated with instrumental or proactive uses of relational aggression (Prinstein & Cillessen, 2003), such as to achieve a social goal. Another recent study found that different forms of relational aggression were used at different stages of social conflict: whereas indirect and behind the back behaviors tended to initiate conflict, more direct verbal forms of relational aggression were used to respond to it (Xie et al., 2002). Thus, socially savvy youth may have an acute awareness of what kinds of behaviors will allow them to disrupt the social hierarchy and the balance of the affiliations within it, and use this to their own advantage. That some of these behaviors have been observed in children as early as the preschool years is amazing in itself, because it implies that even some very young children understand the nature of social power well enough to manipulate their social standing, or at least to attempt to (Crick, 1997; Crick & Grotpeter, 1995).

Although children and adolescents who engage in such behaviors are often actively disliked by their peers and thus can be quite unpopular sociometrically, the benefits of relational aggression appear to outweigh the loss in liking—at least if the stability of this kind of aggression is any indication. Five-year stabilities for relational aggression are in the .40 range, with shorter term stabilities being higher, suggesting that these behaviors are an enduring characteristic of some youth across late childhood and early adolescence (Cillessen & Mayeux, 2004b). Children who enjoy the benefits of high status and social power may be impervious to the level of dislike their peers have for them if their goals are more status-oriented than affiliation-oriented (LaFontana, 2005). Future research should investigate the nature of the social goals of perceived popular versus sociometrically popular youth.

Gender. Issues of gender are difficult to discuss in general terms; it is hard, for example, to untangle gender from the intricate web of interactions between type of status, type of aggression, and developmental period. However, some generalizations can be made. Surprisingly few studies have directly tested for gender effects in the association between status and overt/physical aggression. Many of the early studies of aggression and peer status were done with boys-only groups; data on girls is comparatively limited. Newcomb et al. (1993) acknowledged this lamentable issue in their meta-analysis: so few of the existing studies of sociometric status differences in their review included girls (or, if they did, found no significant gender differences) that including gender as a moderator in their meta-analysis was simply not possible. In general, and without introducing more complex interactions with age and other moderators, overt or physical aggression in both girls and boys is a risk factor for peer rejection. For perceived popularity, physical aggression is certainly not a risk factor, especially for boys for whom it strongly predicts this type of high status (Cillessen & Mayeux, 2004b).

Gender differences have been more consistently addressed in research on the link between peer status and relational aggression, but this remains an understudied research question as well. Speaking specifically of sociometric popularity, the association with aggression is typically negative, and this association has been found to be stronger for girls than for boys in some studies (e.g., Cillessen & Mayeux, 2004b; Rys & Bear, 1997). Further replication of this finding is needed. Why relational aggression may be more strongly linked to disliking for girls than for boys is a meaningful question to be addressed in future studies. The associations between perceived popularity and relational aggression are typically positive for both boys and girls, and again, any real gender difference is in the magnitude. As with sociometric popularity, the relational aggression-perceived popularity link is significantly stronger for girls than for boys in some studies (e.g., Cillessen & Mayeux, 2004b) but not others (Prinstein & Cillessen, 2003; Rose et al., 2004; Xie et al., 2002).

Hints as to the origins of these differences may be found in the dominance research of Charlesworth and colleagues (e.g., Charlesworth & Dzur, 1987; Charlesworth & LaFreniere, 1983). For example, Charlesworth and Dzur found gender differences in the kinds of strategies preschool boys and girls used to gain access to resources. Overall, there were no gender differences in the amount of access to resources the children gained (in this case, the resource was viewing a cartoon movie that only one child could view at a time). However, differences emerged in the kinds of strategies boys and girls used to gain access to the movie. Boys tended to use more physical behaviors, such as blocking, pushing, or pulling at another child, and girls used more verbal behaviors, such as requesting, commanding, and threatening, in order to gain access to the movie. Although methods of gaining access to resources on the one hand and aggression on the other are hardly identical concepts, the link between the boys' preference for behavioral strategies in the Charlesworth studies and physical or overt aggression in others is hard to miss. The same can be said for girls' reliance on verbal strategies as preschoolers and relational aggression (which is often highly verbal, such as spreading rumors or threatening to exclude someone) both in preschool and at later ages (e.g., Archer & Coyne, 2005; Crick, Ostrov, Appleyard, Jansen, & Casas, 2004).

Developmental Trends.   The question of whether aggression is linked to high status or low status also yields different answers depending on the age group being studied. Further complicating the matter, the trends in age tend to differ based on the type of aggression being studied (physical versus relational) and the definition of high or low status being used (sociometric or perceived popularity or unpopularity). Thus, we briefly address developmental trends for all possible combinations of aggression and status. First, we address the relationship between physical and relational aggression and sociometric popularity. We then turn our attention to the relationship between physical and relational aggression and perceived popularity and other measures of social power.

Traditionally, developmental researchers have assumed that physical aggression becomes increasingly unaccepted as a means of conflict resolution as children grow older, with children and adolescents who continue to use aggressive behaviors being the target of disliking because of their increasing deviance from this norm. By this logic, aggression among very young children may not necessarily lead to peer rejection, because aggression is still somewhat typical of this age group and a clear awareness of the norms against it may not yet exist. But as children grow older and learn more socially skilled ways of handling conflict, those who continue to be aggressive in their conflict resolution are disruptive and upsetting to peers because they violate group norms of social behavior and cause harm to others. Thus, in older age groups, aggressive peers would have low acceptance or liking in the peer group and may be actively peer-rejected.

However, most of the data in this area indicate a more complex relationship. It is true that young children (up to first or second grade) who are physically aggressive do not appear to suffer from peer rejection, and in fact, aggression at this age is sometimes associated with high peer status (Coie, Dodge, & Kupersmidt, 1990; Pope, Bierman, & Mumma, 1989). Physical aggression in young children is associated with high levels of play activity (Roper & Hinde, 1978), which is a contributor to high status at young ages, which partly explains the trend. Also, as described earlier, physical aggression is still somewhat normative of this age group. Hawley provides evidence of this trend in her research with "bistrategic controllers" (e.g., Hawley, 2002, 2003b). She found that preschoolers who are good at getting what they want from peers by using a combination of prosocial and coercive strategies (including both physical and relational aggression) were also highly preferred as playmates. In fact, aggressive-prosocial preschoolers (the bistrategic controllers) are as well-liked by their peers as children who use only prosocial means of resource control.

This trend reverses itself in middle childhood, when physical aggression is associated with low peer status around the third and fourth grades (Boivin & Begin, 1989; Newcomb et al., 1993; Pope et al., 1989). The association between aggression and peer rejection is especially strong during this period, with physical aggression being the strongest predictor of low sociometric popularity (Newcomb et al., 1993).

Early adolescence brings another shift in the aggression–status link. Recent evidence suggests that fifth or sixth grade is a transitional period during which physically aggressive and antisocial behavior becomes less negatively associated with peer rejection (Cillessen & Mayeux, 2004b; Pope et al., 1989). Although physical aggression has not been shown to be positively related to sociometric status during any period of adolescence, it does appear to be increasingly accepted and less associated with rejection. For example, in our own data, the relationship between physical aggression and sociometric popularity is moderately negative in fifth grade, but by ninth grade there is no significant relationship between the two variables (Cillessen & Mayeux, 2004b). Over time, physical aggression loses its power to predict who is disliked and rejected by peers.

The relationship between relational aggression and sociometric popularity is not so complex. Relational aggression is positively related to peer rejection at all developmental time points, from the preschool period to adolescence (Cillessen & Mayeux, 2004b; Crick, 1997; Rose et al., 2004). In fact, over developmental time, relational aggression is an increasingly powerful predictor of peer rejection. Although no studies have followed the same group of children from preschool to adolescence, in one 5-year longitudinal study, the magnitude of the relationship between relational aggression and low sociometric popularity more than doubled from fifth grade to ninth grade (Cillessen & Mayeux, 2004b). Children appear to dislike their socially manipulative peers more and more as they get older. Whether this is because those peers become increasingly manipulative as they get older, and thus hurt more people with time, is a question still to be answered.

Knowing what we know about perceived popular and socially central youth, it comes as no surprise that the relationship between these kinds of status and both physical and relational aggression is generally positive at all developmental time points that have been studied (Bagwell et al., 2000; Cillessen & Mayeux, 2004b; Estell et al., 2002; Prinstein & Cillessen, 2003; Rodkin et al., 2000; Rose et al., 2004). Although perceived popularity research with preschoolers is still missing for a number of reasons (both conceptual and methodological), a recent study has found relational aggression to be associated with controversial sociometric status in preschool children (Nelson, Robinson, & Hart, 2005). Children of controversial status are so called because they receive a relatively high number of both positive and negative peer nominations—they are well-liked by some peers, but highly disliked by other peers as well. Studies that have measured both sociometric and perceived popularity find a substantial overlap between perceived popularity and controversial sociometric status, above and beyond the overlap between perceived popularity and any other status category (e.g., Parkhurst & Hopmeyer, 1998). Thus, the Nelson et al. study suggests that the same patterns of association between relational aggression and perceived popularity that are found in later years (see the following discussion) may be present in early childhood.

There is evidence that as early as age 6, some children are able to combine high levels of physical aggression with high social centrality (Estell et al., 2002). Relational aggression is related to perceived popularity as early as third grade (Rose et al., 2004) and the link between relational aggression and perceived popularity grows stronger as children grow older (Cillessen & Mayeux, 2004b). Both levels of relational aggression and the importance of being socially powerful are thought to peak in the middle school years (Youniss, McLellan, & Strouse, 1994), which suggests that the relationship between the two constructs might be strongest in sixth, seventh, and eight grades. This hypothesis has been supported by one longitudinal study that found the relational aggression-perceived popularity link to be strongest in eighth and ninth grades (Cillessen & Mayeux, 2004b). However, links between relational aggression and perceived popularity continue through the high school years (Prinstein & Cillessen, 2003).

Further research is needed to fill gaps in this body of work. Relatively little is known about the associations between the behavior patterns observed in socially dominant preschoolers and perceived popularity and/or social network centrality at older ages. The longitudinal examination of the early precursors of these behavior patterns in older age groups is an exciting avenue for future research.

CONCLUSIONS

In this chapter we have reviewed empirical evidence regarding the association between high social status (both likeability and centrality/popularity) and physical and relational aggression, including factors such as age and gender that moderate this association. We have also highlighted one traditional and two promising theoretical orientations that can be used to explain these findings. Based on this review, several suggestions for future research can be made.

The processes that relate aggression to status and power in the peer group can be further complicated in multiple ways. For example, the majority of the findings discussed pertain to status and power assessed in the peer group at large. The role of smaller networks within the larger peer system needs to be examined further, for example, by identifying the nature of within-clique relations and how they may influence status in the peer group at large. Similar arguments can be made for the role of dyadic relationships, not only friendships, but also enmities and unilateral bully–victim relationships.

A second way to examine the role of aggression further can only come from observational research. Much of the literature reviewed in this chapter is based on global continuous measures of aggression. These measures do not allow us to disentangle the effects of multiple component dimensions of aggression. Aggression can vary according to its duration, intensity, frequency, target person(s), directionality (unilateral or reciprocated), temporal patterns, and conditional probability depending on previous or concurrent other behavior states, relational, and group characteristics. In terms of temporal patterning, for example, social learning theory might suggest that intermittent aggression is the most effective means of asserting power. Is intense aggression toward some accepted if it takes place in the context of beneficial behaviors to others? Does it matter to whom the aggression is directed? Garandeau and Cillessen (2006) presented some conceptual views on such mechanisms to understand bullying aggression and peer group manipulation. Much further research is needed to answer these questions and examine the impact of these other dimensions of aggression on the emergence and maintenance of status and power in the peer group.

One of the most important goals for future research is to distinguish whether there are multiple long-term trajectories associated with perceived popular status in childhood and adolescence. Whereas perceived popularity is clearly associated with positive consequences in adolescence, nothing is known about long-term outcomes or the fate of perceived popular individuals after high school. Two diverging trajectories of popular adolescents into emerging adulthood can be hypothesized. One possibility is a scenario in which youth who are perceived popular and socially central in high school continue to excel socially and academically or professionally, perhaps due in part to their skill in negotiating the social world. Another possibility is that these youth will experience difficulties in their adult social and professional environments, especially if the manipulative and Machiavellian (see Hawley, 2003a) behaviors that were rewarded in high school are no longer effective or acceptable. Simply put, the social success of these adolescents is expected to suffer if the reward contingencies that benefited them in the social ecology of high school cease to exist in later social environments.

It is also important to emphasize that aggression may not always be a risk factor—at least, when it is used without going to extremes by individuals who are of high status. This might be evidenced by the first of the two hypothesized long-term trajectories just described. Individuals who combine their aggressive behaviors with other tendencies that are more prosocially oriented may, in fact, be quite successful over time (Hawley, 2003a, 2003b). The fact that perceived popular youth combine both prosocial and antisocial traits may indicate that this group of high-status adolescents actually has the potential to be highly successful. In this framework, aggression used by high-status adolescents may play an important and useful role in social development. Future research will show the degree to which these adolescents learn to make the best of their "bad" behaviors.

REFERENCES

Adler, P. A., & Adler, P. (1995). Dynamics of inclusion and exclusion in preadolescent cliques. *Social Psychology Quarterly, 58*, 145–162.

Archer, J., & Coyne, S. M. (2005). An integrated review of indirect, relational, and social aggression. *Personality and Social Psychology Review, 9*, 212–230.

Bagwell, C. L., Coie, J. D., Terry, R. A., & Lochman, J. E. (2000). Peer clique participation and social status in preadolescence. *Merrill-Palmer Quarterly, 46*, 280–305.

Bandura, A. (1986). *Social foundations of thought and action. A social cognitive theory.* Englewood Cliffs, NJ: Prentice Hall.

Bandura, A. (1997). *Self-efficacy: The exercise of control.* New York: Freeman.

Bierman, K. L. (2004). *Peer rejection: Developmental processes and intervention strategies.* New York: Guilford.

Bierman, K. L., Smoot, D. L., & Aumiller, K. (1993). Characteristics of aggressive-rejected, aggressive (nonrejected), and rejected (nonaggressive) boys. *Child Development, 64*, 139–151.

Boivin, M., & Begin, G. (1989). Peer status and self-perception among early elementary school children: The case of the rejected children. *Child Development, 60*, 591–596.

Cairns, R. B. (1979). *Social development. The origins and plasticity of interchanges.* San Francisco, CA: Freeman.

Cairns, R. B., Cairns, B. D., Neckerman, H. J., Gest, S. D., & Gariepy, J. (1988). Social networks and aggressive behavior: Peer support or peer rejection? *Developmental Psychology, 24*, 815–823.

Charlesworth, W. R., & Dzur, C. (1987). Gender comparisons of preschoolers' behavior and resource utilization in group problem solving. *Child Development, 58*, 191–200.

Charlesworth, W. R., & LaFreniere, P. (1983). Dominance, friendship, and resource utilization in preschool children's groups. *Ethology and Sociobiology, 4*, 175–186.

Cillessen, A. H. N., & Mayeux, L. (2004a). Sociometric status and peer group behavior: Previous findings and current directions. In J. B. Kupersmidt & K. A. Dodge (Eds.), *Children's peer relations: From development to intervention* (pp. 3–20). Washington, DC: American Psychological Association Press.

Cillessen, A. H. N., & Mayeux, L. (2004b). From censure to reinforcement: Developmental changes in the association between aggression and social status. *Child Development*, 75, 147–163.

Cillessen, A. H. N., & Rose, A. J. (2005). Understanding popularity in the peer system. *Current Directions in Psychological Science*, 14, 102–105.

Coie, J. D., & Dodge, K. A. (1998). Aggression and antisocial behavior. In W. Damon (Series Ed.) & N. Eisenberg (Vol. Ed.), *Handbook of child psychology: Vol. 3. Social, emotional, and personality development* (5th ed., pp. 780–840). New York: Wiley.

Coie, J. D., Dodge, K. A., & Coppotelli, H. (1982). Dimensions and types of social status: A cross-age perspective. *Developmental Psychology*, 18, 557–569.

Coie, J. D., Dodge, K. A., & Kupersmidt, J. B. (1990). Peer group behavior and social status. In S. R. Asher & J. D. Coie (Eds.), *Peer rejection in childhood* (pp. 17–59). New York: Cambridge University Press.

Crick, N. R. (1996). The role of overt aggression, relational aggression, and prosocial behavior in the prediction of children's future social adjustment. *Child Development*, 67, 2317–2327.

Crick, N. R. (1997). Engagement in gender normative versus nonnormative forms of aggression: Links to social-psychological adjustment. *Developmental Psychology*, 33, 610–617.

Crick, N. R., & Grotpeter, J. K. (1995). Relational aggression, gender, and social-psychological adjustment. *Child Development*, 66, 710–722.

Crick, N. R., Ostrov, J. M., Appleyard, K., Jansen, E. A., & Casas, J. F. (2004). Relational aggression in early childhood: "You can't come to my birthday party unless …" In M. Putallaz & K. L. Bierman (Eds.), *Aggression, antisocial behavior, and violence among girls: A developmental perspective* (pp. 71–89). New York: Guilford.

DeRosier, M. E., Cillessen, A. H. N., Coie, J. D., & Dodge, K. A. (1994). Group context and children's aggressive behavior. *Child Development*, 65, 1068–1079.

Dodge, K. A., & Somberg, D. R. (1987). Hostile attributional biases among aggressive boys are exacerbated under conditions of threats to the self. *Child Development*, 58, 213–224.

Estell, D. B., Cairns, R. B., Farmer, T. W., & Cairns, B. D. (2002). Aggression in inner-city early elementary classrooms: Individual and peer-group configurations. *Merrill-Palmer Quarterly*, 48, 52–76.

Fabes, R. A., & Eisenberg, N. (1992). Young children's coping with interpersonal anger. *Child Development*, 63, 116–128.

Farmer, T. W., & Rodkin, P. C. (1996). Antisocial and prosocial correlates of classroom social positions: The social network centrality perspective. *Social Development*, 5, 174–188.

Felson, R. B. (1982). Impression management and the escalation of aggression and violence. *Social Psychology Quarterly*, 45, 245–254.

Forsyth, D. R. (1990). *Group dynamics* (2nd ed.). Pacific Grove, CA: Brooks/Cole.

Garandeau, C. F., & Cillessen, A. H. N. (2006). From indirect aggression to invisible aggression: A conceptual view on bullying and peer group manipulation. *Aggression and violent behavior*, 11, 612–625.

Granic, I., & Dishion, T. J. (2003). Deviant talk in adolescent friendships: A step toward measuring a pathogenic attractor process. *Social Development, 12,* 314–334.

Granic, I., Hollenstein, T., Dishion, T. J., & Patterson, G. R. (2003). Longitudinal analysis of flexibility and reorganization in early adolescence: A dynamic systems study of family interactions. *Developmental Psychology, 39,* 606–617.

Green, V. A., Cillessen, A. H. N., Berthelsen, D., Irving, K., & Catherwood, D. (2003). The effect of gender context on children's social behavior in a limited resource situation: An observational study. *Social Development, 12,* 586–604.

Hawley, P. H. (2002). Social dominance and prosocial and coercive strategies of resource control in preschoolers. *International Journal of Behavioral Development, 26,* 167–176.

Hawley, P. H. (2003a). Prosocial and coercive configurations of resource control in early adolescence: A case for the well-adapted Machiavellian. *Merrill-Palmer Quarterly, 49,* 279–309.

Hawley, P. H. (2003b). Stategies of control, aggression, and morality in preschoolers: An evolutionary perspective. *Journal of Experimental Child Psychology, 85,* 213–235.

LaFontana, K. M. (2005, April). *Concern for popularity: Developmental and motivational perspectives.* Paper presented at the biennial meeting of the Society for Research in Child Development, Atlanta, GA.

LaFontana, K. M., & Cillessen, A. H. N. (1998). The nature of children's stereotypes of popularity. *Social Development, 7,* 301–320.

LaFontana, K. M., & Cillessen, A. H. N. (2002). Children's perceptions of popular and unpopular peers: A multimethod assessment. *Developmental Psychology, 38,* 635–647.

Lewin, K., Lippit, R., & White, R. K. (1939). Patterns of aggressive behavior in experimentally created "social climates." *Journal of Social Psychology, 10,* 271–299.

Merten, J. (1997). Facial-affective behavior, mutual gaze, and emotional experience in dyadic interactions. *Journal of Nonverbal Behavior, 21,* 179–201.

Moffitt, T. E. (1993). Adolescence-limited and life-course-persistent antisocial behavior: A developmental taxonomy. *Psychological Review, 100,* 674–701.

Nelson, D. A., Robinson, C. C., & Hart, C. H. (2005). Relational and physical aggression of preschool-age children: Peer status linkages across informants. *Early Education and Development, 16,* 115–139.

Newcomb, A. F., Bukowski, W. M., & Pattee, L. (1993). Children's peer relations: A meta-analytic review of popular, rejected, neglected, controversial, and average sociometric status. *Psychological Bulletin, 113,* 99–128.

Parker, J. G., & Asher, S. R. (1987). Peer relations and later personal adjustment: Are low-accepted children at risk? *Psychological Bulletin, 102,* 357–389.

Parkhurst, J. T., & Hopmeyer, A. (1998). Sociometric popularity and peer-perceived popularity: Two distinct dimensions of peer status. *Journal of Early Adolescence, 18,* 125–144.

Patterson, G. R., Littman, R. A., & Bricker, W. (1967). Assertive behavior in children: A step toward a theory of aggression. *Monographs of the Society for Research in Child Development, 32*(5, Serial No. 113).

Pope, A. W., Bierman, K. L., & Mumma, G. H. (1989). Relations between hyper-active and aggressive behavior and peer relations at three elementary grade levels. *Journal of Abnormal Child Psychology, 17*, 253–267.

Prinstein, M. J., & Cillessen, A. H. N. (2003). Forms and functions of adolescent peer aggression associated with high levels of peer status. *Merrill-Palmer Quarterly, 49*, 310–342.

Rodkin, P. C., Farmer, T. W., Pearl, R., & Van Acker, R. (2000). Heterogeneity of popular boys: Antisocial and prosocial configurations. *Developmental Psychology, 36*, 14–24.

Roper, R., & Hinde, R. A. (1978). Social behavior in a play group: Consistency and complexity. *Child Development, 49*, 570–579.

Rose, A. J., Swenson, L. P., & Waller, E. M. (2004). Overt and relational aggression and perceived popularity: Developmental differences in concurrent and prospective relations. *Developmental Psychology, 40*, 378–387.

Rys, G. S., & Bear, G. G. (1997). Relational aggression and peer relations: Gender and developmental issues. *Merrill-Palmer Quarterly, 43*, 87–106.

Sherif, M., & Sherif, C. W. (1970). Motivation and intergroup aggression: A per-sistent problem in levels of analysis. In L. Aronson, E. Tobach, D. Lehrman, & J. Rosenblatt (Eds.), *Development and evolution of behavior* (pp. 563–579). San Francisco: Freeman.

Tajfel, H. (1982). Social psychology of intergroup relations. *Annual Review of Psychology, 33*, 1–39.

Thelen, E., & Smith, L. B. (1998). Dynamic systems theories. In W. Damon (Series Ed.) & R. M. Lerner (Vol. Ed.), *Handbook of child psychology: Vol. 1. Theoretical models of human development* (5th ed., pp. 563–634). New York: Wiley.

Underwood, M. K. (2002). Sticks and stones and social exclusion: Aggression among boys and girls. In P. K. Smith & C. H. Hart (Eds.), *Blackwell handbook of childhood social development* (pp. 533–548). Malden, MA: Blackwell.

Wiseman, R. (2002). *Queen bees and wannabes: Helping your daughter survive cliques, gossip, boyfriends, and other realities of adolescence.* New York: Crown.

Wright, J. C., Giammarino, M., & Parad, H. (1986). Social status in small groups: Individual-group similarity and the social misfit. *Journal of Personality and Social Psychology, 50*, 523–536.

Xie, H., Swift, D. J., Cairns, R. B., & Cairns, B. D. (2002). Aggressive behaviors in social interaction and developmental adaptation: A narrative analysis of interpersonal conflicts during early adolescence. *Social Development, 11*, 205–224.

Youniss, J., McLellan, J. A., & Strouse, D. (1994). "We're popular, but we're not snobs:" Adolescents describe their crowds. In R. Montemayor, G. R. Adams, & T. P. Gullotta (Eds.), *Personal relationships in adolescence. Vol. 6. Advances in adolescent development* (pp. 101–121). Thousand Oaks, CA: Sage.

7

PRAISING CORDELIA: SOCIAL AGGRESSION AND SOCIAL DOMINANCE AMONG ADOLESCENT GIRLS

Lorrie K. Sippola
Jaime Paget
Carie M. Buchanan
University of Saskatchewan

Recent media attention in the wake of sensational incidents has the public believing that there is an epidemic of violence sweeping across North America that is infecting adolescent girls. Barron and Lacombe (2005) have suggested that the media has created a moral panic that is epitomized by the Canadian documentary film *Nasty Girls* (Canadian Public Broadcasting Corporation [CBC], 1997). This moral panic is characterized by the distortion and exaggeration of events that include claims of discovering a new phenomenon when it has existed in the past and the manipulation of data to establish the extent of the phenomenon. Barron and Lacombe have also suggested that experts, including some developmental psychologists, have participated in the social construction of the "Nasty girl" by decontextualizing the complexity of girls' aggression from the impact of a culture characterized by sexism, abuse, and inequality. That is, many of the explanations offered for adolescent girls' aggression emphasize individual factors (e.g., lack of social competence, biology, personality traits, etc.) without considering the social and/or cultural context in which this behavior is embedded.

The moral panic regarding girls' physical violence can also be seen in the recent attention given to behaviors that have been variously labeled as indirect, relational, or social aggression. Social exclusion and gossip, in particular, have received increased media attention in the wake of tragic high-school shootings and suicides among teens in the United States and Canada. The post-hoc explanations for these tragic events have frequently suggested that the perpetrators were victims of social exclusion, peer rejection, and/or verbal harassment from peers even when the evidence for the causal relationship between these events is non-existent or weak at best (e.g., see Leary, Kowalski, Smith, & Phillips, 2003). One of the consequences of the media spotlight on social aggression[1] has been an increased demand by parents for drastic actions by school administrators and the legal system to eliminate these types of behaviors. These actions include introducing zero-tolerance policies within schools and criminalizing some behaviors generally associated with social aggression among girls (e.g., "B.C. Girl Convicted," 2002; Galt, 1998; Wittman, 2001). Although research suggests that psychological abuse among girls undoubtedly occurs among adolescents with potentially negative consequences (Casey-Cannon, Hayward, & Gowen, 2001; Owens, Slee, & Shute, 2001), intervention and prevention programs are likely to fail if they do not consider the social and cultural context in which these behaviors occur.

The goal of this chapter is to contribute to an understanding of the experience of social aggression among adolescent girls by examining the social/cultural context for and the adaptive functions of behaviors that are labeled "aggressive." Currently, much of the literature on social aggression has focused on (a) identifying the types of nonphysical behaviors that have negative consequences for victims and perpetrators; (b) examining the correlates of these types of behaviors (i.e., both in terms of characteristics of victims and of perpetrators); (c) debating the question of sex differences in the use of these behaviors; and (d) debating operational definitions of nonphysical forms of aggression. Although this literature has provided important insights into aversive interpersonal behaviors, the context in which these behaviors occur is

---

[1]Although some debate has occurred regarding the terminology used in the literature, a recent review of the literature suggests that indirect, relational, and social aggression are likely to be more similar than different (Archer & Coyne, 2005). Thus, to avoid repetition, we chose to use the term "social aggression" to capture the direct and indirect but nonphysical behaviors that have been associated with aggressive behavior—particularly among girls. These behaviors include malicious gossip, social exclusion, and causing harm to relationships.

frequently overlooked. According to Sameroff (1983), "[t]he study of social development cannot be isolated from the historical context because, depending on the secular period, the meanings and roles associated with society have changed. Even within a single historical context, social development must still be embedded in a larger institutional structure. Attempts to understand the child isolated from context have not produced an understanding of developmental process or outcome" (p. 279).

TOWARD AN UNDERSTANDING OF SOCIAL AGGRESSION AMONG GIRLS

This chapter focuses on two main issues related to social aggression and adolescent girls. First, our focus is on understanding, specifically, social aggression among girls in adolescence. Social aggression fundamentally is a social behavior that occurs within the context of some type of relationship. Previous research has demonstrated that girls are more likely to engage in social aggression against other girls (Cairns, Cairns, Neckerman, Ferguson, & Gariepy, 1989; Crick, et al., 2001) and that social aggression among girls increases during adolescence (Cairns et al., 1989). Moreover, social aggression may be experienced more negatively by adolescent girls than by boys (Crick, 1995, Crick, Grotpeter, & Bigbee, 1999, Paquette & Underwood, 1999). These observations suggest that in order to understand the causes and consequences of social aggression among adolescent girls, we need to better understand the nature of their same-sex relationships during this period of development and the context in which these relationships are embedded.

The second issue addressed in this chapter, and the task assigned to contributors of this volume, is the question regarding the potential adaptive function of social aggression for adolescent girls' social development. In this chapter, we explore the implications of Karen Horney's theory of female development for understanding the experience of social aggression among adolescent girls. Even though Horney wrote about the experiences of girls and women in the 1920–1930s, we suggest that the socialization processes she described continue to influence female development in contemporary North American society. Although social aggression has frequently been viewed as indicative of dysfunction (Crick, 1997; Grotpeter & Crick; 1996, Van Schoiack-Edstrom, Frey, & Beland, 2002), Horney's theory of female development suggests that, under some conditions, aggression may actually be an adaptive response to the social/cultural context in which these behaviors occur.

The central thesis of our chapter is that social aggression among some girls may emerge as a function of increased feelings of competitiveness towards other girls—particularly for the attention of males—during the transition to heterosexual relationships in adolescence.[2] This view is consistent with an evolutionary perspective of adolescent girls' aggression (Campbell, 2004) that posits that the underlying mechanism underlying female–female aggression is reproductive success. However, consistent with Karen Horney's views, we suggest that the expression of competition is influenced by a cultural context that places the needs/desires of males above those of females and objectifies women. From this perspective, social aggression may be viewed as an adaptive response to the "compulsory heterosexuality" (Rich, 2003) inherent in North American society.

We begin this chapter by exploring Karen Horney's theoretical framework for understanding the social/cultural influences of social aggression among adolescent girls. Although other authors have also suggested that North American culture influences social aggression in girls, they have suggested that social aggression reflects an underlying anger that girls are not allowed to express (L. M. Brown, 1998; Underwood, 2003). Moreover, these authors have not specifically focused on girls' relationships with other girls. This approach implies that girls use social aggression primarily in reaction to their cultural environment and fails to examine the nature of the relationship in which much of girls' social aggression occurs. For example, in an interesting and compelling study, L. M. Brown (1998) describes the experiences of a group of White girls as they attempt to resist the pressure to conform to contradictory messages regarding femininity in their communities. However, it is important to recognize that many girls may not resist these messages but rather embrace them because they are perceived as adaptive responses to the pervasive cultural imperatives regarding what it means to be a woman in a patriarchal society. From our perspective, some girls will use social aggression proactively to successfully pursue their social goals because these strategies conform to what they believe in and, based on the cultural messages they process, provide an effective means to a desired goal. Thus, our chapter is intended to complement the efforts of previous writers concerned about girls' well-being.

After examining Horney's theory, we then examine the contemporary context for adolescent development that may influence girls' attitudes toward other girls. We suggest that the socialization processes that she described persist today as reflected by the experience of "compulsory heterosexuality" (Rich, 2003). However, we expand on Horney's theory

---

[2]The developmental path for adolescent girls who identify as lesbian may be quite different. However, a discussion of feelings of competitiveness in lesbian adolescent girls is beyond the scope of this chapter.

to examine the processes of devaluation and sexualization of adolescent girls in the peer group. Finally, we examine cultural representations of socially competent and socially aggressive adolescent girls to illustrate how social aggression may be viewed as an adaptive response to the overwhelming imperatives inherent in the patriarchal structure of heterosexuality in North American culture.

It is important to note an important limitation of this chapter at the outset. Frequently, proposals for interventions are put forth without much regard for the important variables of race or class. However, it is quite likely that the mechanisms underlying the forms of aggression among adolescent girls vary in important ways as a function of race and class and may require quite different intervention approaches. Consequently, it is not our intention in this chapter to propose a universal explanation for social aggression among girls. Consistent with the cultural context from which Horney's theory emerged, our application of her theory to the issue of social aggression is restricted to White, middle-class adolescent girls living in Westernized civilizations.

THE "FEMININE TYPE": HORNEY'S EXEMPLAR OF SOCIAL AGGRESSION AND SOCIAL COMPETENCE IN ADOLESCENT GIRLS

Horney's theory[3] of female development emerged from an attempt to understand the development of the neurotic personality. She argued that the psychological conflicts experienced by her clients were rational responses to the contradictions and dehumanization inherent in Western civilization. "Neurotics" simply experienced these characteristics of society more negatively than others. Furthermore, Horney argued that males' and females' responses to these contradictions and dehumanizing experiences were fundamentally different as a function of the systemic inequalities in Western culture. Thus an important aspect of her work was to critically examine the cultural context for female development.

One of the most negative aspects of North American culture, according to Horney, is the overarching emphasis on competition; individual achievement over others (i.e., superiority) is valued over personal achievement (i.e., mastery). Horney argued that the interpersonal competitiveness that pervades North American culture is also reflected in human relationships. The emphasis on success in relation to others in this competitive climate generates feelings of hostility and fear that undermine self-confidence and self-esteem. This competitive climate also emphasizes the importance of

---

[3]References for this section include: Horney (1964, 1967) and Westkott, (1989).

the "other" as a measure of one's self-worth. Thus, the self-concept of the average North American, according to Horney, is based largely on the evaluations of self provided by others.

Horney suggested that the competitiveness that pervades North American culture is replicated within the family context. Although this competitiveness influences the psychological functioning of both sons and daughters, she suggested that unique socialization processes have distinct consequences for girls' development in this context. Specifically, Horney suggested that devaluation of femininity and sexualization of girls in the family context are important processes influencing the psychological development of girls. These processes reflect a patriarchal culture that inherently views female as inferior and as an object to be used for the pleasure of men. As a result of their inferior status, girls internalize negative feelings toward females that are manifested by feelings of competitiveness. However, girls learn early in childhood that overt competition with other females (i.e., the mother) must be avoided because of the differential power structure of the family. Consequently, when competitive urges emerge, girls may feel that they must adopt strategies to avoid appearing competitive. One strategy may be to avoid competition altogether by being "good," "nice," and "perfect." Another strategy is to engage in competition whenever an opportunity arises, but to do so indirectly by manipulating others who are in a position of power—particularly male family members.

Horney suggested that competitive urges toward other females begin in childhood but become more intense during adolescence. She suggested that the psychological conflicts created by these feelings are the result of cultural definitions of femininity that pit patriarchal ideals against an independent female identity. The patriarchal ideal suggests that women's primary motivation in life is to attract and maintain the love of a man. This motivation is not, according to Horney, the result of a biological drive. Rather, it is a response to the overwhelming cultural imperative of heterosexuality that pervades girls' lives beginning in childhood and intensifying during adolescence. Thus, the cultural context of competitiveness and the socialization processes of devaluation and sexualization of girls provide the foundations for the emergence of the "feminine type." Although Horney described the development of other female personality traits in response to these processes, the feminine type reflects the type of popular, dominant, adolescent girl described by contemporary researchers who may be most likely to engage in social aggression as a means to an end (Eder, 1985; Parkhurst & Hopmeyer, 1998).

According to Horney, the feminine type strives to be the center of attention, particularly from boys. She compares herself, particularly her appearance, against other women and is envious of girls who are attractive to boys or successful in the types of activities that interest boys. Horney suggested that the self-esteem of these girls is based on their ability to attract and maintain the attention of boys. Consequently, they are sensitive to any perceived threat to their status with boys and will react to defend this status. Their competitive strategies in this regard include the humiliation of other girls, the collection of boys who admire and worship them, and managing their image with others so as to be perceived as successful in the social realm. According to Westkott (1986), the feminine type is the cultural ideal of a society in which an imbalance in power favoring male and masculine persists. Whereas the feminine type must repress feelings of competitiveness within the family context, these feelings may emerge at a time when the feminine type becomes able to exercise some power over others. As we discuss in the following section, adolescence may be an important period of development for the feminine type as a function of the developmental changes in the social context occurring during this time that may heighten feelings of competitiveness among girls.

What are the implications of Horney's theory for understanding social aggression among girls in contemporary society? After all, her theory was based on observations made of women at a time in history when social roles for women were primarily restricted to motherhood. Surely, one could argue, times have changed and women have been freed from the constraints placed on them by traditional patriarchal attitudes? Moreover, she was describing the development of neurotic personalities. Consequently, how relevant is her work for understanding social aggression as adaptation? In the following sections, we explore these questions as we expand on Horney's theory to examine the contemporary context for adolescent girls' development.

COMPETITION AMONG GIRLS IN NORTH AMERICA: BEING THE BEST VERSUS BEING "NICE"?

An important limitation of Horney's theory of female development is the exclusive focus on family dynamics as the context in which broader cultural messages regarding the feminine ideal were recreated. However, the peer group becomes increasingly important for development during adolescence for both boys and girls (Youniss & Smollar, 1985). Consistent with Horney, we propose that girls have unique experiences in the peer group that tend to perpetuate the processes she described: competitiveness, devaluation, and sexualization.

Horney suggested that the neurotic behavior she observed in White, middle-class girls was a rational response to the psychological conflicts created by a culture that was fundamentally sick. Similarly, we propose that some socially aggressive girls, particularly those girls who are socially skilled, admired by others, and perceived as leaders among their peers, are the product of a culture that simultaneously tells girls that they can "be all that they can be" while bombarding them with not-so-subtle messages that this only applies if they also adhere to traditional stereotypes of femininity. That is, "successful" girls will be accepted but only if they take care of their physical appearance (i.e., try to look "pretty"), if they are nice to others, and if they are cooperative and not overtly aggressive or competitive. Thus, White, middle-class heterosexual girls in contemporary society are indoctrinated into a false culture of "niceness" while striving to be competitive in a culture that fosters interpersonal competitiveness and an orientation toward achieving superiority over others (Crystal, Watanabe, & Chen, 2000). Some socially aggressive girls are, we propose, responding to the hypocrisy of the culture in which they are embedded in a manner that serves to enhance their self-esteem and assist them in achieving their social goals. Although some girls may experience difficulties in this environment, others will adapt by successfully using the competitive strategies available to them.

Socialization messages that have emphasized "being nice" as a fundamental aspect of good character in young girls and adolescent women have been pervasive in White, middle-class Western society for decades. For example, in numerous advice books from the first half of the 20th century, girls were told that being a good friend meant being loyal, helping other girls to be "good," being cooperative, not expressing anger, and not spreading rumors or gossip (e.g., Gibson, 1941; Miller & Laitem, 1935; Ullmann, 1948).

This tradition of reifying the fundamental goodness of girls and of their relationships with each other could also be seen, to some extent, in the feminist developmental literature that began to emerge in the 1980s. Authors such as Carol Gilligan (1982) and Jean Baker Miller (1991) proposed that adolescent girls' psychological development is grounded in their sense of self-in-relationship. These authors also implied that girls' peer culture had more in common with cooperative, collectivistic cultures when compared to the independent, individualistic peer culture of boys.

The perception that girls' peer culture in North America emphasizes cooperation and niceness has received some empirical support from developmental researchers who have observed that, in childhood, girls are less overtly competitive when compared to boys (Lever, 1976, 1978; Maccoby, 1990, Thorne, 1986) and are more focused on maintaining an egalitarian structure within their same-sex social networks in competitive situations when compared to boys (Maltz & Borker, 1983).

Adolescent girls are also more likely to fear negative repercussions from same-sex peers for overt competition when compared to boys (Benenson & Benarroch, 1998). Interestingly, much of this research has been conducted with participants from middle-class, European (i.e., mainly White) populations. Furthermore, research by Goodwin (1998) suggests that White, middle-class girls engage in the least competitive and conflictual speech forms when compared to working class and poor Latino and African-American children. Thus, White middle-class girls may act as the "culture police" in their social groups by responding negatively to violations of their cultural norms.

Currently, research on the meaning of competition in adolescence for girls or the role that it may play in their interactions with each other is lacking. However, numerous questions about the association between social aggression and feelings of competitiveness emerge from Horney's theoretical framework. What are adolescent girls competing for? How do they understand competition among each other and is it different when they think about competing with boys? Do competitive feelings among girls increase in early adolescence when compared to childhood? Are there developmental differences in the underlying factors influencing competitive behavior among girls from childhood to adolescence? How might the competitive strategies used by girls, including social aggression, be influenced by gender intensification during adolescence? And, finally, what are lessons being learned about female–female competition during adolescence that might be taken into adulthood?

Although it is beyond the scope of this chapter to examine all of these issues, in the following sections we explore two main questions just raised: (a) What are White, middle-class adolescent girls competing for?; and (b) how might the socialization processes of gender intensification influence the competitive strategies used by adolescent girls to achieve their goals? However, before we address these issues, we examine the social/cultural context in which girls' competitive behaviors are embedded. For the purpose of this chapter, we focus specifically on the climate of the peer group.

DEVALUATION AND SEXUALIZATION OF GIRLS BY PEERS

Boys' hate was dangerous, it was keen and bright, a miraculous birthright, like Arthur's sword snatched out of the stone, in the Grade Seven Reader. Girls' hate, in comparison, seemed muddled and tearful, sourly defensive. Boys would bear down on you on their bicycles and cleave the air where you had been, magnificently, with no remorse, as

if they wished there were knives on the wheels. And they would say anything.
They would say softy, "Hello hooers."
They would say, Hey, where's your fuckhole?" in tones of cheerful disgust.
The things they said stripped away freedom to be what you wanted, reduced you to what it was they saw, and that, plainly was enough to make them gag.

(Munroe, 1971, p. 98)

An important limitation of Horney's theory of female development is the exclusive focus on family dynamics as the context in which broader cultural messages regarding the feminine ideal were recreated. Although these observations were consistent with the state of knowledge about human development at the time, since then researchers have learned more about the importance of peer relations for human development particularly during adolescence (Youniss & Smollar, 1985). Consistent with Horney, we propose that adolescent girls have unique experiences in the peer group that tend to perpetuate the processes she described: devaluation, and sexualization. These processes contribute to a climate in which adolescent girls may be viewed as inferior and as the object of boys' sexual attention. This climate forms the context for the emerging competitive feelings that girls have for each other.

Sexual harassment is a form of victimization that becomes increasingly prevalent among peers in adolescence (Berman, Straatman, Hunt, Izumi, & MacQuarrie, 2002; Casella, 2001; Craig, Pepler, Connolly, & Henderson, 2001; Fineran, 2002; Fineran & Bennett, 1998). Although both boys and girls report experiences of sexual harassment in high school, girls are more likely than boys to report being harassed by other-sex peers (American Association of University Women [AAUW], 1993; Stratton & Backes, 1997). Girls are also more likely than boys to experience being the target of sexual comments, jokes, gestures, and looks (AAUW, 1993). Physical forms of sexual harassment are also more likely to be experienced by adolescent girls when compared to boys (AAUW, 1993; Roscoe, Strouse, & Goodwin, 1994). The results of one study indicate that, of those adolescents reporting sexual harassment perpetrated by peers, 45% of the girls and 19% of the boys experienced unwanted physical contact that was sexual in nature (Roscoe et al., 1994). In contrast, boys are more likely than girls to be targets of homophobic name-calling (AAUW, 1993).

Girls tend to perceive acts of sexual harassment as more threatening or upsetting when compared to boys, with the exception of homophobic name-calling and sexual graffiti for which no differences have been detected (Fineran & Bennett, 1999). Consistent with girls' self-reports, research suggests that the outcomes associated with peer-based sexual harassment in adolescence are, indeed, associated with more negative outcomes for girls when compared to boys (AAUW, 1993; Duffy, Wareham, & Walsh, 2004; Lee, Croniner, Linn, & Chen, 1996). For example, girls who are sexually harassed are more likely than boys to report not wanting to attend school, not wanting to talk in class, experiencing difficulty concentrating, staying home or avoiding classes, finding it hard to study, receiving lower grades, and thinking about changing schools (AAUW, 1993). Girls are also more likely than boys to report feeling embarrassed, confused, self-conscious, afraid, less self-confident, less popular, and doubtful about future romantic relationships. In contrast, boys were twice as likely to report feeling more popular in response to experiencing unwanted sexual attention from girls at school. Girls are also more likely than boys to change their behavior in response to sexual harassment. They try to avoid the harasser by avoiding certain areas, activities, and people at school, by changing their seating in class, and by changing their route between home and school.

Clearly, sexual harassment creates a negative environment for girls (and likely for boys, too). However, adolescent girls and boys perceive the gendered nature of sexual harassment as "normal." For example, interviews with adolescent girls (Tolman, Spencer, Rosen-Reynoso, & Porche, 2003) revealed a pervasive belief that adolescent boys are naturally sexual predators and that there is little that girls can do to protect themselves from this behavior particularly if they want a heterosexual relationship. In contrast, adolescent boys reported feeling intense peer pressure to engage in sexually aggressive behavior. Surprisingly, many girls tolerated this behavior recognizing that boys needed to demonstrate their "masculinity" in front of peers. Tolman and her colleagues suggest that these narratives reveal adolescents' complicity with the codified conventions of "compulsory heterosexuality." According to Rich (2003), compulsory heterosexuality involves the socialization of women and men into the belief that male sexual drive is a "right." These socialization processes also denigrate female sexual pleasure or agency, objectifies women, and incites girls to devalue their relationships with other girls. Thus, a patriarchal structure that inherently places greater value and recognition of adolescent boys' needs/desire at the expense of adolescent girls' needs/desires can be identified in contemporary society.

What are the implications of this context for social aggression among girls? Consistent with Horney's theory, rivalry among girls may become more intense during adolescence as a function of their desire to be attractive to the more powerful boys' in their school. They recognize and accept male power and prerogative by internalizing the devaluation and sexualization of girls that pervades the school climate. Although Horney described three main types of responses to this social context, the feminine type is most likely to engage in the aggressive behaviors typically identified as social aggression. These girls are likely to derive the benefits of this behavior through the successful competition for social dominance and access to high status males because they are more likely to conform to social stereotypes at a time when boys become less accepting of equality for males and females (Galambos, Almeida, & Peterson, 1990).

WHAT ARE ADOLESCENT GIRLS COMPETING FOR?

Social Dominance

The formation of peer cliques creates a context in which attaining and maintaining social status becomes increasingly important for adolescents (see Cillessen & Mayeux, chap. 6, this volume). Indeed, researchers have noted that interest in participating in activities that are associated with social influence and prestige among peers (i.e., becoming a cheerleader or joining the football team) is strongest during early adolescence (B. B. Brown, 1989; Eder & Parker, 1987) At the same time, adolescents become increasingly aware of status differences among individuals (Coleman, 1966; Savin-Williams, 1979). Socially dominant individuals are characterized by high social status and visibility. They tend to be focal members of a group, are effective at influencing others, and are perceived as attractive social partners (Hawley, 1999). In contrast to lower status peers, socially dominant adolescents are generally spared from negative teasing or social ridicule by peers (Gavin & Furman, 1989; Weisfeld, Bloch, & Ivers, 1984). We are not speaking here of the friendly banter between friends but, rather, of the negative and unwanted attention that is generally associated with peer victimization. Thus, gaining and maintaining social dominance in the peer network may be an important developmental goal that underlies many of the social interactions between adolescents (B. B. Brown, 1989; Paikoff & Savin-Williams, 1983; Parker & Gottman, 1989; Weisfeld et al., 1983, 1984).

Whereas girls' same-sex friendship networks in childhood have generally been characterized as egalitarian social structures, dominance hierarchies in these networks have been observed to emerge in early adolescence (Eder, 1985). However, individual status within girls' social hierarchies is notably less stable when compared to individual status within boys' hierarchies (Savin-Williams, 1979). Consequently, girls may experience more difficulty adjusting to dominance hierarchies when compared to boys.

Some authors have suggested that girls use different competitive strategies to achieve social dominance when compared to boys (Boulton, 1992; Maccoby, 1998). Indeed, Savin-Williams (1979) found sex differences in the behaviors used to assert dominance among peers. Specifically, he observed that boys used overt dominance behaviors such as physical aggression and arguing more frequently than girls. Hawley (1999) has described these strategies as "coercive" dominance strategies. In contrast, girls were more likely than boys to complement, ask favours, imitate, and solicit advice. Thus, girls appear to use prosocial strategies (Hawley, 1999) that are consistent with traditional stereotypes of femininity. However, ethnographic research suggests that, in adolescence, some girls may achieve social dominance through aversive behaviors that may have negative consequences for other girls (Eder, 1985; Merton, 1997; Owens, Shute, & Slee, 2000). Indeed, stereotypes of the manipulative, dominant, adolescent female are abundant in popular literature (Angier, 1999; Atwood, 1998; Wiseman, 2003; Wolf, 1997). This stereotype is of a girl who, on the surface, appears to be very socially skilled but who is capable of seriously undermining the confidence of other girls around her while avoiding direct blame for the harm inflicted. According to Horney (1967) and Wolf (1997), these girls may be particularly successful in the competition for the attention of high status males. Interestingly, these girls are likely to be successful because they, like girls who adopt prosocial strategies, are also likely to be perceived as conforming to traditional stereotypes of femininity.

Other-Sex Relationships

Adolescence is also notable for the onset of other-sex relationships including romantic relationships. In contrast to the strong segregation of the sexes observed in childhood, the formation of mixed-sex peer networks followed by the onset of dating relationships (Dunphy, 1963) may enhance competitive feelings among adolescent girls that challenge even the closest friendships. These feelings are illustrated by Naomi Wolf (1997) when she described the ritual preparations she and her adolescent friends engaged in for the Friday-night school dances:

> Each one of us looked at herself and the girl standing next to her. She looked with the imagined eyes of a lover, gauging which of the two the imagined lover would choose and why. If there were things the projected boy might prefer, they would be attacked openly and slyly: the threatening charms would have to be slashed way in the mental calculation, no matter how dear the friend who possessed them. This was not the gleeful

curiosity of preadolescence. Instead, we were engaged in something that felt truly Darwinian: organizing ourselves into a pecking order. (p. 84)

Thus, a pervasive and tyrannical heterosexual climate in which competition for the gaze of the other-sex emerges as an important, if not primary, force in life may become an important context for the development of social aggression among some adolescent girls.[4] For these girls, successfully negotiating through this challenging climate may elicit, indeed demand, the development of sophisticated social skills that we generally recognize as social aggression. That is, one strategy for effectively dealing with the strains and stress associated with the pervasive messages regarding female behavior and compulsory heterosexuality may be to develop aggressive but covert skills the goal of which is to enhance self-perceptions at the expense of others in her environment. By doing so, girls may successfully conform to cultural stereotypes of femininity while, at the same time, succeed in what may be an important developmental goal: being the center of attention of the male gaze.

This idea needs further exploration but is beyond the scope of this chapter.

CULTURAL REPRESENTATIONS OF ADOLESCENT GIRLS: GENDER NORMATIVE AGGRESSION

Evolutionary theorists have suggested that natural selection lies at the root of female–female aggression and use the observation that aggression among females is most intense between the ages of 15 to 24 (Campbell, 2004). However, it is important to note that this is also a time of struggle for contemporary young women as they negotiate the transition into "womanhood" and the inherent conflicts that are created by the mixed messages they receive in North American culture about what this means.

Implicit in this chapter, so far, is the idea that social aggression is likely to be perceived as inherently feminine in nature. Indeed, we would argue that even though boys and girls may engage in socially aggressive behaviors, cultural stereotypes about aggression are likely

---

[4]Although we recognize that not all girls may identify as heterosexual, we would argue that the compulsive heterosexuality that pervades the predominant social context of early adolescence (i.e., school) may have similar consequences at this stage of development. That is, in early adolescence the desire to "fit in" may be stronger than one's sexual desires although this conformity may fade with the development of sexual identity.

to exist among North American, Caucasian adolescents. Crick (1997) has suggested that, in childhood, girls who engage in overt aggression violate gender norms and, consequently, are more likely to experience intolerance, rejection, and negativity from their peers when compared to girls who engage in gender "normative" aggression (i.e., social aggression). Normative beliefs about aggression may become particularly evident in adolescence; a time when socialization pressures to conform to cultural stereotypes of gender are posited to be experienced most intensely (Hill & Lynch, 1983). In other words, girls who engage in aggressive behaviors that are viewed as inherently feminine may be more easily accepted by their peers when compared to girls who engage in overt, physical aggression. Currently, however, research on the link between gender stereotypes, aggression, and social status among peers in adolescence is lacking.

For the purpose of illustration, it may be useful to turn to representations of aggression and femininity in popular culture. In view of the increasing socialization role of media in adolescence (Kantrowitz & Wingert, 1999), exploring the cultural messages regarding femininity and social aggression in the media may further help us to understand this behavior during early adolescence.

Researchers have suggested that adolescents' ideals regarding what it means to be a man or a woman in today's society are partly derived from the messages provided by media (J. D. Brown, Childers, & Waszak, 1990). In particular, television series aimed at adolescents are frequently used as a way of defining gender identity especially through discussions about these series with peers (Pasquier, 1996). North American adolescents watch at least 2–4 hours of television per day (Lichty, 1989; Roberts, Foehr, Rideout, & Brodie, 1999). Consequently, television may influence early adolescents' understanding of gender. In view of these observations, we decided to explore the messages regarding aggression and femininity that are contained in a popular television series among 12 to 18 year old girls: "Buffy the Vampire Slayer" ("BtVS": Whedon, 1997).

"BUFFY THE VAMPIRE SLAYER": MEDIA PORTRAYALS OF GENDER AND AGGRESSION IN ADOLESCENCE

The "BtVS" series ran for seven successful seasons from 1997–2003. Over this time, viewers watched the development of an adolescent girl whose destiny was to fight evil supernatural forces such as vampires and demons that threatened the survival of humanity. She was empowered with supernatural strength and a natural skill for hand to hand (or, hand to heart) combat. Interestingly, the director of the series, Joss

Whedon, wanted to use the series to explore adolescent development and aspired to create a cultural representation of this period of development because he saw it as a monumental step to adulthood. As such, he designed Buffy to be a cultural icon (Whedon, 2004).

These goals led to a television series that explored the developmental challenges of adolescence in an entertaining and engaging manner. The success of the series in becoming a cultural representation of adolescence is evident by the plethora of dedicated teen chat-rooms on "Buffy" Web sites around the world (see www.buffysearch.com for a list). The series has also received extensive attention from a diverse range of academic disciplines (see Badman, 2004, for a bibliography) and several books have been written that explore the cultural significance of the series (e.g., South, 2003; Wilcox & Lavery, 2002; Yeffeth, 2003). In the academic literature examining the cultural significance of BtVS, there has yet to be an analysis of the developmental issues that are represented in the series. In addition, much of the discussion about the show has focused on issues of power in male–female relationships (Symonds, 2004) and has not specifically examined the power structure in relationships among teenage girls. Although a number of authors have suggested that the series has empowered a generation of young girls to subvert traditional gender roles (e.g., Dauber, 2003; Pender, 2002; Thompson, 2003; Vint, 2002), we suggest that these perspectives overlook the important role of peer relationships for adolescent social and psychological well-being. Specifically, previous authors have ignored the implications of subverting traditional gender roles for the development and maintenance of peer relationships even when these implications are explicitly revealed in the series. Consequently, for the purpose of this chapter, we focus on the representation of aggression and femininity in the series and the nature of competitive relationships among girls that is portrayed by two significant characters in the series: Buffy (played by Sarah Michelle Geller) and her classmate Cordelia (played by Charisma Carpenter).

The "data" for this analysis are derived from the first three seasons of the series that take place during Buffy's years in high school. We chose to focus on the characters Buffy and Cordelia for two reasons. First, they represent two types of aggressive adolescent girls. Second, the characterization of the tense relationship between Cordelia and Buffy in these seasons reflects the challenges associated with competition among girls in adolescence.

As the series begins, 16-year-old Buffy is beginning a new high school (Sunnydale High) after moving from Los Angeles. Her parents' recent divorce was precipitated, to some extent, by Buffy's initiation into her role as the chosen one that left her former high school (and her reputation among her peers) in ruins. The transition into a new school provides Buffy with an opportunity to improve her social status among peers. Indeed, the most popular girl in Sunnydale, Cordelia Chase, attempts to befriend Buffy during her first days at the new school. Cordelia recognizes that the new kid, Buffy, is physically attractive, socially competent and a potential threat to her position in the social hierarchy. Consequently, her competitive strategy appears to be to situate Buffy into a group in which she, Cordelia, is clearly recognized as a leader and is supported, to a large extent, by the girls who follow her. However, Buffy rejects Cordelia's friendly overtures after observing her mean behavior toward lower status students in the school. Indeed, Buffy chooses the friendship of two of the school's most reputable losers (i.e., Willow and Xander) over the most popular girl in school, Cordelia. Although Cordelia eventually, and reluctantly, becomes a peripheral member of the "Scooby gang" that provides support to the slayer, the relationship between Buffy and Cordelia reflects an uneasy alliance. Their relationship does not have the characteristics that girls typically associated with "friendship" such as mutual support, warmth, and intimacy (Bukowski, Newcomb, & Hoza, 1987; Sharabany, Gershoni, & Hoffman, 1981). Rather, their relationship is best described as a "mutually antipathy" (Hartup & Abecassis, 2002).

What we found most interesting about these two girls is the manner in which they represent cultural stereotypes of girls' aggression. Cordelia is constructed as "the archetypal high-school cheerleader 'bitch'" (Thompson, 2003). She is the most socially dominant girl in her school. She is the leader of the popular group even though she is not very well-liked by many students in the school. She is narcissistic, physically attractive, socially skilled, intelligent, and outspoken. From our perspective, Cordelia represents the archetypical "feminine type" described by Horney. That is, she conforms to (i.e., does not resist) the pervasive stereotypes of femininity while, at the same time, dominating the other girls at her school. She succeeds at being the center of attention of her peers, particularly with the boys. She compares herself, particularly her appearance, against other women and engages in activities that are most likely to attract the interest of boys (e.g., cheerleading). She humiliates other girls, "collects" boys who admire and worship her, and is perceived by others as successful in the social realm. Interestingly, the strategies that Cordelia uses to proactively achieve her goals or in reaction to a threat to her social status (and, inherently, her self-esteem) involves verbal and social aggression: psychological manipulation, gossip, insults targeting her opponent's weaknesses, and social exclusion.

Buffy Somers is also concerned about issues of social status and popularity. She is acutely aware of the culture of the "pops" having been a member of this group at her previous school prior to discovering her destiny as the vampire slayer. She, too, is intelligent, socially skilled, and physically attractive. In contrast to Cordelia, Buffy is also sensitive to the needs of others and is generally kind-hearted. However, Buffy does not hesitate to use physical aggression in response to perceived threats to herself or to her friends. This is not only when responding to vampires and demons, but also when older, more physically powerful boys attempt to bully her or her friends at school. As a result, Buffy becomes an outcast. In contrast to Cordelia, Buffy develops close, intimate friendships with a small group of peers. However, unlike Cordelia, she frequently experiences the pain of social exclusion and rejection by the larger population of students in her high school as a result of her overt, physical, aggression.

Developmental scientists would predict that both Cordelia and Buffy are at risk for developmental problems as a result of their aggressive behavior (not to mention their frequent battles with vampires and demons!). However, unlike Buffy, Cordelia does not appear to experience long-lasting negative social or emotional consequences as a result of her behavior. Indeed, in contrast to Buffy who frequently battles self-doubt, depression, and persistent feelings of loneliness throughout high school, Cordelia generally emerges victorious and with a strong sense of self. For example, after she is dumped by her popular group of girls for dating a "loser" (i.e., Buffy's friend, Xander) she successfully gains control of the situation by confronting the group and asserting her right to date whomever she pleases. When she discovers Xander and Willow in a compromising romantic situation, she overcomes her feelings of sadness by turning her social aggression on Xander. However, she never abandons the group in high school and continues to assist them in their battles against evil. By the end of high school, she has resolved her feelings about Xander, has discovered her ability to confront demons (both external and internal), and is presented as having successfully avoided the negative effects of the trauma of adolescence.

In contrast, Buffy struggles with her sense of identity and feelings of existential angst throughout the first three seasons; from early adolescence (Season 1) into emerging adulthood (Season 3). Although upon graduation, her classmates publicly recognize the unique contributions Buffy has made to student life, literally, at Sunnydale High, it seems to be too little and too late. The psychological scars resulting from not achieving a sense of belonging with the larger peer network at school follow her as she makes the transition into university and then into young adulthood.

The message underlying the representation of aggression in the social and psychological development of girls contained in BtVS is consistent with the views being presented in this chapter. That is, although Cordelia and Buffy are both physically attractive and socially dominant girls in their social networks, Cordelia appears to suffer fewer negative consequences for her aggressive behavior when compared to Buffy. Consequently, although many girls may identify with Buffy, they may also recognize the benefits associated with conformity to cultural stereotypes of femininity that are so clearly represented by Cordelia's social and psychological "success." In other words, although they may resent the "Cordelias" in their world, they may begrudgingly praise them for their social success. For developmental researchers, these cultural exemplars of aggressive girls serve to remind us of the complexity of individuals. Social aggression is embedded in a constellation of individual characteristics/behaviors and is used more or less successfully depending on the particular configuration of that constellation within an individual.

CONCLUSIONS

A commercial has recently aired on Canadian television that is aimed at early adolescent girls. It begins by following a young girl to her locker and then to the water fountain. As she approaches the water fountain, we see a group of three other girls in the empty hallway in the background. They are watching the target girl and whispering. She stops drinking as she becomes keenly aware of being in the line of sight of the three other girls. She stands up, braces herself, and tries to walk quickly past them as they begin to verbally abuse her. As their words become louder they also become visible to the audience as text that first knock the victim's books from her arms, then hit her across the face, and eventually bring her to her knees. As she recovers and runs from the girls who are tormenting her, a narrator tells us "Words hurt as much as fists. Don't be a part of it."

Implicit in the message is the idea that reducing social aggression among girls is as simple as "just say no" to drugs. However, we suspect that, however well intentioned, these types of commercials will be about as successful as the "just say no" commercials of the Reagan era (Braiker, 2003). Aggression is a complex interpersonal phenomenon that occurs in a complex social space. Although these types of commercials may be effective at bringing to the public eye a form of victimization that has, typically, been overlooked in North American society, they are unlikely to help the general public, including adolescent girls, understand and/or cope with the phenomenon.

Currently, however, we know very little about social aggression among girls in adolescence. Artz (1998) has suggested that to understand physically violent girls, we must take a view of the world from their perspective and not from the perspective of the victims. We suggest that her point is relevant, too, for research on socially aggressive girls, particularly in adolescence. We need to know more about their world, about their perceptions of their world, of the expectations placed on them by significant others (including, perhaps, lower status, victimized girls), and of their relationships with other girls as well as with boys. Ethnographic research has begun to shed some light on these issues (e.g., Eder, 1985; Merton, 1997; Owens, Shute, & Slee, 2000). Similarly, recent research using a person-oriented analysis has provided important directions for future research in this area (e.g., Farmer, Estell, Bishop, O'Neal, & Cairns, 2003). However, more research is needed on this topic.

The goal of this chapter has been to expand on some of the ideas that have been touched on by others when attempting to understand the results of research on social aggression. We have tried to expand on the explanations proposed for social aggression among adolescent girls by examining the potential contributions of Karen Horney's classic work on female development. Although she wrote about women's experiences 75 years ago, her voice resonates with many of the experiences that can be observed among early adolescent girls today. We recognize that this perspective may only be relevant for a particular population of adolescent girls (i.e., girls who are embedded within a North American, Westernized culture). However, the ideas expressed throughout the chapter may serve as the point of departure for asking additional questions in our research.

Throughout this chapter, we have suggested that the use of non-physical, covert forms of aggression, or even the threat of this type of aggression, may provide a competitive edge for some adolescent girls in their attempts to achieve social dominance within a rapidly changing social network. However, we have suggested, also, that the success of this type of aggressive strategy depends on the presence of other behavioral characteristics that are consistent with social dominance such as physical appearance, leadership skills, and social skills. Moreover, the behavioral configurations of aggressive girls who are successful in achieving their social goals are likely to be consistent with peer perceptions of femininity in adolescence. That is, aggressive, socially dominant girls are likely to engage in behaviors that are viewed as gender normative and, thus, conform to the peer group's expectations regarding sex role behavior. Finally, although we do not underestimate the negative consequences that the behavior of these girls may have for other girls (and, possibly, boys), we suggest that the outcomes associated with social aggression in girls must be understood in the broader social and developmental context in which it takes place. It is just possible that, for some girls, social aggression is an adaptive response to a social/cultural context that inherently devalues and sexualizes them.

Although we are certainly not advocating a "girls will be girls" attitude toward social aggression, we do suggest that an examination of the social/cultural context of adolescence is essential to designing and implementing effective intervention and prevention programs. In other words, it is important to understand the adaptive function of behaviors that are labeled "aggressive." As suggested by Kowalski (1997), being "nice" does not always result in achieving one's goals in relationships with others and, consequently, there may be situations that evoke aversive, interpersonal behaviors. Some of these situations may be the result of girls' experiences of devaluation and sexualization in the context of the school and in the culture of the peer group. Responses to these experiences can include anger, as other authors have suggested. However, another response may involve conforming to other's expectations overtly while using covert means to achieve one's own goals.

Horney's perspective foreshadowed an emerging literature in developmental science (Bukowski, 2003; Hawley & Vaughn, 2003; Underwood, 2003) and, we suggest, has important implications for understanding social aggression among girls. A cultural approach necessitates a careful examination of the way that social aggression is used by adults in the adolescent's social world. Although aversive interpersonal behaviors may have negative consequences for the social and emotional well-being of children and adolescents in our society, it is important to recognize the hypocrisy of identifying social aggression as a "problem" among girls. Behaviors such as gossip and social exclusion are pervasive in North American culture— in politics, in business, in communities, and even among adults who may be involved in the development or implementation of these intervention programs. Girls are excellent observers of their environment and some are likely to be more sensitive to these role models for behavior than others (L. M. Brown & Gilligan, 1992). Thus, telling adolescent girls that this behavior is unacceptable is likely to be perceived as hypocritical and unrealistic.

Another implication of Horney's perspective for understanding social aggression among girls is the need to improve our understanding of the "Big Girls" (c.f., Underwood, 2003) in the high school. These girls are most likely attuned to and influencing the cultural climate of the peer group. They are most likely to be the leaders and/or initiators of social aggression and the most effective at using it. They are also likely to be the most influential in helping to combat it. Rather than punishing them, we may need to help them understand the larger cultural context that may be influencing their behaviors. However, developmental scientists need to do a better job of understanding this context first. Although simple answers to complex questions (such as "just say no") may be intuitively appealing, particularly to a concerned parent, we are unlikely to be effective agents of change if we settle for these answers.

REFERENCES

American Association of University Women. (1993). *Hostile hallways: The AAUW survey on sexual harassment in America's schools.* Washington, DC: Author.

Angier, N. (1999). *Woman: An intimate geography.* New York: Houghton Mifflin Company.

Archer, J., & Coyne, S. M. (2005). An integrated review of indirect, relational, and social aggression. *Personality and Social Psychology Review, 9,* 212–230.

Artz, S. (1998). Where have all the school girls gone? Violent girls in the schoolyard. *Child and Youth Care Forum, 27,* 77–109.

Atwood, M. (1998). *Cat's eye.* Toronto: McLelland and Stewart.

B.C. girl convicted in school bullying tragedy. (2002, March 26). *CBC News.* Retrieved September 22, 2005, from http://www.cbc.ca/story/canada/national/2002/03/25/ wesley020325.html

Badman, D. A. (2005). *Buffy bibliography.* Retrieved September 20, 2004, from http://www.madinkbeard.com/buffyology/buffybibliog.html

Baker Miller, J. (1991). The development of women's sense of self. In J. V. Jordan, A. G. Kaplan, J. Baker Miller, I. P. Stiver, & J. L. Surrey (Eds.), *Women's growth in connection: Writings from the stone center* (pp. 11–26). New York: Guilford.

Barron, C., & Lacombe, D. (2005). Moral panic and the nasty girl. *Canadian Review of Sociology & Anthropology, 41,* 51–69.

Benenson, J. F., & Benarroch, D. (1998). Gender differences in responses to friends' hypothetical greater success. *Journal of Early Adolescence, 18,* 192–208.

Berman, H., Straatman, A. L., Hunt, K., Izumi, J., & MacQuarrie, B. (2002). Sexual harassment: The unacknowledged face of violence in the lives of girls. In H. Berman & Y. Jiwani (Eds.) *In the best interest of the girl child: Phase II report* (pp. 17–44). London, ON: Centre for Research on Violence Against Women and Children.

Boulton, M. J. (1992). Rough physical play in adolescents: Does it serve a dominance function? *Early Education & Development, 3,* 312–333.

Braiker, B. (2003). "Just say know": An advocate of drug law reform says D.A.R.E. is a 20-year old failure. *Newsweek, April 15.*

Brown, B. B. (1989). The role of peer groups in adolescents' adjustment to secondary school. In T. J. Berndt & G. W. Ladd (Eds.), *Peer relationships in child development* (pp. 188–215). New York: Wiley.

Brown, J. D., Childers, K.W., & Waszak, C. S. (1990). Television and adolescent sexuality. *Journal of Adolescent Health Care, 11(1),* 62–70.

Brown, L. M. (1998). *Raising their voices: The politics of girls' anger.* Cambridge, MA: Harvard University Press.

Brown, L. M., & Gilligan, C. (1992). *Meeting at the crossroads: Women's psychology and girls' development.* Cambridge, MA: Harvard University Press.

Bukowski, W. M. (2003). What does it mean to say that aggressive children are competent or incompetent? *Merrill-Palmer Quarterly, 49,* 390–400.

Bukowski, W. M., Newcomb, A. F., & Hoza, B. (1987). Friendship conceptions among early adolescents: A longitudinal study of stability and change. *Journal of Early Adolescence, 7,* 143–152.

Cairns, R. B., Cairns, B. D., Neckerman, H. J., Ferguson, L. L., & Gariepy, J. (1989). Growth and aggression: 1. Childhood to early adolescence. *Developmental Psychology, 25,* 320–330.

Campbell, A. (2004). Female competition: Causes, constraints, content, and contexts. *Journal of Sex Research, 41,* 16–26.

Canadian Broadcasting Corporation. (Producer). (1997, March 5). *Nasty girls* [Documentary].

Casella, R. (2001). What is violent about "school violence"? The nature of violence in a city high school. In J. N. Burstyn & G. Benders (Eds.), *Preventing violence in schools: A challenge to American democracy* (pp. 15–46). Mahwah, NJ: Lawrence Erlbaum Associates.

Casey-Cannon, S., Hayward, C., & Gowen, K. (2001). Middle-school girls' reports of peer victimization: Concerns, consequences, and implications. *Professional School Counseling, 5,* 138–147.

Coleman, J. S. (1966). *The adolescent society.* New York: Free Press.

Craig, W. M., Pepler, D. J., Connolly, J., & Henderson, K. (2001). Developmental context of peer harassment in early adolescence. In J. Juvoen & S. Graham (Eds.), *Peer harassment in school: The plight of the vulnerable and victimized* (pp. 242–261). New York: Guilford.

Crick, N. R. (1995). Relational aggression: The role of intent attributions, feelings of distress, and provocation type. *Development and Psychopathology, 7(2),* 313–322.

Crick, N. R. (1997). Engagement in gender normative versus nonnormative forms of aggression: Links to social-psychological adjustment. *Developmental Psychology, 33(4),* 610–616.

Crick, N. R., Grotpeter, J. K., & Bigbee, M. A. (2002). Relationally and physically aggressive children's intent attributions and feelings of distress for relational and instrumental peer provocations. *Child Development, 73,* 1134–1142.

Crick, N. R., Nelson, D. A., Morales, J. R., Cullerton-Sen, C., Casas, J., & Hickman, S. E. (2001). Relational victimization in childhood and adolescence: I hurt you through the grapevine. In S. Graham & J. Juvonen (Eds.), *Peer harassment in school* (pp 192–214). New York: Guilford.

Crystal, D. S., Watanabe, H., & Chen, R. S. (2000). Preference for diversity in competitive and cooperative contexts: A study of American and Japanese children and adolescents. *International Journal of Behavioral Development, 24,* 348–355.

Dauber, S. (2003, May 30). Talk about the end of girl power. *The Christian Science Monitor.* Retrieved March 15, 2004, from http://www.csmonitor.com/2003/0530/p25s01-altv.html

Duffy, J., Wareham, S., & Walsh, M. (2004). Psychological consequences for high school students of having been sexually harassed. *Sex Roles, 50,* 811–821.

Dunphy, D. (1963). The social structure of urban adolescent peer groups. *Sociometry, 26,* 230–246.

Eder, D. (1985). The cycle of popularity: Interpersonal relations among female adolescents. *Sociology of Education, 58(3),* 154–165.

Eder, D., & Parker, S. (1987). The cultural production and reproduction of gender: The effect of extracurricular activities on peer-group culture. *Sociology of Education, 60,* 200–213.

Farmer, T. W., Estell, D., Bishop, J. L., O'Neal, K. K., & Cairns, B. D. (2003). Rejected bullies or popular leaders? The social relations of aggressive subtypes of rural African American early adolescents. *Developmental Psychology, 39*, 992–1004.

Fineran, S. (2002). Adolescents at work; Gender issues and sexual harassment. *Violence against Women, 8*, 953–967.

Fineran, S., & Bennett, L. (1998). Teenage peer sexual harassment: Implications for social work practice in education. *Social Work, 43*, 1–8.

Fineran, S., & Bennett, L. (1999). Gender and power issues of peer sexual harassment among teenagers. *Journal of Interpersonal Violence, 14*, 629–641.

Galambos, N., Almeida, D. M., & Petersen, A. C. (1990). Masculinity, femininity, and sex role attitudes in early adolescence: Exploring gender intensification. *Child Development, 61*, 1905–1914.

Galt, V. (1998, January 13). Handbook to address bullying by girls: Recent attacks lend urgency to project. *The Globe and Mail.* 31 January, p. A3.

Gavin, L. A., & Furman, W. (1989). Age differences in adolescents' perceptions of their peer groups. *Developmental Psychology, 25*, 827–834.

Gibson, J. E. (1941). *On being a girl.* New York: The MacMillan Company.

Gilligan, C. (1982). New maps of development: New visions of maturity. *American Journal of Orthopsychiatry, 52*, 199–212.

Goodwin, M. J. (1998). Cooperation and competition across girls' play activities. In J. Coates (Ed.), *Language and gender* (pp. 121–146). Oxford, UK: Blackwell.

Grotpeter, J. K., & Crick, N. R. (1996). Relational aggression, overt aggression, and friendship. *Developmental Psychology, 67*, 2328–2338.

Hartup, W. W., & Abecassis, M. (2002). Friends and enemies. In P. K. Smith & C. H. Hart (Eds.), *Blackwell handbook of childhood social development. Blackwell handbooks of developmental psychology* (pp. 286–306). Malden, MA: Blackwell Publishing.

Hawley, P. (1999). The ontogenesis of social dominance: A strategy-based evolutionary perspective. *Developmental Review*, 97–132.

Hawley, P., & Vaughn, B. E. (2003). Aggression and adaptive functioning: The bright side to bad behaviour. *Merrill-Palmer Quarterly, 49*, 239–242.

Hill, J. P., & Lynch, M. E. (1983). The intensification of gender related expectations during early adolescence. In J. Brookes-Gunn & A. C. Petersen (Eds.), *Girls at puberty: Biological and psychological perspectives* (pp. 201–228). New York: Plenum.

Horney, K. (1994). *The neurotic personality of our time.* New York: Norton. (Original work published 1964)

Horney, K. (1967). *Feminine psychology.* New York: Norton.

Kantrowitz, B., & Wingert, P. (1999, October 18). The truth about teens. *Newsweek*, pp. 62–72.

Kowalski, R. (1997). The underbelly of social interaction: Aversive interpersonal behaviors. In R. Kowalski (Ed.), *Aversive interpersonal behaviors* (pp. 1–9). New York: Plenum.

Leary, M. R., Kowalski, R. M., Smith, L., & Phillips, S. (2003). Teasing, rejection, and violence: Case studies of the school shootings. *Aggressive Behavior, 29*, 202–214.

Lee, V. E., Croniner, R. G., Linn, E, & Chen, X. (1996). The culture of sexual harassment on secondary schools. *American Educational Research Journal, 33,* 383–417.

Lever, J. (1976). Sex differences in the games children play. *Social Problems, 23,* 478–487.

Lichty, L. W. (1989). Television in America: Success story. In P. S. Cook, D. Gomery, & L. W. Lichty (Eds.), *American media* (pp. 159–176). Los Angeles, CA: Wilson Centre Press.

Maccoby, E. (1990). Gender and relationships: A developmental account. *AmericanPsychologist, 45,* 513–520.

Maccoby, E. (1998). *The two sexes: Growing up apart, coming together.* Cambridge, MA: Harvard University Press.

Maltz, D. N., & Borker, R. A. (1983). A cultural approach to male–female miscommunication. In J. Gumperz (Ed.), *Language and social identity* (pp. 195–216). New York: Cambridge University Press.

Merton, D. (1997). The meaning of meanness: Popularity, competition, and conflict among junior high school girls. *Sociology of Education, 70,* 175–191.

Miller, F. S., & Laitem, H.H. (1935). *Personal problems of high school girls.* New York: Wiley.

Munroe, A. (1971). *Lives of girls and women.* Toronto: McGraw-Hill Ryerson.

Owens, L., Shute, R., & Slee, P. (2000). "Guess what I heard!": Indirect aggression among teenage girls in Australia. *Aggressive Behavior, 26,* 67–83.

Owens, L., Slee, P., & Shute, R. (2001). Victimization among teenage girls: What can be done about indirect harassment? In J. Juvonen & S. Graham (Eds.), *Peer harassment in school: The plight of the vulnerable and victimized* (pp. 215–241). New York: Guilford.

Paikoff, R. L., & Savin-Williams, R. C. (1983). An exploratory study of dominance interactions among adolescent females at a summer camp. *Journal of Youth & Adolescence, 12,* 419–433.

Paquette, J. A., & Underwood, M. K. (1999). Gender differences in young adolescents' experiences of peer victimization: Social and physical aggression. *Merrill-Palmer Quarterly, 45,* 242–266.

Parker, J. G., & Gottman, J. M. (1989). Social and emotional development in a relational context: Friendship interaction from early childhood to adolescence. In T. J. Berndt & G. W. Ladd (Eds.), *Peer relationships in child development. Wiley series on personality processes* (pp. 95–131). Oxford, UK: Wiley.

Parkhurst, J. T., & Hopmeyer, A. (1998). Sociometric popularity and peer-perceived popularity: Two distinct dimensions of peer status. *Journal of Early Adolescence, 18,* 125–144.

Pasquier, D. (1996). Teen series' reception: Television, adolescence and culture of feelings. *Childhood: A Global Journal of Child Research, 3,* 351–373.

Pender, P. (2002). "I'm Buffy and you're . . . history": The postmodern politics of *Buffy the Vampire Slayer.* In R. V. Wilcox & D. Lavery (Eds.), *Fighting the forces: What's at stake in Buffy the Vampire Slayer* (pp. 35–44). Lanham, MD: Rowman Littlefield.

Rich, A. C. (2003). Compulsory heterosexuality and lesbian existence. *Journal of Women's History, 15,* 11-48.

Roberts, D. F., Foehr, U. G., Rideout, V. J., & Brodie, M. (1999). *Kids and the media at the new millennium: A comprehensive national analysis of children's media use.* New York: Henry J. Kaiser Family Foundation.

Roscoe, B., Strouse, J. S., & Goodwin, M. P. (1994). Sexual harassment: Early adolescents' self-reports of experiences and acceptance. *Adolescence, 29,* 515–523.

Sameroff, A. J. (1983). Developmental systems: Contexts and evolution. In W. Kessen (Ed.), *History, theory, and methods* (4th ed., Vol. 1, pp. 237–294). New York: Wiley.

Savin-Williams, R. C. (1979). Dominance hierarchies in groups of early adolescents. *Child Development, 50,* 923–935.

Sharabany, R., Gershoni, R., & Hoffman, J. E. (1981). Girlfriend, boyfriend: Age and sex differences in intimate friendship. *Developmental Psychology, 17,* 800–808.

South, J. B. (2003). *Buffy the Vampire Slayer* and Philosophy: Fear and Trembling in Sunnydale. *Popular Culture and Philosophy, Vol. 4.* Chicago, IL: Open Court Publishing.

Stratton, S. D., & Backes, J. S. (1997). Sexual harassment in North Dakota public schools: A study of eight schools. *High School Journal, 80,* 163–172.

Symonds, G. (2004). "Solving problems with sharp objects": Female empowerment, sex and violence in *Buffy the Vampire Slayer. Slayage: The Online International Journal of Buffy Studies, 11–12.* Retrieved June 16, 2004, from http://slayage.tv/essays/ slayage11_12/Symonds.htm

Thompson, J. (2003). "Just a girl": Feminism, Postmodernism and *Buffy the Vampire Slayer. Refractory: A Journal of Entertainment Media, 2.* Retrieved July 3, 2004, from http://www.refractory.unimelb.edu.au/journalissues/vol2/ jimthompson.html

Thorne, B. (1986). Girls and boys together . . . but mostly apart: Gender arrangements in elementary schools. In W. W. Hartup & Z. Rubin (Eds.), *Relationships and development* (pp. 167–184). Hillsdale, NJ: Lawrence Erlbaum Associates.

Tolman, D., Spencer, R., Porche, M., & Rosen-Reynoso, M. (2003). Sowing the seeds of violence in heterosexual relationships: Early adolescents narrate compulsory heterosexuality. *Journal of Social Issues, 59,* 159–178.

Ullmann, F. (1948). *Girl alive!* New York: The World Publishing Company.

Underwood, M. K. (2003). The comity of modest manipulation, the importance of distinguishing among bad behaviours. *Merrill-Palmer Quarterly, 49,* 373–389.

Underwood, M. K. (2003). *Social aggression among girls.* New York: Guilford Press.

Van Schoiack-Edstrom, L., Frey, K. S., & Beland, K. (2002). Changing adolescents' attitudes about relational and physical aggression: An early evaluation of a school-based intervention. *School Psychology Review, 31,* 201–216.

Vint, S. (2002). "Killing us softly?" A feminist search for the 'real' Buffy. *Slayage: The Online International Journal of Buffy Studies, 5.* Retrieved July 3, 2004, from http://www.slayage.tv/essays/slayage5/ vint.htm

Weisfeld, G. E., Bloch, S. A., & Ivers, J. W. (1983). A factor analytic study of peer-perceived dominance in adolescent boys. *Adolescence, 70,* 229–243.

Weisfeld, G. E., Bloch, S. A., & Ivers, J. W. (1984). Possible determinants of social dominance among adolescent girls. *Journal of Genetic Psychology, 144,* 115–129.

Westkott, M. (1986). *The feminist legacy of Karen Horney.* New Haven, CT: Yale University Press.

Whedon, J. (Executive Producer). (1997). *Buffy the Vampire Slayer.* [Television series]. Los Angeles: United Paramount Network.

Whedon, J. (2004). Retrieved May 15, 2004, from www.slayage.tv

Wilcox, R. V., & Lavery, D. (2002). *Fighting the forces: What's at stake in* Buffy the Vampire Slayer. Lanham, MD: Rowman & Littlefield Publishers, Inc.

Wiseman, R. (2003). *Queen bees & wannabes.* New York: Three Rivers Press.

Wittman, J. (2001, March 13). A common sense proposal for ending violence on campus? *Los Angeles Youth Supportive Services.* Retrieved on September 24, 2005, from http://www.la-youth.org/Zero_tolerance_press_release1.html

Wolf, N. (1997). *Promiscuities: The secret struggle for womanhood.* Toronto: Random House of Canada.

Yeffeth, G. (2003). *Seven seasons of Buffy: Science fiction and fantasy writers discuss their favorite television show.* Dallas, TX: BenBella Books.

Youniss, J., & Smollar, J. (1985.) *Adolescent relations with mothers, fathers, and friends.* Chicago: University of Chicago Press.

8

SELF, OTHER, AND AGGRESSION: THE NEVER-ENDING SEARCH FOR THE ROOTS OF ADAPTATION

William M. Bukowski
Concordia University

Maurissa Abecassis
Colby-Sawyer College

It seems as if there are two parallel universes, each taking a different view of the association between aggression and competence during childhood and adolescence. In one universe, aggression is seen as antithetical to adaptation and positively correlated with all things bad and negatively correlated with all things good. In the other universe, aggression is seen to coexist with, or even promote, competence and adaptation. How can the perspectives of these two universes— one claiming that aggression is a negative factor for healthy development while the other claims it can be linked to competent functioning—be reconciled? In this chapter, we outline the evidence from the two universes and propose that recent findings argue for the need to reconsider how aggression and adaptation are inter-related. We propose that the two universes can be reconciled by reframing many of the questions that have been asked about aggression and development. At the base of our thoughts is the idea that the typical ways that we have studied and considered aggression need, at least in part, to be reconsidered. The most challenging part of this sort of re-analysis derives from the highly differentiated and complex nature of the concepts of aggression and adaptation.

In this discussion, we take a largely functional approach to aggression, especially as it is associated with children's experiences with peers. Our goal is not to show where aggression comes from or why one child might be more aggressive than another. Instead, we wish to discuss a few ideas about why aggression appears to be so bad from some vantage points, but not so bad from others.

There is no doubt that the view that aggression is a negative correlate of healthy development has dominated the study of developmental psychology. According to this perspective, aggression in childhood is a marker of maladjustment and it impedes adaptation and development. Accordingly, children who are aggressive have been identified as being at risk for multiple forms of concurrent and subsequent maladaptation. There is no shortage of information to justify this perspective. To be sure, measures of aggression are typically positively correlated with measures of all things "bad." Children who exhibit high levels of aggression are at risk for a long list of maladaptive outcomes, including criminality, limited levels of academic and occupational achievement, and unhappiness. In general, measures of aggression are observed to be negatively correlated with nearly every concurrent measure of adjustment that one can think of, including measures of happiness, measures of being liked by same- and other-sex peers during childhood, measures of friendship, and measures of psychological health. There is also plenty of evidence that measures of aggression in childhood predict measures of well being in adulthood. If one wants to know who will have a troubled adulthood, one need only to find out who is aggressive in childhood. A closer look at this evidence, however, shows that the association between aggression and well-being is not as consistent or as powerful as one might think and that it is far from monolithic. The strength of the association between aggression and well being often varies across studies and, in some cases, appears to be weak.

The perspective of the second universe is that to some extent, aggression can be a feature of the process of adaptation. This view claims that, regardless of whether we like it or not, aggression can, in some forms, be positively associated with social functioning, competence and adaptation. At the heart of this view is the argument that association between aggression and adaptation is more complex than a simple "aggression-is-bad" formulation would allow.

A variety of findings support this view. For example, although well-liked children tend to be less aggressive than are disliked children, they are not less aggressive than children of average likeableness, indicating that liking can co-occur with aggression (Newcomb, Bukowski, & Pattee, 1993). Also, children who are aggressive can have as many friends as children who are not aggressive (Cairns, Xie, & Leung, 1998) and aggressive boys and girls can, at some points during development, be attractive to their peers (Bukowski, Sippola, & Newcomb, 2000). There is evidence also that the association between aggression and measures of adaptation appears to be substantially smaller among children who are sociable or altruistic than among those who are not (Hawley, 2003). In other words, the adaptation of children whose behavior includes both aggression and prosocial acts is not lower than that of the average child. Other evidence shows that the association between aggression and adaptation is not the same for all forms of aggression (Little, Brauner, Jones, Nock, & Hawley, 2003; Poulin & Boivin, 2000). For example, measures of proactive aggression are less strongly associated with measures of negative outcomes than are measures of reactive aggression.

It may be that there are easy and superficial explanations for the existence of the two universes. One explanation may be that studies of aggressive behavior are often concerned with different facets of aggression, have different goals and research strategies, and arrive at different conclusions about the role of aggression in the lives of human beings. Moreover researchers are concerned with different parts of the "distribution"—some are interested in the normal range, however broadly defined, whereas others are primarily concerned with extreme groups and how they differ from the norm. The usual tensions also exist between those who study aggression from a categorical approach and those who measure it as a continuous dimension. Finally, there is the ever-present interpretive issue of how to make sense of the findings from empirical studies and how to ascribe meaning to our measures and observations. We draw on some of these differences in our discussion.

We also try to see aggression from a particular frame, specifically from the perspective of the dialectic between self and other. This dialectic concerns the struggle for individuals to work out the inherent contradictions between striving for individual achievements that bring resources and rewards to the self and functioning within a group and promoting the group's well-being. The self–other dialectic is an essential theme woven across and within multiple aspects of development. Central to this dialectic is the notion of autonomy, that is, how one can be sensitive to one's own needs and desires and to those of others at the same time. We use this perspective to explain why aggression can, in some cases, be a positive correlate of competence, whereas in others it is a negative correlate. We claim that the diverse challenges of being an individual in a social group means that there is a time and place for a broad range of behaviors including, in some cases, some forms of aggression. More importantly, we claim that non-additive and nonlinear models are needed to understand how aggression is linked to functioning with peers. This view parallels the person-centered approaches advocated by Bergman and others (Laursen & Hoff, 2006).

THE COMPLEXITY OF AGGRESSION

Although there is no universally agreed-on definition of aggression, the basic point of many definitions is that aggression is an act that by intention harms another person or group of persons. This definition seems to be clear, but its application can be tricky as many factors need to be considered including (a) the type of aggression being examined, (b) how one assesses intentionality, (c) what constitutes harm, and (d) the outcome of an aggressive act (i.e., "are all aggressive acts bad?"). We discuss each of the points, especially as they are related to the self/ other dialectic in the following sections.

Does the Type of Aggression Matter?

It is well known that the lion's share of the work on aggression, adaptation, and various aspects of physical aggression have been studied. In many of the studies, peer nominations, self-reports and some teacher reports are used to identify children who are deemed physically aggressive. Typical questions used to identify aggressive children include questions like: "Name three peers who are … mean, hit, shove, bully." From a developmental perspective, it is known that physical aggression tends to decrease across childhood so that being a physically aggressive adolescent is more non-normative than being a physically aggressive school-age child, which, in turn, is more non-normative than showing aggression in the toddler and preschool years. By this metric, it is not a surprise that if aggression is a preferred response or method of coping then it may be associated with poorer adaptation as it is a less advanced means of coping. Think of the typical preschool teacher's admonition to children to "use your words" instead of behaving in a physically aggressive manner.

However, it is also well known that one needs to go beyond an assessment of physical aggression only so as to assess more internalized and psychologically complex aspects of aggression. In contrast with physical aggression, there is an increase with age in the use of more internalized, and, in many respects, more complex forms of aggression such as verbal aggression (name calling, insults, back-handed comments, aggressive humor), relational aggression, and lying. The success of these forms of aggression (i.e., to cause harm), may depend on a child having good reasoning abilities, including planning, intellect, and even social skills.

Consider a few examples: Verbal aggression is a wide category that includes a range of behaviors that asserts its impact by causing psychological/mental/emotional, rather than physical harm. Even in this area, there is a clear developmental trend with name-calling and some insults as less sophisticated than back-handed remarks and aggressive humor. What makes aggressive humor, for example, psychologically "sophisticated"? Aggressive humor involves one child making a joke at a peer's expense— often poking fun at some aspect of the peer. If there is an audience of peers, the insult contained within the joke is amplified as others laugh at the peer who is the butt of the joke. In some ways, this kind of aggression is socially sanctioned—peers are expected to "roll with the punches," "to not take it seriously," or to "not let it get to you." What makes this type of aggression especially challenging is in designating it as aggressive. As described in a subsequent section—judging a punch as designed to "intentionally harm" is easy; judging an aggressive joke as designed to "intentionally harm" another is more difficult. Humor, by definition, is meant to entertain, and although some may laugh at a joke, the peer who is the subject of the joke may feel hurt or harmed by it. The peer telling the joke can deny the intentionality by claiming that he or she was not being serious. Long ago, Freud argued that humor is, in fact, aggressive and often expresses unconscious conflicts and otherwise unexpressed feelings (Freud, 1976). In general, peers' assessment of at least some verbal forms of aggression is more complex—raising the question of whether peers might deem the child who makes aggressive jokes and back-handed comments as funny and clever or mean and aggressive—or all of these things?

Turning to relational aggression, although it is apparent in preschool-aged children, it is more common in girls and increases in prevalence among both boys and girls in adolescence. Less is known about the long-term implications of involvement in this form of aggression, though there is some suggestion that children who use relational aggression on friends tend to have poorer adjustment later in childhood (Crick & Grotepeter, 1996). By definition, relational aggression includes the desire to psychologically harm another by causing injury to and damaging another's relationships. The tactics linked to relational aggression include actual or threatened social exclusion, gossiping and spreading rumors, and additional threats designed to coerce a peer (e.g., "if you don't play with me now, I won't be your friend anymore"). Although children recognize and report that they find relational aggression and its tactics to be mean and aggressive (Crick, 1995), threatening to ruin another's relationship for example, is predicated on a fairly complex understanding of social interaction. A child must understand that this particular peer values her social relationship, that one can ruin or seriously harm a relationship by spreading false information, and that just by threatening to engage in such an act one can induce fear and anxiety in another, and gain control of another's behavior.

Finally lying and truth-telling are important, if not controversial, examples of potentially aggressive acts. Social lies have been defined as lies designed to "spare another's feelings" (Bussey, 1992). Another way of defining social lies includes lies that are designed to help a person avoid being in an uncomfortable circumstance, sharing a difficult truth, or covering up an act of harm. Imagine the following scenario: A friend shares a personal secret with you and you agree not to tell anyone. You happen to tell the secret to another person and it gets back to your friend. Your friend asks you if you told the secret to anyone and you lie by denying it. One could argue that disclosing the secret was a deliberate act of harm and the lie further perpetuates the harm already caused. The truth in this case, will be painful and could cause greater distress in the moment, but that would not be the intention. Consider now difficult truths. In this case, you might be in the midst of a disagreement with a friend. You feel hurt by your friend and want to talk about your recent conflict. This will require you to talk about aspects of the interaction and actions by your friend that made you feel hurt. Your friend may have a difficult time accepting what you say in a nondefensive fashion. If your friend perceives your comments as hurtful and assumes the worst of you (i.e., that you intended to hurt her) does this make your honest disclosure an aggressive act? The point of this discussion is that aggression and defining an act as aggressive are necessarily complex and depend on perceptions of intent and experience of harm or hurt that can vary widely from person to person.

An important question to consider is whether manipulation constitutes a form of aggression. Manipulate is defined as "manag(ing) a person or situation to one's own advantage especially unfairly and unscrupulously" (*Oxford English Dictionary,* 1971, p. 1031). What is common between manipulation and troubling aspects of aggressive behavior is (a) the self-focus involved in behaving aggressively or manipulating, and (b) the co-opting or taking physically or psychically from another. Insofar as all acts of manipulation do not cause harm to another, then not all manipulation is "aggressive" in the sense of causing harm. But, manipulation, at its core, has the quality of influencing and asserting control over another through a variety of devices that can include threats of aggression (as in relational aggression) and lies. In one study, children and adults were asked to convince a peer that a poor tasting drink tasted good and that a peer should sample it (Keating & Heltman, 1994). Children received a reward if they could convince peers that the drink tasted good. The most successful children in this study showed a variety of positive behaviors toward peers (smiling and positive comments) and often lied about the taste of the drink to try and convince peers to believe it tasted good. Children who were effective at "convincing" or "manipulating" children more rarely used overtly aggressive tactics such as threats. In this case, children intended to convince peers that the drink tasted good, not to cause harm to the peers per se but for a rather self-centered reason—to get more of a reward. The point behind describing this study is to show once again that identifying what constitutes aggression—particularly effective, complex and sophisticated aspects of aggression—is not clear-cut.

Does the frequency of involvement in aggression tell us something about adaptation? Peer nominations give us a sense of which children typically engage in aggressive acts and their associated adjustment. As described in the opening section, the findings on this are variable. Beyond the type of aggression, one must also consider the severity and not just the frequency of engaging in aggressive acts. It is also possible that some children may engage in aggressive acts less frequently but when they do engage in these acts, they tend to cause greater harm or more serious harm to another. Most studies looking at the link between aggression and adaptation have not assessed this issue. As a result, little is known about the quality or the impact of serious but infrequent aggressive acts on adjustment. In much of the literature looking at aggression and adaptation, the frequency of engaging in aggression is what is studied, but we know little about children who act out aggressively only infrequently but do so more severely. This issue is not an idle concern. Indeed, some of the children who have engaged in shootings at schools appear to fit this profile.

How do we determine intentionality? One of the critical aspects of the definition of aggression is the idea that aggressive acts are intentional. But, who judges the intentionality of an act? What if the child asserts that he did not intend to harm another? Do we take the child at his word? Or do we use the peer group's view of intentionality? To our knowledge few (if any) studies have actually assessed the "alleged" aggressor's perception of his behavior. Crick and Dodge's (1994) work on the social information-processing model asks the victim how he/she perceives acts under accidental, ambiguous, and intentional circumstances, but no work has reported on a child's perception and view of their own real behavior toward a peer. In practice, most studies of aggression between children implicitly rely on the peer group's implicit judgment of intentionality. In other words, children nominate peers who, over time, they perceive as behaving aggressively. In these nominations, children are not explicitly asked to assess intentionality with questions like: "Who meant to hit and behave aggressively?" Nominations of children who are aggressive express the peer group's assumptions and attributions about a peer's behavior and liking of the peer may be confounded with this kind of judgment. As Hymel (1986) has shown, the actions of children who are well liked are judged more generously than the acts of peers who are disliked. Similarly, Ray, Norman, Sadowski, & Cohen's (1999) work on enemies informs us about the extent to which an enemy's actions in ambiguous and accidental circumstances are attributed to a desire to harm another. The point here is that liking (or disliking) may sway attributions of intentionality and that behavior may sway liking (or disliking) and then attributions. Perception of the "intent to harm" is often predicated on another's attribution for the behavior.

Taken together, this work suggests that attribution of the "intention to harm" is left to the judgment of the peer group. When one is unfamiliar with a peer, it can be especially difficult to assume intentionality behind behavior. It is likely that peers who are not well liked may be given little lee-way in how their behavior might be viewed and "intention to harm" might be assumed more readily. Another consideration in determining or attributing "intention to harm" is related to the type of aggression (i.e., physical, as opposed to more psychologically/verbal forms of aggression). It is easier to judge physical acts of aggression than it is to judge some aspects of verbal aggression such as aggressive humor, lying, or back-handed comments. With the exception of name-calling and direct insults, other forms of verbal aggression may be harder to observe, easier to cover up, harder for peers to judge the "intent to harm" and easier for aggressors to deny their "intent to harm."

Finally, a judgment about a child's "intent to harm" in committing aggressive acts can also be swayed by knowledge of the child's emotional state and emotional coping. It is unlikely to be adaptive if a child, in response to a range of feelings, always selects aggression as their preferred response. Children who characteristically respond to a variety of emotions by acting aggressively probably have a narrow repertoire and limited set of problem-solving skills. Furthermore, some emotions that precede or motivate the "intent to harm" (e.g., frustration, fear, anxiety) may involve self-oriented emotion regulation, although other emotions (e.g., jealousy, envy, revenge, or anger with another) have a more dyadic/relational or other-oriented quality. In essence, a judgment of aggression as adaptive or maladaptive depends on a contextualized understanding of the aggression, which includes an understanding of emotionally based coping.

WHAT CONSTITUTES HARM AND IS ALL AGGRESSION BAD?

The harm that aggression causes for others is one of the primary reasons why aggressive acts are deemed as bad. This criterion gives us an opportunity to evaluate acts according to how much they are driven by a desire to cause harm, and how much harm they cause. In this way, the question of whether aggression is related to adaptation can be assessed for acts that fit this criterion well and those that do so poorly.

One could begin by asking whether some types of aggression are "more harmful" than others. In large part, the answer to this depends on the severity of the aggression. A bruise will heal but a gunshot can kill. An off-beat joke at the expense of another can feel bad, but an insult that touches on an area of vulnerability can be remembered and replayed until one's dying day. Another way of looking at this issue is through the self-other dialectic. How much does an act of aggression harm another and benefit the self, or harm another and benefit others? Consider the following scenario:

> Albert sees his friend Henry in a disagreement with Tim. Henry had been taking turns playing with a truck with several other children. Tim approached the children and didn't want to wait his turn in line, got angry and grabbed the truck from Henry's hands. Albert sees this, walks up to Tim, pushes him over, and takes the truck back telling Tim "what you did isn't fair—you aren't playing nicely." Albert returns the truck to his friend Henry and joins the other children in the game.

In this scenario, Tim's act of aggression benefits himself and not others. Albert behaves aggressively in response to Tim's aggression toward Albert's friends. How do we judge Albert's behavior—did he behave aggressively and cause harm intentionally? Yes—he pushed over a peer and took a toy away. Is this act of aggression adaptive or maladaptive? Although Albert intended to harm Tim, he did so for prosocial reasons—to defend his friend and to address a situation he perceived as unfair. All at once, Albert's act is both aggressive and prosocial. To be sure, Albert could have asked Tim to return the truck, thus avoiding aggression, but the fact that he behaved aggressively to defend a friend would be regarded as an other-oriented act. In fact, he defends the value of "fair-play" and benefits by joining his friends in the game. Clearly some aggression may involve good social skills, when used in moderation.

There are other compelling examples of ways in which aggression may benefit others more than it harms. From the literature on bullying, we know that children who are victimized but who have friends who are strong and will defend them (i.e., potentially acting aggressively on their behalf) are less victimized over time (Hodges, Malone, & Perry, 1997). In this case, we assume that peers act aggressively for an "other-oriented" reason—that is to defend a friend. The basis for war is another compelling large-scale example of the ways in which not all aggression is necessarily "bad." Imagine a war that is initiated solely to capture land. In this case the aggression of a war causes the death of others because of a desire for land. Compare this type of war with one in which a nation engages in war to stop genocide and ethnic cleansing. In both war examples, people would be killed but in the latter example, in the service of putting a halt to the killing of innocent people. It goes without saying that it is clearly preferable not to have to go to war and to be able to use more prosocial strategies for stopping genocide (see Walzer, 2004). However, in the absence of workable prosocial strategies, aggression and harm may be necessary to stop a larger evil, specifically the slaughter of innocent people.

SUMMARY

The concept of aggression, judging the intentionality behind an act, assessing the harm an act causes, and deciding on the adaptiveness or maladaptiveness of an aggressive act are necessarily complex and multifaceted matters. A basic premise of our analysis is that the overuse of aggression is maladaptive as is its complete absence. To some degree, aggression or negative thoughts or behaviors more generally may be part of the human response repertoire. Who has not felt the need to return an insult when insulted first, to make a joke at another's expense, to tell a lie, gossip a little, or to engage in some private glee when a disliked other has experienced a setback? Nevertheless, people vary in the extent to which they use aggression and in the types of aggression that they use. Central to any assessment of aggression needs to be a consideration of the "intent to harm." In some cases, intent can be hard to detect (e.g., humor compared to hitting), making it an often subtle aspect of human exchange. We propose that the adaptiveness or the maladaptiveness of an aggressive act can be judged according to its repercussions for the self, the other, and the balance between them. Aggression is most maladaptive when it (a) subjects others to harm, and is intended to do so, and does not serve the larger group's goals; (b) is used consistently as one's preferred strategy for protection; and (c) when its intent and impact is unambiguous and especially harsh. Our goal is to show that an answer to the question of whether aggression is adaptive or maladaptive is necessarily complex. This complexity derives from basic questions about what it means to be a well-adapted person who can look out for the self and the other at the same time.

NEW THOUGHTS AND THREE CRITICAL FINDINGS

Three findings from the current debate about aggression and competence during early adolescence are especially intriguing. They are (a) that there

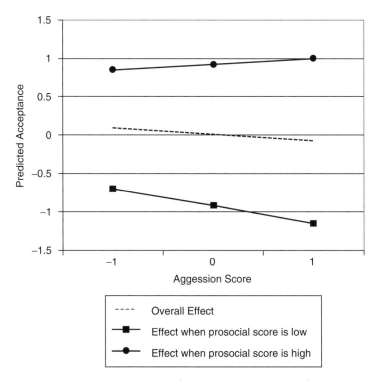

FIGURE 8.1.   Univariate and interactive associations between
aggression and acceptance among peers as a function of the
measure of prosocial tendencies.

is a curvilinear relationships between aggression and adaptation (Prinstein & Cillessen, 2003); (b) that children who are aggressive and prosocial are reasonably successful in their functioning with peers (Hawley, 2003); and (c) that measures of proactive aggression are less strongly associated with indices of adjustment than are measures of reactive aggression (Little et al., 2003; Poulin & Boivin, 2000). We use these findings as the empirical point of departure for some analyses of our own followed by some interpretation of these results using the self–other dialectic as our conceptual base.

The curvilinear function reported by Prinstein and Cillessen (2003) showed that the association between aggression and perceived popularity was defined by an inverted J curve. This curve showed that perceived popularity was highest among individuals who were a bit above the midpoint of a measure of aggression. It showed also that children who were highest in aggression were lowest in perceived popularity and that children who were lowest in aggression were a bit lower in

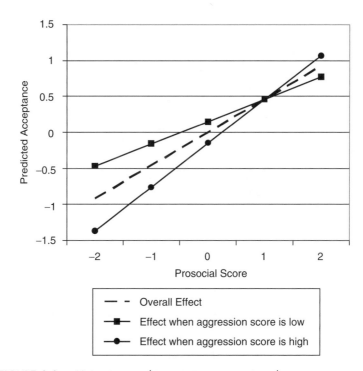

FIGURE 8.2.   Univariate and interactive associations between prosocial tendencies and acceptance among peers as a function of the measure of aggression.

perceived popularity than children at the midpoint of the aggression distribution. There are two important aspects of this finding: first, persons who study peer relations may wish to look beyond their nearly universal interest in linear effects. The second is that although high levels of aggression are accompanied by low levels of perceived popularity, low levels of aggression are not necessarily accompanied by high levels of popularity. Among the interpretations of these findings is that, to achieve a level of competence among peers, one needs to be able to engage in at least a minimal level of self-assertion. In contrast to interpretations based on linear results or extreme group comparisons, functioning with peers was not linked most directly with an absence of aggression. These findings confirm the idea that a balance between self and other promotes competence. Moreover, they imply that perhaps at one point along the distribution of aggression the level of harm that is committed surpasses a tolerable set point. In other words, self-assertion appears to be tolerated, or even valued, until it reaches a "tipping point" after which it has negative consequences.

The findings of Patricia Hawley (2003) regarding the association between aggression, prosocial tendencies and competence provide are an even more direct index that a balance of self and other may explain the factors underlying competence. Essentially, what she showed was that children who were aggressive were seen as competent if they were also prosocial. That is, even if a child commits acts that have negative consequences for others, the child would still be seen by peers as "acceptable" if they also did things to promote the well-being of others. This report that the presumably negative effects of aggression on competence can be mitigated by other-oriented tendencies is important as it shows that the significance of aggression needs to be considered from a contextual perspective. Apparently aggression can be part of the process underlying competence, so long as it occurs in the context of positive features.

In an attempt to replicate Hawley's results, we took a preliminary look at the association between measures of prosocial tendencies, aggression and peer acceptance in a study the first author is conducting. Using a sample of children and early adolescents (ages 9- to 12-years-old) from Montreal, in Quebec, and from Barranquilla, a large city on the Caribbean coast in northern Colombia in Latin America (N = ~900), we examined how perceptions of aggression and prosocial tendencies were related to a measure of acceptance among peers. Aggression and prosocial tendencies were measured with a nomination-based peer-assessment technique in which there were three items for aggression ("Someone who is mean," "Someone who hurts others," and "Someone who causes trouble") and two for prosocial tendencies ("Someone who cares about others," and "Someone who helps others"). The measure of acceptance was the number of times a child was chosen as a friend in an unlimited choice nomination-based sociometric questionnaire. All of these measures were based on same-sex assessment and were standardized within sex within classrooms.

Our findings very much confirmed Hawley's findings and maybe added a bit to them. Regression analyses revealed univariate associations and an interaction between the aggression and prosocial scores and the measure of acceptance. The findings are shown in Figures 8.1 and 8.2. The first figure shows that although the overall association between aggression and acceptance is negative, this association was positive among children whose prosocial scores were high (i.e., 1 s.d. above the mean)! That is, aggression is positively associated with peer acceptance for children who are also prosocial. The next figure shows that the overall association between the prosocial score and the measure of acceptance was positive, but that it was stronger for children whose aggression scores were high rather than low. In other words, aggression increased the strength of the association between acceptance and being prosocial. From within the frame of the self–other dialectic, these findings imply that perhaps a balance of self-assertion and concern for others is the royal road to being liked by peers.

A third finding deserves our attention because it shows that not all forms of aggression are related to measures of being accepted by peers. Again we propose that this observation can be explained by the notion of the balance between self and other. The finding is that measures of reactive aggression (i.e., that one acts aggressively following provocation) are more strongly negatively related to measures of functioning with peers than are measures of proactive aggression (i.e., acting aggressively to achieve instrumental goals and without have been provoked). This observation has been made in several independent studies (e.g.; Little et al, 2003; Poulin & Boivin, 2000; see Little & Card, 2005 for a review of this literature). From one perspective, this finding appears to be counterintuitive. If one presumes that an unprovoked act of aggression would be seen as less justifiable than an act that followed provocation, then one would expect that proactive aggression would be seen more negatively than an act of reactive aggression. But the database implies that the reverse of this pattern is true. Individuals who engage in reactive aggressions appear to be at higher risk for social maladjustment than individual who engage in proactive aggression.

Perhaps the critical distinction between these two forms of aggression does not derive directly from whether the aggressive act was provoked or not provoked. Instead, an important difference may be whether the aggressive act is specifically aimed at another person and was intended as a form of harm. To use language from the military, the damage from proactive aggression may be "collateral" or incidental rather than direct. That is, proactive aggression typically is motivated by a goal other than harm, although these acts may be harmful. In this way the harm associated with proactive aggression is not the intended outcome of the act, but is, instead, the unfortunate result of an effort to achieve an instrumental goal. In this way it was not directly aimed at a person (i.e., the other) with the intent to harm the person. Reactive aggression, however, is almost by definition aimed at another and is intended to harm. As an intentionally self-protective and other-directed harmful act, reactive aggression is apparently seen as a more negative form of behavior than is proactive aggression. Moreover, it is likely that in many cases reactive aggression could be the result of emotional regulation deficiencies that give the perpetrator the reputation as an undercontrolled and unpredictable person.

We have tried to explain these three sets of findings from the frame of the self/other dialectic and the related concept of harm. We have proposed that variation exists across the continuum of aggression and between measures of aggression in the extent to which acts are motivated by a self-focused instrumental concern or by a specific desire to harm others. This distinction between a self-focused or other-focused orientation can also be used to distinguish between measures of adaptation. For example, whereas some forms of adaptation refer to the control of resources, others refer to one's ability to function within social or interpersonal contexts. The repercussion of this delicate balance between the self–other dialectic is clear. Up to a certain point, the association between aggression and adaptation varies as a function of how much aggression disrupts the most critical aspects of someone's functioning, particularly their ability to function within groups and to form close relationships. For example, a child's ability to obtain and control the toys in his preschool classroom through the use of aggression is of little advantage if none of the child's peers wish to play with him.

"SURVIVOR," "BIG BROTHER," AND "THE APPRENTICE": REALITY TV AND AGGRESSION

The complexity of the association between aggression and well-being can be seen in places other than the research studies of social scientists. One of these is the ubiquitous domain of pop culture. The television shows that have drawn the attention of many teenagers give us one means of seeing the view of aggression in the lives of adolescents. Consider for example, the adolescent fondness for competitive reality television programs. In the past 5 years, teenage (and adult) audiences swarmed like locusts to shows where contestants stepped on each other, sometimes literally, to see who could survive, avoid being fired, or get the brass ring that holds the keys to the executive office. One could charitably imagine that the attraction of these shows derived from their postmodernist application of an ironic stance intended to expose the fundamental and inherent flaws of the dog-eat-dog sensibility of the capitalist system. Certainly the use of satire as a form of social commentary has always drawn attention. Nevertheless, the magnetic power of these shows appears to be due to their depiction, albeit exaggerated, of the subtle and not-so-subtle competitive processes that underlie the dynamics of social groups and interpersonal relationships. Perhaps the adolescents (of all ages!) who make up the audiences of these shows see the competitive and multidimensionally aggressive acts of the contestants/participants as very real manifestations of the Darwinian nature of social experience in the peer group. These shows offer viewers an "insider perspective" about how contestants truly feel about one

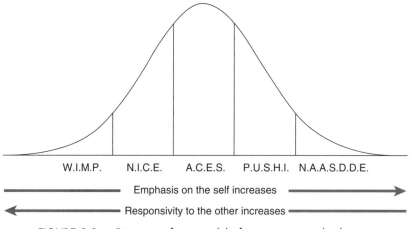

FIGURE 8.3.   Diagram of our model of aggression and adaptive
functioning using concepts of self and other.

another, their negative feelings and views, and their plans for developing alliances, and fostering doubt and rumor about rivals and the development of planned aggressions toward housemates or challengers.
Viewers see how contestants reason, manage, and manipulate feelings
and relationships with others to insure their continued survival. To win
at these games, one must show competence, social skill, aggression,
manipulation, and assertiveness when needed, while still being liked or
respected by competitors. The link between adaptation and aggression
is clearly evident in these shows.

There are, of course, other interpretations that do not directly invoke
notions of self and other and of harm. For example, an alternative explanation for the observation that children can be drawn to peers who are
above-average in aggression is that completely nonaggressive children
are simply boring. One does not need to be a devotee of Tolstoy to
believe that "all happy families are alike, all unhappy families are
unhappy in their own way" (Tolstoy, 1937, p. 1). In other words, the
unrelenting inhibited sameness and predictability of utterly non-aggressive people may make them hopelessly dull and uninteresting. The lack
of skill and vitality that likely prevents them from being able to "get up
and do what needs to be done" probably does not help them win friends
or be liked. On the other hand, it may be that the restlessness and non-
alikeness that is characteristic of highly assertive people can at times
give them an attractive dynamism that draws others to them. Utterly
nonaggressive people are no doubt deserving of our praise, but their
monotony may lead to habituation and a loss of interest from peers.

An explanation that the aggressive/prosocial child is liked more than a child who is prosocial only, can be found in the work of a literary critic (Howe, 1994). He claimed that among the most challenging Tasks for novelists is to portray goodness. Characters who have been portrayed as examples of goodness (in his words those who "hunger for a purpose, for a goal, beyond the mere gratification of ego"; 1994, p. 154)) are uninteresting to readers and need to be bolstered by other features in order to make them attractive. Apparently, extreme goodness alone is not enough to make someone attractive to others. Anyone who has ever seen the film the *Wizard of Oz* knows this already. The two witches in the film are literally black and white representatives of sweetness and nastiness. To us, at least, the "good witch" is a source of much genuine wise counsel and guidance for Dorothy and her little dog. But at times, this good witch is so sappy and sugar-coated that one can hardly imagine that hanging around with her would be very much fun. All of this is to say that the observation that moderately aggressive children can be attractive to peers may be due to the relative dullness and unattractiveness of peers who are utterly lacking in any self assertiveness.

A(NOTHER) TAXONOMY OF AGGRESSION

In this next-to-last section, we would like to propose a new taxonomy of aggression. Built on the ideas we have discussed so far, the purpose of this taxonomy is to organize our thinking about the association between aggression and adaptation. One can, of course, reasonably ask whether we really need another taxonomy of aggression. After all, several taxonomic schemes exist already. Currently, we can categorize aggression according to multiple systems. These systems can distinguish between forms of aggression (e.g., physical or relational), and the reasons that motivated it (e.g., proactive or reactive). Systems can also distinguish between individuals according to whether the individual's level of aggression is high, medium, or low, and how it changes—or doesn't change—over time. In spite of the categorical and taxonomic richness that exists already, we propose that another one may be needed.

The taxonomy we propose is largely descriptive. Its descriptions are functional rather than based on characteristics or features of particular acts. Specifically, it describes the people who fall at different places along a distribution according to how they have resolved the self–other dialectic. The categories we propose divide the "normal distribution" of aggression into five sections. Each section represents a different resolution of the self–other dialectic and shows how this resolution is manifested in aggression.

From the outset, we need to admit that this taxonomy is speculative but serious. To be sure, the labels that we give to our categories rely in a small way on terminological whimsy. Nevertheless, our proposed system has an empirical and conceptual base and our intentions are serious even when we inject some fun into our terminology. Our goal is to provide a taxonomy that has conceptual utility rather than an immediate empirical application. At some point, this approach might have a direct empirical value or application. At this point though, our goal is to present a provocative model that would encourage a view of aggression from a new light.

A schematic representation of our taxonomy is shown in Figure 8.3. The distribution is divided into five sections that differ in the extent to which the individuals in each group resolve the self–other dialectic by emphasizing the self or being responsive to the other. The categories are organized so that an emphasis on the self and the view of the self as entitled increases from left to right in the model. Along this same continuum, responsiveness to the other and the view of the other as entitled decreases. Accordingly, the least self-involved individuals who are most responsive to others are found in the far right-hand side of the distribution whereas the most self-involved and least other-oriented individuals are found on the right side. Individuals who fall at the midpoint of the distribution are those who balance the demands of self and others. In keeping with the findings presented earlier in this chapter, an explicit point of this system is that the best-adjusted children would be found at the midpoint of the distribution.

We have given a descriptive acronym to each of the five sections created in the distribution. As our readers will see, we composed these acronyms to evoke particular images. Our attempt at evocation should not imply that we are not serious in our effort to create a valuable taxonomic system. In our model the group to the far left (i.e., those who put little emphasis on the self and are overly sensitive to the demands of others) are known by the titular acronym W. I. M. P. These letters stand for "Without Immediate Means of Protection." These children are utterly lacking in aggressive tendencies and, as a result, are at considerable risk for being pushed around by others. It is likely that they feel anxious in the presence of others. Their sensitivity to others and to the entitlement of others is so strong that it overwhelms them and they run away from it. As members of groups, they let others "do the talking;" and they would rather "go with the flow" rather than be leaders or assert themselves. This group is likely to show elevated levels of passive withdrawal.

The second group from the left is given the title N. I. C. E. This acronym stands for "Non-Intrusive, Compromising, Egalitarian." These children are more likely to assert themselves than is the first group, but they still restrain themselves when it comes to getting what they want. They are oriented towards compromises and egalitarian circumstances even when it means that their goals are treated as less critical than those of others. Although their positive emphasis on values such as equality and self-restraint is admirable, this responsiveness to others may come at some cost to themselves. The children in this group tend to have some success in the domain of social achievement. According to findings shown in Figure 8.1, the children in this group are likely to experience reasonably strong levels of social acceptance from their peers.

The title A. C. E. S. is given to the middle group. The initials in this acronym represent the words "Assertive, appropriately Competitive, Effective, Sociable and sensitive." The children in this group have been able to find a balance between their own needs and desires and their sensitivity to the perspectives and rights of others. They can assert themselves while still recognizing the needs of others. They can be competitive without being driven by a need for dominance. Their aggression is manifested as assertiveness. Although this assertiveness helps them achieve their own goals, it does not interfere with or impede the activities of others. In this way, they are effective in accomplishing their own goals and can function as positive members of a group.

The fourth group is called P. U. S. H. I. The letters stand for "Pugnacious, Undercontrolled, Self-centered, Hubris, and Irritating." These children have their own agenda and wish that others would follow it. They either fail to see the needs and goals of others or simply choose to overlook them or regard them as less important than their own objectives. Their resolution of the self–other dialectic puts more emphasis on the self than the other. They like having their own way and will boldly go after it even if it means "getting into other people's faces." They are wont to complain and act out when their self-involved goals are not met. They show some level of sociability in the sense that they are motivated to be involved in relations with others, but they like these relations to conform to their personal objectives. Some of their peers may like them, but overall they are not well-liked and their constant self-focus and standard disregard for others is irritating.

The fifth group, found at the far right, is titled N. A. A. S. D. D. E. The letters in this acronym are the initials for "Negative Actions and Attitudes, Smug self-involvement, Destructive, Dysregulated, and Externalizing." This group places far more emphasis on the self than the other. They have a condescending view toward others, seeing them as undeserving or whose actions and goals are trivial or illegitimate. They maintain a very positive view of themselves and regard themselves as justified to act in aggressive ways, including both instrumental or proactive acts and reactive acts as a form or retaliation. Their actions are literally antisocial in the sense that they act against others. These are the children who are furthest to the right on the curve shown in Figure 8.1. Very few peers, if any, like them.

As we have stated already, the system we have proposed is intended to be provocative. The three points that we hope to convey in this system are (a) that the concepts of self and other can be used to describe children at different points along the continuum of aggression; (b) that one can use these concepts to explain why adaptation is highest at moderate points along this continuum; and (c) that the quality of aggression changes across the continuum. This system calls out for further elaboration and empirical scrutiny.

HARRY POTTER AND THE SOCIAL SCIENTIST'S TALE

In this final section of this chapter, we return to the world of popular culture, as we refer to a highly popular character who is not free of aggressive acts. This example shows that one does not need to turn to the ideas of social scientists to find ways of understanding how aggression and adaptation are interrelated. Instead, sometimes one can turn to the list of "best-sellers" to find stories that enlighten. Of all the stories ever told about a young person, few have captured a world-wide audience as thoroughly as the story of Harry Potter (Rowling, 1998, 1999a, 1999b, 2000, 2005). Millions and millions of readers, many of them young and all young at heart, have followed the adventures of the bespectacled English early-adolescent as he has made his way through life in his school. It is true that some recalcitrant Muggles continue to see the multivolume story about Harry and his schoolmates as a simple tale about magic, wizardry, and witchcraft. Some writers, such as Stephen King (2000) and Alison Lurie (1999), have gone so far as to make this claim in print. Over time though, most enlightened persons have come to see the story about Harry as a parable about friendship, goodness, and the process of growing up in the company of one's peers. By nearly any definition, Harry is competent, if not extra-competent. He is well-liked, helpful, appropriately competitive, clever, smart, engaging, funny, loyal, sociable, and, yes, at times, a bit aggressive (at least by some definitions). He revels in the warmth of the active, chaotic, and dynamic energy of the Weasley home, his adoptive family. At school, Harry is willing to fight for the good when circumstances call for it. His aggression is regulated and serves functions that most people would regard as acceptable. On our proposed taxonomy, Harry would likely fall into the A.C.E.S. category. He is not excessive, self-centered, or indiscriminately harmful. Harry uses aggression as a means of self assertion to achieve goodness when all else has failed. These moments of aggression are not antithetical to the many traditionally positive features we all see in Harry. Instead, they complement them. No one objects when he stands up, even aggressively, to the dreaded and nasty (or N.A.A.S.D.E.E.) members of Slytherin, or to Voldemort. The unbridled aggression of Harry's foes confirms the existence of the first universe that we described at the outset of this chapter (i.e., that aggression is negative); the actions of Harry and his friends confirm the existence of the second universe. Harry's readers are with him as they wait, anxiously, for the anticipated moment of his fateful face-to-face encounter with Snape, and, of course, with the extra-evil and horrid Voldemort. Will Harry be aggressive, or even destructive, when these moments arrive? We don't know yet, but many of us, in our least-pretentious moments, probably hope so and we wouldn't blame him if he were.

CONCLUSIONS

The association between aggression and adaptation is neither simple nor linear. The complex nature of this association derives from the complex nature of both aggression and adaptation. Each of these phenomena is multifaceted and has multiple manifestations and meanings across a broad continuum. The conceptual point of departure for our inquiry into the association between adaptation and aggression is the dialectic between self and other. We argue that, to some degree, self-assertion and competitiveness are necessary for adaptation, as they promote one's ability to achieve personal goals. Perhaps by definition, however, acts of aggression contradict one's capacity to function with others. Insofar as aggression has been often defined as intent to harm, being aggressive means that one is acting against others. According to the view we discuss, adaptation and aggression are related to each other in a curvilinear manner. We propose that individuals who do not assert themselves are at risk for being taken advantage of by others and they fail to garner critical resources. Persons who engage in self-assertion to the point of hurting others, however, not only disrupt group functioning but, in doing so, they deny themselves opportunities for basic forms of human relationship. The study of the association between aggression and adaptation needs to be sensitive to many processes and constraints. Although aggression should be discouraged in many cases, at some times it may be an adaptive or even necessary response. If you don't believe us, ask Harry Potter instead.

ACKNOWLEDGMENTS

Work on this chapter was supported by a grant to the first author from the Social Sciences and Humanities Research Council of Canada and by a faculty release time award granted to the second author from Colby-Sawyer College. Direct correspondence to the first author at Department of Psychology and Centre for Research in Human Development, Concordia University, 7141 rue Sherbrooke Ouest, Montréal, Québec, CANADA, H4B 1R6.

REFERENCES

Bukowski, W. M., Sippola, L., & Newcomb, A. F., (2000). Variations in patterns of attraction to same- and other-sex peers during early adolescence. *Developmental Psychology, 36,* 147–154.

Bussey, K. (1992). Lying and truthfulness: Children's definitions, standards, and evaluative reactions. *Child Development, 63,* 129–137.

Cairns, R., Xie, H., & Leung, M. (1998). The popularity of friendship and the neglect of social networks: Toward a new balance. In W. M. Bukowski & A. H. Cillessen (Eds.), *Sociometry then and now: Building on six decades of measuring children's experiences with the peer group* (pp. 25–53). San Francisco: Jossey-Bass.

Crick, N. (1995). Relational aggression: The role of intent attributions, feelings of distress and provocation type. *Development and Psychopathology, 7,* 313–322.

Crick, N. R. & Dodge, K. A. (1994). A review and reformulation of social information-processing mechanisms in children's social adjustment. *Psychological Bulletin, 115,* 74–101.

Crick, N., & Grotpeter, J. (1996). Children's treatment by peers: Victims of relational and overt aggression. *Development and Psychopathology, 7,* 313–322.

Freud, S. (1976). *Jokes and their relation to the unconscious.* Harmondsworth, NY: Penguin. (Original work published in 1905)

Hawley, P. (2003). Prosocial and coercive configurations of resource control in early adolescence: A case for the well-adapted Machiavellian. *Merrill-Palmer Quarterly, 49,* 279–309.

Hodges, E. V. E., Malone, M. J., & Perry, D. G. (1997). Individual risk and social risk as interacting determinants of victimization in the peer group. *Developmental Psychology, 33,* 1032–1039.

Hymel, S. (1986). Interpretations of peer behavior: Affective Bias in childhood and adolescence. *Child Development, 57,* 321–447.

Howe, I. (1994). Absolute goodness and the limits of fiction. In N. Howe (Ed.), *A critic's notebook* (pp. 127–139). New York: Harcourt Brace.

King, S. (July 23, 2000). Wild about Harry. *New York Times Book Review,* Section 7, p. 134.

Keating, C., & Heltman, K., (1994). Dominance and deception in children and adults: Are leaders the best misleaders? *Personality and Social Psychology Bulletin, 20,* 312–321.

Laursen, B., & Hoff, E. (2006). Person centered and variable centered approaches to longitudinal data. M*errill-Palmer Quarterly, 52,* 377–389.

Little, T. D., Brauner, J., Jones, S. M., Nock, M. K., & Hawley, P. H. (2003). Rethinking aggression: A typological examination of the functions of aggression. *Merrill-Palmer Quarterly, 49,* 343–369.

Little, T. D., & Card, N. A. (2005). On the use of social relations and actor-partner interdependence models in developmental research. *International Journal of Behavioral Development, 29*(2), 173–179.

Lurie, A. (December 16, 1999). "Not for muggles." *The New York Review (of books),* pp. 6–9.

Newcomb, A. F., Bukowski, W. M., & Pattee, L. (1993). Children's peer relations: A meta-analytic review of popular, rejected, neglected, controversial, and average sociometric status, *Psychological Bulletin, 113,* 99–128.

Oxford English Dictionary. (1971). *The compact Oxford English Dictionary.* Oxford, UK: Clarendon Press.

Poulin, F., & Boivin, M. (2000). Reactive and proactive aggression: Evidence of a two-factor model. *Psychological Assessment, 12,* 115–122.

Prinstein, M., & Cillessen, M. (2003). Aggression to protect one's status among peers: Forms and functions of adolescent aggressive behavior in a social context. *Merrill-Palmer Quarterly, 49,* 310–342.

Ray, G., Norman, M., Sadowski, C., & Cohen, R., (1999). The role of evaluator–victim relationships in children's evaluations of peer provocations. *Social Development, 8*(3) 380–394.

Rowling, J. K. (1998). *Harry Potter and the philosopher's stone.* London: Bloomsbury.

Rowling, J. K. (1999). *Harry Potter and the chamber of secrets.* London: Bloomsbury.

Rowling, J. K. (1999). *Harry Potter and the prisoner of Azkaban.* London: Bloomsbury.

Rowling, J .K. (2000). *Harry Potter and the goblet of fire.* London: Bloomsbury.

Rowling, J. K. (2005). *Harry Potter and the half blood prince.* London: Bloomsbury.

Tolstoy, L. (1937). *Anna Karenina.* New York: Random House. (Original work published 1877)

Walzer, M. (2004). *Arguing about war.* New Haven, CT: Yale University Press.

9

SOCIAL SYNCHRONY, PEER NETWORKS, AND AGGRESSION IN SCHOOL

Thomas W. Farmer
The Pennsylvania State University

Hongling Xie
Temple University

Beverley D. Cairns
Bryan C. Hutchins
University of North Carolina at Chapel Hill

> In the course of living, all individuals must serve two masters simultaneously: the need to maintain internal consistency and personal integration through independent action, and the need to synchronize these actions with those of other persons. Given that the needs of two persons are rarely identical, the potential for mutual disruption is enormous.
>
> —Cairns, Neckerman, and Cairns (1989, p. 281)

The quote just cited captures three important concepts in development. First, it recognizes that factors both internal and external to the individual contribute to social interchanges and interactional patterns. Second, it suggests that children develop within dynamic and fluid social contexts. Third, it implies that developmental adaptation naturally arises from the possibility for conflict and aggression as persons must calibrate their individual needs with social demands. To understand the adaptive functions of aggression in development, it is helpful to consider how these three concepts come together to guide the establishment, maintenance, and reorganization of behavior patterns in childhood and adolescence. By focusing on social synchrony and social networks in school, the goal of this chapter is to elucidate key ways in which aggressive expression contributes to adaptation at the individual, social structural, and institutional levels.

SOCIAL INTERCHANGES AND INTERACTIONAL PATTERNS

The Self and Social Interactions

The development of the child's personality could not go on at all without the constant modification of his sense of himself by suggestions from others. So, he himself, at every stage, is really in part someone else, even in his own thoughts of himself. (Baldwin, 1897, p. 30)

As children develop, their interactions with others play an important role in their beliefs, values, and behaviors (Youniss, 1980). The immediate controls of the actions of a child in a social interchange rests in the behavior of the other person or persons involved in the interaction (Sears, 1951). Yet, social actions are multi-determined and involve the contributions of genetic, neurobiological, endocrinological, cognitive, social network, and cultural factors (Cairns, 1979). Therefore, when a child interacts with others there is necessarily an ongoing coordination or calibration between the capacities and propensities of the self and the needs of others (Cairns, 2000). When the needs of the self are counter to the demands of the context, the outcome may be adaptation in the behavior and internal states of the child, accommodations within the social ecology, or disruption of the interchange and, perhaps, the relationship (Cairns & Cairns, 1994).

Given that social interactions during childhood are often between children with competing needs and desires, it is reasonable to expect that conflict and disagreements would be commonplace. This discord is not necessarily undesirable. On the contrary, the development of the self involves a number of safeguards such that interpersonal discord and even aggression may be viewed as normative developmental processes that support adaptation (Cairns & Cairns, 2000; Cairns, Neckerman, & Cairns, 1989; Hood, 1996). These safeguards include social norms and adult guidance, peer co-construction of beliefs and values, social organization and social structures, and institutional supports.

As Youniss (1980) describes, children experience two distinct social worlds. One world involves interactions with adults, particularly parents.

A central focus of interchanges between adults and young children is to teach the child the expectations, norms, and rules of the culture and society in which the child is embedded. In adult–child relations, the two individuals are on unequal footing. The adult operates from a position of authority and her or his role is to impart critical information to the child. The child's role is to learn from the adult. Although they are not on equal footing with adults, a child's engagement in adult–child interchanges is critical for her or his understanding of societal norms and rules. Therefore, the adult typically attempts to pace their own behavior to correspond with and extend the abilities of the child. The second social world of the child involves interactions with peers. Unlike interchanges with adults, children of the same age come to the interaction on equal footing (cf. Hawley, this volume). Rather than adopting the rules and expectations of the other as in adult–child interactions, participants in child–child interactions are free to exert their own will and views. In so doing, they are in a position where, to achieve their own needs and goals, they must align their behavior with the goals and needs of the other. Thus, within these two worlds, the child receives two different supports for promoting their behavioral adaptation. One support involves adopting general social values and norms as directed by adults, whereas the other involves the co-construction of social rules and beliefs in interchanges with peers. These two interactional patterns reflect different safeguards for promoting adaptive social behaviors and involve distinct forms of social synchrony.

Social Synchrony

The concept of social synchrony refers to interchanges in which the behaviors of two individuals are mutually coordinated so that the actions of each support the actions of the other (Cairns, Neckerman, & Cairns, 1989). Cairns (1979) describes two forms of social synchrony: reciprocity and complementarity.

Reciprocity. The term reciprocity refers to social interchanges in which the acts of two or more persons support each other in a relationship and their actions become similar to each other. With reciprocal interactions, the actors tend to have equal status and are free to respond to each other in a similar fashion. Therefore, with reciprocity the action of one individual is likely to produce a similar action from the other individual.

Complementarity. The term complementarity refers to social interchanges in which the acts of two individuals are distinct from the acts of the other. However, the actors are mutually dependent in that the actions of each person are necessary to support the actions of the other. Examples include follower–leader, teacher–student, and bully–victim. The critical component of complementarity is that the actors are of unequal status, but the role of each requires the role of the other. Therefore, although the two individuals act in distinct ways, the meaning or impact of the behavior is not realized without the behavior of the other.

Adult–child interactions reflect complementary interchanges and serve as one form of social safeguard against frequent expressions of aggression. When children interact with adults they typically learn generally accepted social norms and rules (Youniss, 1980). When children interact with other children of similar status they bring these norms and rules to the interchange. When they are from similar backgrounds and cultures, rules and expectations serve to provide children with a common or similar base for their interactions and likely include strategies to handle or reduce conflict. However, when the rules or norms do not mesh or the children do not accurately enact what they have been taught, there is a strong probability of disagreement as each child attempts to exert their will and needs over the other. Reciprocity can serve as a second safeguard in such circumstances. As the interchange becomes more heated, children may recognize that if they act on their own volitions, they run the risk of escalating the situation to aggressive conflict. The possibility of the aggressive disruption of the interchange and the relationship may serve as an outer boundary that prompts the actors to reconsider their actions and adapt their behaviors. In turn, each participant may develop new social cognitions that they co-construct as they coordinate their behaviors (Cairns, Neckerman, & Cairns, 1989; Youniss, 1986). Thus, the possibility of aggression may promote interpersonal coordination and social growth.

Organizational and Institutional Supports

In early childhood, young children need direct support and guidance in their actions with same-age mates (Youniss, 1980). During the preschool years, adult caregivers in organized day-care settings tend to provide a range of supports for toddlers and young children depending on the children's abilities to synchronize and regulate their behavior with others (Holmberg, 1980). In the preschool and early elementary school years, young children form social structures that include dominance hierarchies and the formation of distinct peer groups (Estell, Cairns, Farmer, & Cairns, 2002; Farver, 1996; Strayer & Santos, 1996). The propensity for children to organize themselves into complex social structures grows directly from their efforts to synchronize and coordinate their behaviors across a broad pool of potential playmates and associates (Cairns & Cairns, 1986).

Both reciprocity and complementarity come into play as children organize their social world. Reflecting processes of reciprocity, children are attracted to others who are similar to them (e.g., Cairns, Xie, & Leung, 1998). As they develop stable affiliations, children who associate together are likely to become more similar as they interact with each other and co-construct new beliefs and viewpoints during their social interchanges. However, some children may bring skills and characteristics to the interchange that place them in positions of higher status. These youth are likely to take on dominant or leadership positions within the peer group and the general social structure (Strayer & Noel, 1986; Strayer & Trudel, 1984). Reflecting processes of complementarity, such youth may use a range of social behaviors including social manipulation and aggression to influence the behaviors of their peers. In this regard, dominant children may engage in conflictual and negative interchanges that nonetheless directly impact the behaviors of others and support their leadership roles (Hawley, 1999; 2003; Vaughn, Vollenweider, Bost, Azria-Evans, & Snider, 2003). Through processes of reciprocity, group boundaries may be established and consolidated as group members interact more frequently and positively with other group members and engage in more conflictual and negative patterns and relationships with peers who are not in their group (Gest, Farmer, Cairns, & Xie, 2003; Haselager, Hartup, van Lieshout, & Riksen-Walraven, 1998; Nangle, Erdley, Zeff, Stanchfield, & Gold, 2004, Rodkin, Pearl, Farmer, & Van Acker, 2003; Rose, Swenson, & Carlson, 2004). Through complementary relationships, dominant group leaders may use both prosocial and aggressive strategies to build support of followers within the group and to protect possible challenges to their leadership from others both within and outside the group (Adler & Adler, 1998; Farmer, Estell, Bishop, O'Neal, & Cairn, 2003; Hawley, Little, & Pasupathi, 2002).

The offshoot is that episodes of conflict and aggression may help facilitate interpersonal growth, social organization, and the establishment of a social order that ultimately serves to reduce the frequency and severity of aggressive expression (e.g., Pellegrini & Bartini, 2001; Strayer & Noel, 1986). Leaders of schools and other social institutions that group children together are often aware of the need to provide guidance and monitoring on one hand and the need for children to develop their own social order on the other (Cairns & Cairns, 1994). Aggression becomes both a boundary and a marker for the give and take between natural social dynamics and institutional intervention. Therefore, although concern about children and youth who develop consolidated patterns of antisocial behavior is warranted, aggressive expression appears to have a variety of important functions in human development (Cairns & Cairns, 2000; Strayer & Noel, 1986). The commonplace role of aggression in social development comes into better focus by a careful examination of the contributions of aggression to classroom and school social dynamics.

SCHOOL SOCIAL NETWORKS, SOCIAL STRUCTURES, AND AGGRESSION

Social structures naturally develop as children establish synchronous relationships with others. Children who frequently interact with each other tend to share the same preferences for activities and to have similar patterns of interactions with the available pool of peers (Gest et al., 2003; Strayer & Trudel, 1984). Consequently, efforts to synchronize behavior across a large pool of classmates result in the formation of distinct peer groups. As groups develop within classrooms and schools, hierarchical social structures emerge with some groups and individuals having greater influence and status than others (Adler & Adler, 1996; Cairns, Perrin, & Cairns, 1985; Farmer & Rodkin, 1996). Hierarchical social structures can promote order and reduce the overall level of conflict and aggression as children navigate their social worlds (Strayer & Noel, 1986). However, expressions of aggression also arise out of children's efforts to establish and maintain social positions that support and promote their own needs and goals (see Card & Little, this volume; see also, Adler & Adler, 1995; Hawley, 2003). The complex role of aggression in children's social relations can be clarified by examining the interplay between peer groups, hierarchical social structures, and strategies of influence within the peer social system.

Peer Affiliations and Hierarchical Social Structures

Peer Group Homophily.   Children have a tendency to associate with peers who are similar to them on key interpersonal variables including academic achievement, aggression, leadership, and popularity (Cairns, Cairns, Neckerman, Gest, & Gariépy, 1988; Edwards, 1994; Espelage, Holt, & Henkel, 2003; Estell et al., 2002; Farmer & Hollowell, 1994; Farver, 1996; Leung, 1996; Rose, Swenson, & Carlson, 2004; Xie, Cairns, & Cairns, 1999). This propensity is known as homophily and it reflects two different aspects of social synchrony. First, it suggests that as children develop relationships, they tend to select associates with whom they can easily coordinate their activities and needs. The selection of similar peers facilitates the reciprocal coordination of interactions. Second, reciprocal interchanges result in the co-construction of social beliefs and the coordination of behavior patterns as children affiliate together over time (Berndt, 1979; Cairns & Cairns, 1994; Kandel, 1978; Kindermann, 1993). As a result, many classrooms have groups that are composed of high concentrations of aggressive children who support each others' behavior (Cairns et al., 1988; Farmer & Hollowell, 1994; Farver, 1996).

Peer group heterogeneity.   Although there is a propensity for youth to develop affiliations with similar peers, there is also considerable heterogeneity in children's peer groups. Recent work indicates that children who affiliate together may be similar on some characteristics but not on all of the characteristics. For example, a significant proportion of children and adolescents who are characterized as Model (i.e., high teacher ratings for studious, prosocial, popular) tend to associate with peers who are rated as Tough (i.e., popular, aggressive). In turn, non-aggressive children who are not popular and who have few positive characteristics tend to affiliate with aggressive unpopular peers (Estell, Farmer, Pearl, Van Acker, & Rodkin, 2003; Farmer et al. 2003; Farmer et al., 2002). In such groups, children with different characteristics may have distinct but mutually supportive social roles.

These findings suggest that complementarity as well as homophily are likely to be involved in the formation and maintenance of peer groups. That is, children are likely to not only associate with peers who are similar to them but also with peers who complement their behaviors and skills. Otherwise, it would be difficult for children to find their own unique social roles and positions within the peer group. Further, with complementary social roles, children are able to foster alliances and mutually dependent relationships that can help to consolidate and sustain their own social positions.

Social Network Centrality and Social Roles.   Some children are more influential than others, both within the peer group and the broader social structure (Adler & Adler, 1996; Cairns, Leung, Buchanan, & Cairns, 1995; Corsaro & Eder, 1990). Such youth are viewed as having nuclear centrality and are core members of the peer group. The most central members tend to be leaders within the peer group and, in some cases, may be viewed as leaders for the classroom in general. Other nuclear youth are typically in supportive roles to the leader but sometimes they may actually vie for status and influence with the leader (Adler & Adler, 1995; Eder, 1985; Merten, 1996). Some group members have secondary levels of centrality. These children are clearly part of the group but typically in the role of a follower, and their influence depends on their relationship with the leaders of the group. Still other group members may be viewed as peripheral. Although some may make frequent attempts to interact with group members and be part of the group, their identity with the group is often not acknowledged by nuclear members (Adler & Adler, 1995; Cairns et al., 1995). Others may float among several groups, or form groups with marginal salience. Finally, a small proportion of children are not members of peer groups. These youth are viewed as being socially isolated and are vulnerable to being bullied and victimized by peers (Evans & Eder, 1993).

Social Influence Within the Peer System

As just indicated, children who are most influential in the social structure are considered to be nuclear and tend to be leaders of their peer groups. However, different leaders may have very different roles within the social structure depending both on their own skills and characteristics and the characteristics of their peer group. Often the activities of the individuals in this role center around consolidating their power, maintaining their influence over their closest associates, and protecting the boundaries of the peer group (Adler, Kless, & Adler, 1992; Eder, Evans, & Parker, 1995; Merten, 1997). Likewise, other children within the group may be focused on maintaining or improving their own social positions. This includes trying to stay in good favor with the group leaders while simultaneously protecting against be displaced by others either from within or outside of the group. During uncertain times when the social hierarchy is not clearly defined (i.e., the beginning of preschool, the transition to middle school), the social context may be particularly susceptible to various expressions of aggression (Merten, 1997; Pellegrini & Bartini, 2001; Strayer & Noel, 1986).

Protecting Social Positions and Group Boundaries. Peer groups tend to be gender specific and usually take on distinct identities within the social structure. The more salient peer groups are identifiable by the prominent features of their nuclear members such as the "popular" groups, the "athletes or jocks," and the "good students" or "nerds" (Eder, Evans, & Parker, 1995; Farmer & Farmer, 1996; Kinney, 1993). By late childhood or early adolescence, the characteristics of a child's peer group and the position that the child has in the group can be an important part of her or his identity. Many children are concerned with gaining favor with higher status peers and associating with peers in higher status groups. Accordingly, they may attempt to enhance their social positions by building coalitions and by prompting the demotion or social ostracism of rivals. This is done through such strategies as gossiping, starting rumors, manipulation of friendships, abandoning existing friendships for higher status peers, or developing friendships with peers who will help to challenge the social power of one's adversaries.

This can be a high-stakes game as youth approach early adolescence. On one hand, many children feel compelled to establish as many close associations as possible to ensure a strong base of peer support and acceptance. On the other hand, they must be careful not to compromise the boundaries of their peer group and jeopardize their own status by associating with others who do not fit within the parameters of the group's identity (Adler & Adler, 1995; Eder & Parker, 1987; Evans & Eder, 1993). This balancing act results in some interesting paradoxes as youth who are viewed as popular leaders may become highly disliked by their peers, and youth who are not considered to be popular may be able to reinvent themselves and achieve higher status in the social structure (Eder, 1985; Farmer et al., 2003; Kinney, 1993). This reflects the fact that late childhood and early adolescence is a period of high social vulnerability and opportunity and a time when all youth may be susceptible to involvement in various forms of aggressive expression.

Social Dominance, Physical Aggression, and Bullying. Studies that use social network centrality, peer nominations of popularity, or teacher ratings of popularity to measure students' social status indicate that some highly aggressive children (particularly boys) have high positions in the classroom or school social structure (Farmer & Rodkin, 1996; LaFontana & Cillessen, 2002; Lease, Kennedy, & Axelrod, 2002; Rodkin, Farmer, Pearl, & Van Acker, 2000). These findings are consistent with naturalistic observations of boys' playground behavior. Pellegrini (1995) found that boys used rough-and-tumble play to establish dominance in the social hierarchy as they began middle school. Rough behavior on the playground was negatively correlated with peer nominations for being liked but, positively correlated with peer ratings of social dominance. Boys who were nominated by peers as tough systematically chose less tough boys to exploit during rough play. Pellegrini and Smith (1998) suggest that rough-and-tumble play may be used to assess the strength and toughness of others in the peer group and to display one's prowess publicly to establish dominance. This is consistent with ethnographic work that suggests that children selectively identify targets that are not able to challenge them and that they use such episodes to consolidate their dominance in the social structure (Adler & Adler, 1996; Evans & Eder, 1993).

Social dominance and influence in the social structure also come into play in bullying. Although some bullies are themselves aggressive victims, many have high social positions and are able to engage peers to support their behavior (Atlas & Pepler, 1998; Pepler, Craig, & Roberts, 1998). In fact, bullying episodes in elementary school tend to involve several peers as onlookers, helpers, and encouragers. Although some children (particularly girls) come to the aid of the targeted child, many youth appear to respond in ways that are aimed at protecting their status in the social structure. The work by Salmivalli and colleagues (Salmivalli, Huttunen, & Lagerspetz, 1997; Salmivalli, Lagerspetz, Björkqvist, Osterman, & Kaukiainen, 1996) suggest that some classroom's social structures promote bullying behavior. These researchers found that bullies associated with peers who assisted or reinforced their behavior, and they had larger social networks than peers who were victims, defenders, or outsiders. Other work suggests that bullies are more likely to be nominated as group leaders than are other boys, particularly when they are members of aggressive peer groups (Estell, Farmer, & Cairns, in press). Collectively, the research on social dominance and bullying suggests that aggression is related to social power and that highly aggressive leaders are able to use both aggressive strategies and their ability to influence others as a means to sustain dominant positions in the school social structure. This corresponds with the view that some bullies have high levels of social competence (e.g., Sutton, Smith, & Swettenham, 1999).

Social Aggression and Social Network Centrality. In early adolescence, youth begin to develop a more sophisticated understanding of social relationships. During this period, girls show a significant decrease in the use of physically aggressive responses to interpersonal conflict and begin to use more concealed strategies that involve the social network (Cairns, Cairns, Neckerman, Ferguson, & Gariépy, 1989; Xie, Swift, Cairns, & Cairns, 2002). The term social aggression has been used to refer to actions whereby interpersonal damage is achieved by nonconfrontational and largely concealed methods that employ the social community. These strategies include starting rumors, gossiping, social ostracism, and character defamation (Xie, Cairns, & Cairns, 2002). Youth who are adept at social aggression tend to have high social network centrality and a relatively good understanding of the dynamics of the classroom or school social context (Xie, Cairns, & Cairns, 2005; Xie, Farmer, & Cairns, 2003; Xie, Swift, et al., 2002). This seems to be a logical requirement as it would be difficult for low-status youth with little understanding of classroom social relations to effectively activate the social network (Xie, Cairns, & Cairns, 2002).

Research on social aggression contributes three important points for understanding the linkages between aggression and adaptation. First, it suggests that aggression does not always involve physical force but that it can also be expressed by more subtle forms that may (by virtue of being concealed) protect the identity and security of the aggressor. Second, it suggests that aggression sometimes involves sophisticated cognitive processes and requires the ability to influence others within the social community. Third, the fact that social aggression is concealed and can be employed without someone's knowledge may actually serve as a significant deterrent to more physical forms of aggressive transgressions. Rather than relying on physical forces, physically weaker children may employ social aggression to negotiate their social relationships and maintain social status (Little, Brauner, Jones, Nock, & Hawley, 2003). The advantage of being able to conceal one's identity with social aggression can be also seen in the decreased likelihood of punishment and retaliation (Xie, Swift et al., 2002). Given societal sanctions against physical aggression, some children may opt to use social aggression rather than physical aggression. These three points converge to suggest that social aggression may be a highly adaptive form of aggressive expression (Cairns & Cairns, 2000).

When aggression is considered in light of processes of social synchrony and the negotiation of school social networks, its adaptive functions come into focus. During childhood and early adolescence, aggression is a natural part of peer relationships and school dynamics. As children develop relationships with others, there is a tendency for considerable jockeying for new relationships and higher status. Although clear social structures develop as early as preschool, peer groups and social positions are highly dynamic and fluid throughout childhood and adolescence (Cairns & Cairns, 1994). As children establish their identities through their relationships with others, they learn to use aggressive strategies to both protect and enhance their standing in both the peer group and the broader social structure. Rather than being viewed as a basis for psychopathology, it is likely that these experiences can become an opportunity to learn more sophisticated skills for managing conflict and relationships (Cairns & Cairns, 2000; Vaughn et al., 2003). This concept is reflected in the high social centrality of girls who adeptly use the social network as a means of expressing aggression (Xie, Cairns, & Cairns, 2005) and in the characteristics of the well-adapted Machiavellian who uses both prosocial and aggressive strategies to meet their social needs (Hawley, 2003). The adaptive functions of aggression can be more fully understood by examining how social interactions contribute to developmental reorganization at the individual, social structural, and institutional levels.

SOCIAL INTERACTIONS, SYSTEMS REORGANIZATION, AND ADAPTATION

As suggested in the previous discussion, aggressive expression can play an important role in the development and change of children's social networks in the classroom and school. As children learn to coordinate their behaviors with others, there will be missteps along the way that may escalate toward aggressive episodes. Further, many children will experience significant shifts in their peer affiliations and social positions as social networks develop and evolve both over the course of the school year and across school years (Cairns & Cairns, 1994; Cairns et al., 1995). Changes in an individual's behavior patterns and her or his position within the school social structure tend to go hand in hand. In many cases, such changes may involve various forms of aggression. In considering the role of aggression in adaptation, it is important to recognize the primacy of social interactions in the realignment of behavior patterns and the calibration of developmental systems (Cairns, 2000):

> Developmental science presupposes integration of influences within and without the individual. On this score, social interactions occur at the interface between individuals and their context. Hence the analysis cannot be reduced to one without information from the other. This methodological assumption leads inevitably to the implication that social interactions require a level of mutual analysis that is radically different from the one traditionally endorsed in psychology. Rather than focus exclusively on individual states or individual variables, the organizing units over time become the dynamic interactions in which persons are involved in particular contexts. A new set of theoretical and design considerations—for example, the bidirectionality of feedback between internal states and external stimulation, the need to include level of analyses that describe interactional units rather than persons—must come into play. (p. 55)

Accordingly, changes in the developmental trajectories and behavior patterns of individuals should be examined in relation to the alignment of internal and external influences. Various factors in development operate in a correlated and bidirectional fashion (Cairns, 1979). Because it is highly malleable and open to rapid reorganization in response to changes in other developmental factors (e.g., biophysical, cognitive, contextual), behavior operates as a leading edge in individual adjustment (Cairns & Cairns, 2000). That is, change in one factor may prompt a change in behavior. In turn, this may prompt changes in other factors and the reorganization of the entire developmental system (Cairns & Cairns, 1994; Farmer & Farmer, 2001). Therefore, in considering the role of aggression in adaptation, it is necessary to take into account changes at the individual, social structural and institutional levels.

Social Synchrony, Social Networks, and Individual Adaptation

To understand change in individual functioning it is necessary to first understand continuity in behavior patterns (Cairns, 1979). From a developmental science perspective, patterns of behavior are established and maintained when internal and external factors become calibrated and support each other. This means that internal factors such as social cognitions and emotional regulation are coordinated with external factors including the child's social networks and social roles. When the developmental system is well calibrated, the child's social interchanges are synchronized with others in the social context in ways that promote stability in behavioral expression.

However, individual capacities and social contexts are dynamic. As a child matures and social systems evolve, synchronous relationships that have supported continuity in a child's behavior may become disrupted. This disruption may occur because of family relocation, changes in classroom assignment, changes in the child's interest and abilities, changes in the interests and abilities of the child's associates, or changes in the social relations and social roles of others in the social context. However, picking new friends does not appear to be random. Often times, the new friends resemble a child's old friends in many aspects (Cairns & Cairns, 1994; Neckerman, 1996). Despite the changes in faces, continuity in the key characteristics of one's friends is maintained. As a result, a child's behavior is continuously supported by his or her friends in the midst of changes.

Such changes in friendship and/or peer groups are necessary for a person's unique developmental pathway. Aggression is sometimes hard to avoid during the process, but in the long run, it may serve positive functions. Consider the relationship between a bully and a victim who are in the same peer group, or two rivals who don't particularly like each other but who hang around with the same crowd. In both situations, the dissolution of the relationship can be viewed as a favorable outcome. Yet, there is a strong potential for considerable harm as these relationships are being dissolved. However, in the long run, some expressions of aggression may contribute to more productive relationships and help to promote patterns of adaptive behavior.

This brings us to the question "Is aggression adaptive?" From a developmental science perspective, the answer cannot be divorced from the unique circumstances of the individual or the conditions of the social context in which the aggressive behavior occurs (Cairns & Cairns, 2000). Therefore, a general response is not appropriate. Nor can adaptation be inferred from immediate or proximal consequences.

Rather, to assess the impact of aggressive expression on adaptation, it is necessary to consider if the behavior contributed to systems reorganization and whether it is linked to consolidated patterns of adaptive functioning.

To illustrate, consider a high school freshman in a rural area who has an hour-long bus ride to school twice a day with peers from a poor community that takes considerable pride in its reputation for being rough and tough. The boy did not go to elementary school with the other kids on the bus, is fairly studious, and, though large in stature, comes across as gawky and vulnerable. He quickly becomes a target for taunts and teasing. After a week of pushes and punches, he responds to being tripped with a couple of punches that drew blood. The episode did not escalate into a full fight, but both parties received a warning from the bus driver that the next incident would be reported. The next day, the kids on the bus treated the boy a bit differently and the toughest boy welcomed him to the back seat area where the tough kids hung out. Over time, the boy found himself managing the complexity of maintaining friendships with the tough kids on his bus and being friends with kids at school who were considered to be the nerds. Although the boy's developmental system did not reorganize to support aggressive behavior patterns, he did expand his social relations and social network in ways that promoted his social competence. In the long run, the aggressive episode may have prevented more insidious problems.

As this illustration depicts, aggression can be a way to escape deleterious relationships or one tool in the management of the complexity of one's life. Undoubtedly, numerous examples could be provided to demonstrate how aggression is related to the problematic reorganization of the developmental system and long-term patterns of maladaptive behavior. But the point here is to clarify that even in non-extraordinary circumstances, aggression may help realign maladaptive synchronous relationships that, in turn, may support the adaptive recalibration of the developmental system. The important contributions of aggression to adaptation do not stop at the individual level, but should also be considered at the social structural and institutional levels.

Social Structural Modifications

Just as aggressive expression can help individuals to modify deleterious social roles and to escape problematic synchronous relationships, it can also promote the management of social boundaries and help maintain a social order (Pellegrini, 1999; Strayer & Strayer, 1976).

As suggested in our review on school social networks and social structures, various forms of aggression are involved in both the formation of social hierarchies and the maintenance of peer group boundaries. Children who become leaders tend to be skillful at using aggressive strategies to consolidate their power (Estell, Farmer, & Cairns, in press; Farmer et al., 2003; Xie, Swift, et al., 2002). Yet, in efforts to maintain their influence and social positions, youth who are in leadership roles may act in ways that are harmful to others or that significantly limit the social opportunities and roles of peers (Adler & Adler, 1995). In other cases, youth who are marginalized may engage in bullying and socially aggressive strategies as a way to deflect negative actions directed toward them (Atlas & Pepler, 1998; Evans & Eder, 1993). In these circumstances, it may be difficult for children who receive the brunt of such transgressions to escape the synchronous relationships that sustain their victimization or that prevent them from developing more productive social roles. Yet, peer groups and social structures tend not to be monarchies and must be responsive to the collective will. Therefore, such strategies as social aggression and public displays of defiance and actual confrontation can sometimes serve as a means of modifying the social structure and of maintaining a balance of power that promotes the opportunities of many rather than the desires of a few (Farmer, 2000; Rodkin & Hodges, 2003).

Consequently, as youth become too powerful or abusive toward others, peers may sometimes step up—not necessarily as an act of benevolence but as a means of promoting their own influence or to protect their own status. As many veteran teachers know, the natural ebb and flow of classroom and school social dynamics can sometimes be self-righting and at, other times, benefit from the support of an "invisible hand" (Cairns & Cairns, 1994). Establishing institutional strategies that clarify when to intervene and when to allow natural developmental processes to support adaptation is an important consideration for teachers and school administrators (Cairns & Cairns, 2000; Farmer, 2000).

Institutional Adjustments and Accommodations

As we have maintained throughout this chapter, aggression can be an outward boundary for the maintenance or reorganization of social roles and synchronous relationships. That is, as patterns of social interactions and relationships extend beyond a threshold that is manageable for one or more individuals, the possibility and actual expression of aggression may be necessary to recalibrate or terminate the relationship, depending on the capacities and needs of the individuals involved. In these situations, aggression is momentary and is in response to the need of one or more children to escape from synchronous relationships that inhibit their own productive patterns of development. In such cases, it would be short-sighted for schools and other institutions to summarily punish aggressive acts without being responsive to the broader issues that contributed to the aggressive interchanges. This does not mean that such behavior should be excused. Rather, it means schools should place themselves in a position where they are able to learn from each episode of aggression and make modifications that serve to not only to address the immediate issue but to also be responsive to broader contextual and institutional factors.

The need for institutional modifications is even more pronounced when there are chronic patterns of aggression. Chronic patterns of aggression may include repeated incidents from the same child or group of children or it may refer to aggression that occurs at the same time of the day or in particular places or contexts within the school. Frequently repeated patterns of aggression may be a marker for problematic social structures or institutional practices that support maladaptive rather than productive patterns. The point here is that school officials must be careful not to respond to just to the surface behavior (i.e., aggression). Instead, it is necessary for them to identify the peer social dynamics that are contributing to the issue. In turn, they must respond not only to the immediate situation, but also focus on the establishment of practices sensitive to peer social dynamics so that the likelihood of future problems is likely to be reduced (Baker, 1998; Swearer & Doll, 2001). In this way, students' aggression becomes a marker to help schools calibrate their policies and practices with the developmental needs and social growth of students.

Again, it is not possible to come up with general guidelines or responses because different schools, communities, and the characteristics of the individuals within the school community make for an exponential possibility of scenarios. However, a few examples are provided in order to illustrate how aggression can serve to mark the need for the change of institutional practices. One example is the transition to middle school. As children move from elementary school to middle school, they are likely to experience considerable reshuffling of peer relations in the midst of other key changes including puberty, increased freedom and responsibilities, and more demanding academic expectations (Cairns & Cairns, 1994; Eccles, 1999). During this same time, they are often moving from an environment where they had one or two teachers whom they are with all day to one in which they have a different teacher each hour. In elementary classes, many teachers are fairly aware of classroom social dynamics and can monitor and unobtrusively intervene with problematic social roles and peer group relations. In middle school settings, most teachers see more than 100 students a day and have very little opportunity to observe children's peer interactions or to provide support for youth who are having difficulties. Chronic patterns of aggression at the individual or peer group level serve as a marker for the need for adult support and guidance for the particular students involved and for more general monitoring of the school social dynamics (Farmer, 2000). In addition, such problems may indicate that other institutional practices such as limited extracurricular activities and the grouping of students for classes need to be more carefully considered and addressed (Eder & Parker, 1987; Kinney 1993). The point here is that patterns of aggression may help schools to adapt their policies and practices to ensure that they are responsive to the social needs of students.

A second example involves the identification of problematic areas and times in the school day where conflict and aggression are likely to occur. Depending on the school and the practices for monitoring students, these may include hall transitions, lunch time, and the end of the day while students are waiting for buses. When schools examine discipline referrals for aggression they can often identify settings or areas where students are not adequately monitored and are not receiving the adult supports that they need (Baker, 1998; Lewis, Sugai, & Colvin, 1998; Nelson, 1996). In such cases, problems of aggression can point to a more general lack of supervision and adult monitoring. By demonstrating a need for careful adult guidance during particular activities and times, problems of aggression serve to promote the development of institutional practices that prevent other safety concerns and that provide students with a generally more secure and supportive school environment (Baker, 1998; Furlong, 1996).

A third example involves institutional policies and practices for grouping students who have behavioral difficulties. In recent years, there have been growing concerns about behavioral contagions and deviancy training as schools and other agencies group together students with conduct problems (Arnold & Hughes, 1999; Dishion, McCord, & Poulin, 1999). Such concerns are legitimate and point to the need for schools to be aware of how grouping practices contribute to social dynamics that support behavioral difficulties. However, our work suggests that the issue is not one of how such children are grouped per se, but rather the types of supports and contexts that are provided for them (Farmer, Farmer, & Gut, 1999). We have found inclusive classrooms in which students with emotional and behavioral disorders take control and create contexts that are highly coercive and disruptive, but we have also identified inclusive classrooms where such students are well integrated into productive social networks with nondisabled peers (Farmer & Farmer, 1996; Farmer & Hollowell, 1994; Pearl et al., 1998). Likewise, we have found special classrooms and alternative schools where highly aggressive youth develop productive roles and relationships while grouped together, and we have found other contexts and circumstance where such youth create a world of chaos and violence (Farmer & Cairns, 1991; Farmer, Clemmer, & Farmer, 2001; Farmer, Farmer, & Clemmer, 2003; Farmer, Stuart, Lorch, & Fields, 1993). The critical issue here is that there cannot be blanket policies or practices regarding the placement of such students. Rather, their behavior must be viewed as a guide for intervention efforts. When a child's problems continue or escalate in a particular setting, there is a need to consider additional interventions and a possible change of placement. If, however, a treatment setting supports the positive reorganization and adaptation of a student's behavior patterns, there is also a need to consider a new placement and set of supports that allow the student to build new supportive relationships that help her or him maintain positive patterns of adjustment (Farmer & Farmer, 2001). In sum, the behavior of children with conduct problems serves as a critical guide for understanding their adaptive needs.

Whether the focus is on policies and practices for promoting productive school transitions, the prevention of violence, the grouping of youth with behavior problems, or myriad other issues that schools encounter, aggressive expression often serves as a marker and guide for understanding how well students' needs are being met. Although it is important to have efforts in place to reduce aggression in school, it is also important to have procedures in place that support the reasoned and rationale analysis of why aggression is occurring and to focus on what can be learned from it. When this is done in a careful and thoughtful manner, it is likely to result in practices and policies that not only reduce aggression at the surface level, but that also address students' broader developmental needs and promotes their productive engagement in school.

In conclusion, aggressive expression is a natural part of synchronous and dynamic social interchanges that occur as children navigate their social world. Rather than necessarily being an indicator of pathology, aggression can serve as an important tool in normal development. This is clearly demonstrated as children establish a social order when they are aggregated together in school. But it doesn't stop there. We can see various forms of aggression playing out in boardrooms, workplaces, and even the political arena as children turn into adults. Accordingly, it is perhaps most productive and appropriate to view aggression as a form of behavior expression that serves as a boundary for the modification of social roles and relationships or as a marker to indicate that there may be a need to monitor and adjust social structural factors or institutional practices that are not responsive to the needs of individuals. At times, some children will develop synchronous relationships and social roles that impede their broader developmental needs. In such cases, aggression may serve as a way to rectify this situation. Yet, in other cases, the concerns and issues may be beyond the capacities of an individual child or group of children to negotiate and may require some form of adult support or intervention. In either case, there is a strong need for teachers and school administrators to be aware of classroom and school social dynamics and to have ways of monitoring and supporting students without overly interfering with their abilities to work through their difficulties and to manage conflict. At the core of the matter, adults must work to prevent the harm and injury that can be caused by aggression without constraining the productive functions that aggression can serve in development.

CONCLUSIONS

Social behavior is the leading edge of development (Cairns, 2000). By linking a complex system of developmental factors, behavior plays a critical role in calibrating the internal needs and states of children and youth with the demands and opportunities of the contexts in which they develop. Accordingly, as youth interact with each other and with adults within their social worlds, their behaviors can become synchronized in ways that support sustained patterns across time. At times, expressions of aggression may function within the social system in ways that prevent disorganization and more destructive or harmful patterns. A social structure with productive patterns of dominance is likely to be viewed more favorably than a chaotic system of children constantly competing and vying for control and resources. In other cases, aggression may help prompt the reorganization of a system of factors in ways that promote the adjustment of the individual. Standing up to a bully may have consequences that go well beyond the escape of a maladaptive synchronous relationship. It may help to realign patterns of behavior, social roles, and the child's self-esteem in ways that prompt new opportunities and trajectories. In still other situations, aggression may serve as a marker to others that there is a need to provide support and to help reorganize factors that are deleterious for the child or for children in general. In conclusion, by overlooking the productive functions of aggressive behavior and focusing only on maladaptive consequences, researchers run the risk of denying the complexity of developmental systems and the critical role that aggression can sometimes play in the calibration of various developmental factors and the possible amelioration of problems within the system.

ACKNOWLEDGMENTS

This chapter was supported by grants U81CCU416369 and R49CCR419824 from the Centers for Disease Control and Prevention, grants R305L030162 and R305A040056 from the Institute of Education Sciences, and grant H324C040230 from the Office of Special Education Programs to Thomas W. Farmer (Principal Investigator). The views expressed in this article are ours and do not represent the granting agencies.

REFERENCES

Adler, P. A., & Adler, P. (1995). Dynamics of inclusion and exclusion in preadolescent cliques. *Social Psychology Quarterly, 58*, 145–162.

Adler, P. A. & Adler, P. (1996). Preadolescent clique stratification and the hierarchy of identity. *Sociological Inquiry, 66*, 111–142.

Adler, P. A., & Adler, P. (1998). *Peer power: Preadolescent culture and identity.* New Brunswick, NJ: Rutgers University Press.

Adler, P. A., Kless, S., & Adler, P. (1992). Socialization to gender roles: Popularity among elementary school boys and girls. *Sociology of Education, 65*, 169–187

Arnold, M. E., & Hughes, J. N. (1999). First do no harm: Adverse effects of grouping deviant youth for skills training. *Journal of School Psychology, 37*, 99–115.

Atlas, R. S., & Pepler, D. J. (1998). Observations of bullying in the classroom. *Journal of Educational Research, 92*, 86–99.

Baker, J. A. (1998). Are we missing the forest for the trees? Considering the social context of school violence. *Journal of School Psychology, 36*, 29–44.

Baldwin, J. M. (1897). *Social and ethical interpretations in mental development: A study in social psychology.* New York: Macmillan.

Berndt, T. J. (1979). Developmental changes in conformity to peers and parents. *Developmental Psychology, 15*, 608–616.

Cairns, R. B. (1979). *Social development: The origins and plasticity of interchanges.* San Francisco: W. H. Freeman.

Cairns, R. B. (2000). Developmental science: Three audacious implications. In L. R. Bergman, R. B. Cairns, L-G. Nilsson, & L. Nystedt (Eds.), *Developmental science and the holistic approach* (pp. 49–62). Mahwah, NJ: Lawrence Erlbaum Associates.

Cairns, R. B., & Cairns, B. D. (1986). On social values and social development: Gender and aggression. In L. Frederick-Cofer (Ed.), *Human nature and public policy: Scientific views women, children, and families,* (pp. 17–201). New York: Praeger.

Cairns, R. B., & Cairns, B. D. (1994). *Lifelines and risks: Pathways of youth in our time.* New York: Harvester Wheatsheaf.

Cairns, R. B., & Cairns, B. D. (2000). The natural history and developmental functions of aggression. In A. Sameroff, M. Lewis & S. Miller (Eds.), *Handbook of Developmental Psychopathology* (2nd ed., pp. 403–429). New York: Kluwer Academic/ Plenum Publishers.

Cairns, R. B., Cairns, B. D., Neckerman, H. J., Ferguson, L. L. & Gariépy, J-L. (1989). Growth and aggression: I. Childhood to early adolescence. *Developmental Psychology, 25,* 320–330.

Cairns, R. B., Cairns, B. D., Neckerman, H. J., Gest, S. D., & Gariépy, J-L. (1988). Social networks and aggressive behavior: Peer support or peer rejection? *Developmental Psychology, 24,* 815–823.

Cairns, R. B., Leung, M.-C., Buchanan, L. & Cairns, B. D. (1995). Friendships and social networks in childhood and adolescence: fluidity, reliability, and interrelations. *Child Development, 66,* 1330–1345.

Cairns, R. B., Neckerman, H. J., & Cairns, B. D. (1989). Social networks and the shadows of synchrony. In G. R. Adams & R. Montemayor (Eds.), *Biology of adolescent behavior and development. Advances in adolescent development: Vol. 1. An annual book series* (pp. 275–305). Thousand Oaks, CA: Sage.

Cairns, R. B., Perrin, J. E., & Cairns, B. D. (1985). Social structure and social cognition in early adolescence: Affiliative patterns. *Journal of Early Adolescence, 5,* 339–355.

Cairns, R. B., Xie, H., & Leung, M.-C. (1998). The popularity of friendship and the neglect of social networks: Toward a new balance. *New Directions in Child Development, 80,* 25–53.

Corsaro, W. A., & Eder, D. (1990). Children's peer cultures. *Annual Review of Sociology, 16,* 197–220

Dishion, T. J., McCord, J., & Poulin, F. (1999). When interventions harm: Peer groups and problem behavior. *American Psychologist, 54,* 755–764

Eccles, J. S. (1999). The development of children ages 6–14. *Future of Children, 9,* 30–44.

Eder, D. (1985). The cycle of popularity: Interpersonal relations among female adolescents. *Sociology of Education, 58,* 154–165.

Eder, D., Evans, C. C., & Parker, S. (1995). *School talk: Gender and adolescent Culture.* New Brunswick, NJ: Rutgers University Press.

Eder, D., & Parker, S. (1987). The cultural production and reproduction of gender: The effect of extracurricular activities on peer-group culture. *Sociology of Education, 60,* 200–213.

Edwards, C. A. (1994). Leadership in groups of school-age girls. *Developmental Psychology, 30,* 920–927.

Espelage, D. L., Holt, M. K., & Henkel, R. R. (2003). Examination of peer-group contextual effects on aggression during early adolescence. *Child Development, 74,* 205–220.

Estell, D. B., Cairns, R. B., Farmer, T. W., & Cairns, B. D. (2002). Aggression in inner-city early elementary classrooms: Individual and peer-group configurations. *Merrill-Palmer Quarterly, 48,* 52–76.

Estell, D. B., Farmer, T. W., & Cairns, B. D. (in press) Bullies and victims in rural African American youth: Behavioral characteristics and social network placement. *Aggressive Behavior.*

Estell, D. B., Farmer, T. W., Pearl, R., Van Acker, R., & Rodkin, P. C. (2003). Heterogeneity in the relationship between popularity and aggression: Individual, group, and classroom influences. *New Directions for Child and Adolescent Development, 101,* 75–85.

Evans, C., & Eder, D. (1993). "No exit": Processes of social isolation in the middle school. *Journal of Contemporary Ethnography, 22,* 139–170.

Farmer, T. W. (2000). The social dynamics of aggressive and disruptive behavior in school: Implications for behavior consultation. *Journal of Educational and Psychological Consultation, 11*, 299–322.

Farmer, T. W., & Cairns, R. B. (1991). Social networks and social status in emotionally disturbed children. *Behavioral Disorders, 16*, 288–298.

Farmer, T. W., Clemmer, J. T., & Farmer, E. M. Z. (2001). *Interim report on the connection between the identification of minority and at-risk students as students with behavior or emotional disabilities and the gap in student achievement.* A report to the North Carolina Department of Public Instruction.

Farmer, T. W., Estell, D. B., Bishop, J. L., O'Neal, K. K., & Cairns, B. D. (2003). Rejected bullies or popular leaders? The social relations of aggressive subtypes of rural African-American early adolescents. *Developmental Psychology, 39*, 992–1004.

Farmer, T. W., & Farmer, E. M. Z. (1996). The social relationships of students with exceptionalities in mainstream classrooms: Social network centrality and homophily. *Exceptional Children, 62*, 431–450.

Farmer, T. W., & Farmer, E. M. Z. (2001). Developmental science, systems of care, and prevention of emotional and behavioral problems in youth. *American Journal of Orthopsychiatry, 71*, 171–181.

Farmer, T. W., Farmer, E. M. Z., & Clemmer, J. T. (2003). *Alternative learning programs in North Carolina: Findings from telephone surveys and site visits.* Report to the North Carolina Department of Public Instruction.

Farmer, T. W., Farmer, E. M. Z., & Gut, D. M. (1999). Implications of social development research for school-based interventions for aggressive youth with EBD. *Journal of Emotional and Behavioral Disorders, 7*, 130–136.

Farmer, T. W., & Hollowell, J. L. (1994). Social networks in mainstream classrooms: Social affiliations and behavioral characteristics of students with emotional and behavioral disorders. *Journal of Emotional and Behavioral Disorders, 2*, 143–155.

Farmer, T. W., Leung, M. -C., Pearl, R., Rodkin, P. C., Cadwallader, T. W., & Van Acker, R. (2002). Deviant or diverse groups? The peer affiliations of aggressive elementary students. *Journal of Educational Psychology, 94*, 611–620.

Farmer, T. W., & Rodkin, P. C. (1996). Antisocial and prosocial correlates of classroom social positions: The social network centrality perspective. *Social Development, 5*, 176–190.

Farmer, T. W., Stuart, C., Lorch, N., & Fields, E. (1993). The social behavior and peer relations of emotionally and behaviorally disturbed students in residential treatment: A pilot study. *Journal of Emotional and Behavioral Disorders, 1*, 223–234.

Farver, J. A. M. (1996). Aggressive behavior in preschooler's social networks: Do birds of a feather flock together? *Early Childhood Research Quarterly, 11*, 333–350.

Furlong, M. J. (1996). Tools for assessing school violence. In S. Miller, J. Brodine, & T. Miller (Eds.), *Safe by design: Planning for peaceful school communities* (pp. 71–84). Seattle, WA: Committee for Children.

Gest, S. D., Farmer, T. W., Cairns, B. D., & Xie, H. (2003). Identifying children's peer social networks in school classrooms: Links between peer reports and observed interactions. *Social Development, 12*, 513–529.

Haselager, G. J. T., Hartup, W. W., van Lieshout, C. F. M., & Riksen-Walraven, J. M.
    A. (1998). Similarities between friends and nonfriends in middle childhood.
    Child Development, 69, 1198–1208.
Hawley, P. H. (1999). The ontogenesis of social dominance: A strategy-based
    evolutionary perspective. *Developmental Review, 19*, 97–132.
Hawley, P. H. (2003). Prosocial and coercive configurations of resource control
    in early adolescence: A case for the well-adapted Machiavellian. *Merrill-
    Palmer Quarterly, 49*, 279–309.
Hawley, P. H., Little, T. D., & Pasupathi, M. (2002). Winning friends and influenc-
    ing peers: Strategies of peer influence in late childhood. *International Journal
    of Behavioral Development, 26*, 466–473.
Holmberg, M. C. (1980). The development of social interchange patterns from
    12 to 42 months. *Child Development, 51*, 448–456.
Hood, K. E. (1996). Intractable tangles of sex and gender in women's aggressive
    development: An optimistic view. In R. B. Cairns & D. Stoff (Eds.), *Aggression
    and violence: Genetic, neurobiological, and biosocial perspectives*, (pp
    309–335). Mahwah, NJ: Lawrence Erlbaum Associates.
Kandel, D. (1978). Similarity in real-life adolescent friendship pairs. *Journal of
    Personality and Social Psychology, 36*, 306–312.
Kindermann, T. A. (1993). Natural peer groups as contexts for individual devel-
    opment: The case of children's motivation in school. *Developmental
    Psychology, 29*, 970–977.
Kinney, D. A. (1993). From 'nerds to normals': The recovery of identity among
    adolescents from middle school to high school. *Sociology of Education, 66*, 21–40.
LaFontana, K. M., & Cillessen, A. H. N. (2002). Children's perceptions of popular
    and unpopular peers: A multi-method assessment. *Developmental
    Psychology, 38*, 635–647.
Lease, A. M., Kennedy, C. A., & Axelrod, J. L. (2002). Children's social construc-
    tions of popularity. *Social Development, 11*, 87–109.
Leung, M. -C. (1996). Social networks and self-enhancement in Chinese children:
    A comparison of self reports and peer reports of group membership. *Social
    Development, 6*, 146–157.
Lewis, T. J., Sugai, G., & Colvin, G. (1998). Reducing problem behavior through
    a school-wide system of effective behavioral support: Investigation of a
    school-wide social skills training program and contextual interventions.
    School Psychology Review, 27, 446–459.
Little, T. D., Brauner, J., Jones, S. M., Nock, M. K., & Hawley, P. H. (2003).
    Rethinking aggression: A typological examination of the functions of aggres-
    sion. *Merrill-Palmer Quarterly, 49*, 343–369.
Merten, D. E. (1996). Visibility and vulnerability: Responses to rejection by nonag-
    gressive junior high school boys. *Journal of Early Adolescence, 16*, 5–26.
Merten, D. E. (1997). The meaning of meanness: Popularity, competition, and
    conflict among junior high school girls. *Sociology of Education, 70*, 175–191.
Nangle, D. W., Erdley, C. A., Zeff, K. A., Stanchfield, L. L., & Gold, J. A. (2004).
    Opposites do not attract: Social status and behavioral-style concordances
    and discordances among children and the peers who like or dislike them.
    Journal of Abnormal Child Psychology, 32, 425–434.

Neckerman, H. J. (1996). The stability of social groups in childhood and adolescence: The role of the classroom social environment. *Social Development, 5,* 131–145.

Nelson, J. R. (1996). Designing schools to meet the needs of students who exhibit disruptive behavior. *Journal of Emotional and Behavioral Disorders, 4,* 147–161.

Pearl, R., Farmer, T. W., Van Acker, R., Rodkin, P. C., Bost, K. K., Coe, M., & Henley, W. (1998). The social integration of students with mild disabilities in general education classrooms: Peer group membership and peer-assessed social behavior. *Elementary School Journal, 99,* 167–185.

Pellegrini, A. D. (1995). A longitudinal study of boys' rough-and-tumble play and dominance in early adolescence. *Journal of Applied Developmental Psychology, 19,* 165–176.

Pellegrini, A. D. (1999). Risky business: Making inferences about risk and its value [Review of the book: *Risk and our pedagogical relation to children: On the playground and beyond*]. *Early Childhood Research Quarterly, 14,* 435–438.

Pellegrini, A. D., & Bartini, M. (2001). Dominance in early adolescent boys: Affiliative and aggressive dimensions and possible functions. *Merrill-Palmer Quarterly, 47,* 142–163.

Pelligrini, A. D., & Long, J. D. (2002). A longitudinal study of bullying, dominance, and victimization during the transition from primary school through secondary school. *British Journal of Developmental Psychology, 20,* 259–280.

Pellegrini, A. D., & Smith, P. K. (1998). Physical activity play: The nature and function of a neglected aspect of play. *Child Development, 69,* 577–598.

Pepler, D. J., Craig, W. M., & Roberts, W. L. (1998). Observations of aggressive and nonaggressive children on the school playground. *Merrill-Palmer Quarterly, 44,* 55–76.

Rodkin, P. C., Farmer, T. W., Pearl, R., & Van Acker, R. (2000). The heterogeneity of popularity in boys: Antisocial and prosocial configurations. *Developmental Psychology, 36,* 14–24.

Rodkin, P. C., & Hodges, E. V. E. (2003). Bullies and victims in the peer ecology: Four questions for psychologists and school professionals. *School Psychology Review, 32,* 384–400.

Rodkin, P. C., Pearl, R., Farmer, T. W., & Van Acker, R. (2003). Enemies in the gendered societies of middle childhood: Prevalence, stability, associations with social status, and aggression. *New Directions in Child and Adolescent Development, 102,* 73–88.

Rose, A. J., Swenson, L. P., & Carlson, W. (2004). Friendships of aggressive youth: Considering the influences of being disliked and of being perceived as popular. *Journal of Experimental Child Psychology, 88,* 25–45.

Salmivalli C., Huttunen A., & Lagerspetz, K. (1997). Peer networks and bullying in schools. *Scandinavian Journal of Psychology, 38,* 305–312.

Salmivalli, C., Lagerspetz, K., Björkqvist, K., Osterman, K., & Kaukiainen, A. (1996). Bullying as a group process: Participant roles and their relations to social status within the group. *Aggressive Behavior, 22,* 1–15.

Sears, R. R. (1951). A theoretical framework for personality and social behavior. *American Psychologist, 6,* 476–483.

Strayer, F. F., & Noel, J. M. (1986). The prosocial and antisocial functions of aggression: An ethological study of triadic conflict among young children. In C. Zahn-Waxler, E. M. Cummings, & R. Iannotti (Eds.), *Altruism and aggression* (pp. 107–131). New York: Cambridge University Press.

Strayer, F., & Santos, A. J. (1996). Affiliative structures in preschool peer groups. *Social Development, 5,* 117–130.

Strayer, F. F., & Strayer, J. (1976). An ethological analysis of social agonism and dominance relations among preschool children. *Child Development, 47,* 980–989.

Strayer, F. F., & Trudel, M. (1984). Developmental changes in the nature and function of social dominance among young children. *Ethology and Sociobiology, 5,* 279–295.

Sutton, J., Smith, P. K., & Swettenham, J. (1999). Bullying and "theory of mind": A critique of the "social skills deficit" view of anti-social behaviour. *Social Development, 8,* 117–127.

Swearer, S. M., & Doll, B. (2001). Bullying in schools: An ecological framework. *Journal of Emotional Abuse, 2,* 7–23.

Vaughn, B. E., Vollenweider, M., Bost, K. K., Azria-Evans, M. R., & Snider, J. (2003). Negative interactions and social competence for preschool children in two samples: Reconsidering the interpretation of aggressive behavior for young children. *Merrill-Palmer Quarterly, 49,* 245–278.

Xie, H., Cairns, R. B., & Cairns, B. D. (1999). Social network centrality and social competence among inner-city children. *Journal of Emotional and Behavioral Disorders, 7,* 147–155.

Xie, H., Cairns, R. B., & Cairns, B. D. (2002). The development of social aggression and physical aggression: A narrative analysis of interpersonal conflicts. *Aggressive Behavior, 28,* 341–355.

Xie, H., Cairns, B. D., & Cairns, R. B. (2005). The development of aggressive behaviors among girls: Measurement issues, social functions, and differential trajectories. In D. Pepler, K. Madsen, C. Webster, & K. Levene (Eds.), *Development and treatment of girlhood aggression* (pp. 103–134). Mahwah, NJ: Lawrence Erlbaum Associates.

Xie, H., Farmer, T. W., & Cairns, B. D. (2003). Different forms of aggression among inner-city African-American children: Gender, configurations, and school social networks. *Journal of School Psychology, 41,* 355–375.

Xie, H., Swift, D. J., Cairns, B. D., & Cairns, R. B. (2002). Aggressive behaviors in social interaction and developmental adaptation: A narrative analysis of interpersonal conflicts during early adolescents. *Social Development, 11,* 205–224.

Youniss, J. (1980). *Parents and peers in social development: A Sullivan-Piaget perspective.* Chicago: University of Chicago Press.

Youniss, J. (1986). Development of reciprocity through friendship. In C. Zahn-Waxler, E .M. Cummings & R. Iannotti (Eds.), *Altruism and aggression: Biological and social origins* (pp. 88–106). New York: Cambridge University Press.

10

AGGRESSION AND ADAPTATION: PSYCHOLOGICAL RECORD, EDUCATIONAL PROMISE

Philip C. Rodkin
Travis Wilson
University of Illinois at Urbana-Champaign

Scholars from a variety of theoretical perspectives have agreed that aggression can be an adaptive solution to social problems. Sustained research into aggression and adaptation has lagged behind because of societal values, and also because the usefulness to society of stressing dysfunctions of aggression is much better established. In this chapter we lay out the psychological record and suggest some empirical approaches and educational strategies that take into account that aggression can sometimes be adaptive for some children (cf. Pellegrini, this volume).

PSYCHOLOGICAL RECORD ON AGGRESSION AS ADAPTATION

Instinct Theories

Instinct theorists of all stripes held views consistent with the adaptability of aggression, at least under some circumstances. These early scholars who searched for defining dimensions of human and nonhuman experience could not help but point out powerful proclivities toward aggression. The moral values placed on the aggressive wellspring, however, varied across accounts and were always embedded in some cultural and historical matrix. The instinct theorist par excellence, William McDougall

(1908/1914), devoted a chapter of his social psychology textbook to the instinct of "pugnacity." McDougall, a Briton who heartily endorsed the imperialistic tendencies of his day, wrote plainly that "the instinct of pugnacity has played a part second to none in the evolution of social organization" (p. 279). McDougall thought that aggression would increase with civilizing tendencies. Proclaiming with satisfaction that the pugnacious instinct was "stronger in the European peoples than it was in primitive man" (p. 279), McDougall advocated that "in the nursery and the school righteous anger will always have a great and proper part to play in the training of the individual for his life in society" (p. 293). From its earliest days, powerful voices in psychology found the adaptability of aggression an obvious fact of life and had no compunctions saying so.

Psychoanalytic instinct theory is harder to pin down. The clinical focus of psychoanalysis inherently means that it emphasizes the dysfunctional and maladaptive, whether in regards to aggression or any other class of behaviors. Freud has been read as landing on both sides of the aggression–adaptation issue. Cairns (1979) writes that Freud conceptualized the aggressive instinct of Thanatos as "socially nonfunctional and without redeeming features … the very antithesis of survival. The individual and the species persisted despite the operation of this inborn tendency" (p. 164). Bukowski (2003), however, interprets the 1932 Einstein–Freud correspondence (in which Einstein asks Freud, "Is there any way of delivering mankind from the menace of war?") as suggesting that "Freud concluded that if one were to eliminate aspects and processes of human nature that led to war, one would also eliminate the possibility of love" (p. 391).

So where did Freud stand? One of his most highly reproduced statements on aggression, from chapter V of *Civilization and Its Discontents*, goes like this:

> Men are not gentle creatures who want [only] to be loved … their neighbor is for them not only a potential helper or sexual object, but also someone who tempts them to satisfy their aggressiveness on him, to exploit his capacity for work without compensation, to use him sexually without his consent, to seize his possessions, to humiliate him, to cause him pain, to torture and kill him. *Homo homini lupus* [Man is a wolf to man]. Who, in the face of all his experience of life and of history, will have the courage to dispute this assertion? (Freud, 1930/1961, pp. 68–69)

Freud's metaphysical, near-theological insight is that aggression and evil are close cousins residing within each one of us and across the human species. Aggression is adaptive insofar as it is ubiquitous and effective. But as a European Jew whose life reached across two World Wars, Freud never sanitizes the destruction that human aggression brings, nor does he attempt to justify the usefulness of horrific behaviors that work too well and too often. As an "indestructible feature of human nature" that is "not easy ... to give up" (p. 72), Freud thought that aggression was adaptive and highly evolved, but this adaptability is in the context of a view of human nature past and present that is anything but triumphalist, where the naturalistic fallacy could never apply. Freud's boiler-room theory of instinctual drives and mechanisms of sublimated release have long been discarded, but the questions he leaves us with resonate in our 21st century world.

Freud's *Civilizations and Its Discontents* quote is often juxtaposed against an equally notable passage from Lorenz's *On Aggression* (1963):

> [A]ggression, far from being the diabolical, destructive principle that classical psychoanalysis makes it out to be, is really an essential part of the life-preserving organization of instincts. Though by accident it may function in the wrong way and cause destruction, the same is true of practically any functional part of any system. (pp. 44–45)

Lorenz here uses what today might seem like the rhetoric of precision bombing—dysfunctional only in the rare accidental case. The difference with Freud, though, is largely one of tone and life experience, particularly during the rise of Nazi Germany (Lehrman, 1953). The two are not far apart on the substance of the adaptability of aggression. Like Freud, Lorenz (1963) quotes Plautus' *Homo homini lupus* in arguing that through his mastery of aggression, man has exterminated the "bear and the wolf" (p. 38) and so now is a wolf unto himself. In what seems to be a contradiction to the epigraph just quoted, Lorenz writes that "aggressive behavior, more than most other qualities and functions, becomes exaggerated to the point of the grotesque and inexpedient ... a hereditary evil" (p. 39). The solutions to aggression that Freud and Lorenz propose are similar, not surprising given their emphasis on instincts and drives. For example, Lorenz writes of the importance of "redirecting discharge" from aggressive drives into ritualistic competitions such as sport (pp. 270–271). Lorenz also stresses laughter and humor as an antidote to violence. One difference between Lorenz and both McDougall and Freud is that Lorenz professes optimism in cultural evolution away from the suitability of aggression. Reason shall overcome, concludes Lorenz, and future societies will have only a "tolerable" amount of aggression thanks to the "great constructors [the power of natural selection]" (pp. 289–290).

Early Behaviorism

When you creak open the pages of Carl Murchison's *Psychologies of 1925*, intended from its preface to plainly show a "genuine cross-section of contemporary theoretical psychology ... up-to-date through the year 1925," you get placed in the middle of a debate between McDougall and John Watson over the reality of instincts. Watson is winning; this is shown most clearly in hindsight from the immortality of his "dozen healthy infants" boast (p. 10). McDougall fights a losing battle in the war between nature and nurture and is bewildered from the start. "This is a strange and embarrassing position for any man of science ... an absurd procedure" (p. 273), to have to defend human instincts, purpose, and will, he blustered. McDougall's star was fast-fading. His 1920 book, *The Group Mind*, which promoted a psychology of groups that would over-lay a psychology of individuals, suffered ridicule within the behavioris-tic social psychology emerging in American universities (e.g., Allport, 1924). McDougall and his instincts were on the way out (Kuo, 1922).

What is important for us is that views on whether aggression could be adaptive did not shift with the paradigm change within psychology from instincts to behavior, from nature to nurture. Murphy, Murphy, and Newcomb's (1937) *Experimental Social Psychology* includes a 130-page chapter on the development of aggression, skewed toward the early and middle childhood periods (see also Goodenough, 1931). The chapter title is called: "Characteristic Social Behavior of Children in Our Culture: Aggression and Competition," emphasizing both the nor-mative aspect of aggressive behavior ("characteristic") and the sensi-tivity of aggression to context. Despite the title of their text, Murphy, Murphy, and Newcomb did not completely represent the behavioristic social psychology that Watson and Floyd Allport foretold. Murphy et al. (1937) retained McDougall's interest in motivation and tried to con-nect social psychology with other social sciences like sociology and anthropology. As you would expect from its length, their coverage of childhood aggression is extensive and pertinent to research today. For instance:

> ... [W]e have two distinct types of aggressiveness: one that is socially approved of, namely, self-assertiveness and ability to make contacts with children; and one which is socially obnoxious, consisting of jealousies, overt attacks on other children, criticizing others unfavorably—a general pattern of making oneself not liked. Though both of these things have been called aggressiveness, it is clear that from a social point of view they reveal very different forms of adaptation. (p. 379)

What is refreshing about Murphy, Murphy, and Newcomb's chapter is how they recast aggression as a problem for adults as much as for children. Although Freud goes unmentioned, the theme of conflict between the individual and society is prominent. Aggression here is, in part, children's frustrated response to obstacles placed in the way of their goals by adults and other children (see also Barker, Dembo, & Lewin, 1941). Murphy et al. shine a spotlight on how adults use aggression by endorsing competitive values, maintaining authority over children, and through institutional mechanisms such as police and armies. Many children are constantly dominated by adult regulations and strictures that "may have an inner value to the child equivalent to aggression from the adult" (p. 405). Murphy et al. recognized early that although adults may think and act as if only one message about aggression is being sent to the child—"aggression is bad"—from the child's point of view reality is less clear.

Dollard et al.'s (1939) *Frustration and Aggression* is an interesting contrast to Murphy et al.'s volume published 2 years earlier. *Experimental Social Psychology* is an alternative voice in the developmental social psychology of its day—motivational and mentalistic. *Frustration and Aggression* is the dominant voice, carrying forward Clark Hull's drive-based behavioristics into the study of significant social behaviors such as aggression (and attachment). Dollard et al. famously meld Hull and Freud into a singular empirical research program, covering topics ranging from childhood aggression to the wanton killings of African Americans in the U.S. South. Their alloy of frustration and aggression marked the high-water point of Freudian psychoanalysis within American universities; subsequent shortcomings of frustration–aggression theory helped usher out Freud and Hull from social development research.

Frustration and aggression and its progenitors in the social cognition and learning traditions often adopt an aggression-is-dysfunctional point of view. After all, a common cause of behaviorism and psychoanalysis is changing undesired, unfortunate behavior. Dollard et al. open their monograph by calling aggression a "problem," and so obviously not an adaptive solution. But as with Freud versus Lorenz, the difference between *Experimental Social Psychology* and *Frustration and Aggression* is one of perspective and value rather than theory. Dollard and his Yale group clearly agree that aggression can be adaptive and that adults aggress more than children. Like McDougall, they are unabashed that aggression should be used by those who have it for socially desired ends. For example, Dollard et al. argue that criminals and those who would soon grow up to be criminals need to anticipate that their behavior will be punished. They go on to write that:

> ... [P]unishment is no less a form of aggression than is crime. The fact that the latter is "anti-social" and the former is what may be called "pro-social," i.e., is aligned with and directed towards the enforcement and perpetuation of the mores of a group, does not alter the essentially aggressive character of both. (pp. 110–111)

Like Murphy et al., Dollard et al. recognize that aggression is always a judgment, dependent on point of view (Cairns, 1979). But where Murphy et al. encourage you to step into the child's world, Dollard et al. generally stay on the side of authorities such as parents and police to reduce problem behavior. They end their volume with a vivid chapter on Ashanti culture, concluding that aggression is permitted when "the expression of aggression serves a socially useful end" (p. 190). There are other passages in *Frustration and Aggression* in which the functional value of aggression in children is recognized. Parents are warned not to suppress the aggressive responses of their children too severely, or else they won't make it either on the playground or in adult life (p. 83). Whereas Murphy et al. ponder the irony of both children and adults putting value on aggression, Dollard et al. have few reservations about building a society and socialization processes that use aggression and social regulation effectively to wipe out problem behavior and create a better common good. On a conceptual level neither Dollard et al. nor Murphy et al. have any issue with the proposition that aggression can be adaptive.

Aggression After World War II

World War II changed how psychologists studied aggression. How could it not? Awful questions in the war's aftermath had to be addressed: How could a leader like Hitler arise? Are there limits to the potential of human evil and aggressive destruction? American psychology (or at least psychologists in America, after the emigration of Kurt Lewin, Fritz Heider, and others) took the lead as Europe rebuilt. The preeminent theory, frustration–aggression, had been in place since the late 1930s. Dollard et al. (1939) wrote in the bold, conquer-the-world-prose of early psychological texts, presenting a unifying theory from a new, fast-developing behavioral science that could explain phenomena as varied as "suicides, race prejudice ... sibling jealousy ... street fights ... and war" (p. 26) fortified by Freud's subterranean insights. Frustration–aggression theory and its hybrid, psychoanalytic behavioral drive architecture, were put to the test during the 1950s and 1960s. It didn't take long to determine that too many frustration–aggression predictions were empirically unsupported (Eron, 1994). With regards to the psychological study of aggression, Sears (1959) put it best: "since World War II, it has been anybody's game" (pp. iv–v).

This game was sponsored by the U.S. government (cf., Smith, this volume), which expanded the depth of aggression research and placed a guiding hand over its direction. The 1950 act that created the National Science Foundation included social science as a legitimate "other science" only after much backroom dealing. Leading figures like sociologist Talcott Parsons successfully lobbied for social science participation by sweeping under the rug nonpositivistic models of psychology so as to stress the unity of natural and social sciences. Social science in the tradition of John Dewey and Gunmar Myrdal, directed towards social critique and reconstruction, was hushed in favor of behavioral technologies that could improve societal effectiveness as society viewed it (Solovey, 2004). This was this case for aggression and for other socially significant human behaviors (Rappaport, 2005).

There was no shift in scientific thinking during the years following World War II against the idea that aggression could be an adaptive behavior. Perspectives stressing the functions or adaptations of aggressive behavior were accepted but not pursued as a fruitful starting-point for investigation. Sears (1961) asked 12-year-olds about their acceptance of prosocial aggression or "moral righteousness," defined as "aggression used in a socially approved way for purposes that are acceptable to the moral standards of a group" (p. 471). Almost 50 years later, this prosocial aggression distinction has been dropped from the literature while many other aggression subtypes flourish. Maybe it was lost in the general miasma of the Sears group's nonfindings, an uninteresting follow-up of the children featured in Sears, Maccoby, and Levin's (1957) failure to find connections between parents' reports of how they parent and their children's behavior. Sears (1961) went no further than to say that prosocial aggression was correlated with "aggression anxiety," or dislike of aggression, and was higher in girls than in boys. Bandura (1969) clearly recognized that aggression can be adaptive for the aggressor and have "positive social consequences" (Card & Little, this volume). "In many instances," he writes, "aggressive behavior eventually succeeds in securing desired goals and, like any other efficacious, modeled behavior, it is widely emulated as a method of achieving social change" (p. 381). Even Fred Skinner (1985), that nurturist non pareil, noted that:

> Probably we are all to some extent instinctively aggressive. Skillful aggressive maneuvers that hurt others should have had great survival value, even as recently as a few thousand generations ago, and I don't think that has all been wiped out by subsequent evolution. ... [T]here are many reasons why we so often turn to punitive measures. (pp. 22–23)

Thus, even those most associated with an aggression-as-maladaptive point of view recognized that aggression can be adaptive.

Research on the dysfunctional characteristics of aggressive persons and aggressive behavior became a thriving modern enterprise in the post-World War II environment. Links between aggression and adaptation were neither denied nor emphasized. The national zeitgeist and its guiding hand were on the side of social order and quiet. Daniel Courtwright (1996), in an historical analysis of male American violence premised on evolutionary thinking, writes that the 1950s were an exceptional time because it was marked by "a potent force for social order, welcome in a country that had been through a lot" (p. 224). Postwar parenting literature, a smiling Dr. Spock firmly at the helm, took hold of the ideal that children are best when they are sociable, adaptable, cooperative, and consensus-oriented (Mintz, 2004, p. 280). One U.S. senator proclaimed in 1954 that juvenile delinquency was a scourge greater than Communism; federal funds earmarked for the reduction of aggressive and antisocial behavior grew markedly during the Eisenhower administration (Mintz, 2004, pp. 293–294). This was not a propitious time, as Murphy et al. might have suggested, to question how aggression promotes adaptation in individual–environment fits (cf., Farmer, Xie, Cairns, & Hutchins, this volume). During the 1950s and 1960s, aggressive behavior was studied experimentally (Hartup, 2005) with the larger goal of reducing problem behavior as so viewed by the larger society. It is during this time, according to the Cairns and Cairns (2001) recollection of the postwar research environment, that the "view that aggressive acts are by definition dysfunctional" (p. 36) became dominant.

Prominent research literatures of the time reflect the increasing emphasis on aggression-as-dysfunction. Much effort was placed on showing that authoritarianism characterized bad people, bad places, and bad styles. The J-Type was discovered in 1938 by German personality psychologist E. R. Jaensch and lauded as a Nazi archetype. In 1950 the J-Type was rediscovered by Adorno, Frenkel-Brunswik, Levinson, and Sanford in sinister garb as The Authoritarian Personality (Brown, 1965). The authoritarian personality was stuffed to the gills with dysfunction: aggressive, frustrated (Berkowitz, 1962), cold, prejudiced (Allport, 1954), mercilessly harsh to those below him, and pathetically submissive to those above him. The massive original study of the authoritarian personality was funded privately by the American Jewish Committee. Autocratic summer camps, stressing competition and domination, produced children prone towards aggression and scapegoating innocent victims (Lewin, Lippitt, & White, 1939; Lippitt, Polansky, Redl, & Rosen, 1952; Sherif, 1956). Authoritarian parenting, in particular maternal coldness and punitive punishment, were linked to unhappy, aggressive young children (Sears, Maccoby, & Levin, 1957). Aggressive youth, according to Bandura's early writings, suffered from "a lack of affectional nurturance" in childhood and a disruption of normal dependency (or attachment; Bowlby, 1950) relationships (Bandura & Walters, 1959, p. 32). The collective judgment of this work is that aggression is connected to a plethora of undesirable characteristics: poor parenting followed by peer rejection in middle childhood and the emergence of deviant peer groups in adolescence (Dishion, Patterson, & Griesler, 1994).

The conceptual framework of research on childhood aggression was upgraded to social learning and social cognition in the 1960s (Eron, 1994) but the underlying emphasis on aggression-as-dysfunction has remained strong to the present day. Most every societal response to childhood aggression is based on the premise that aggression is deficient. For instance, Berkowitz's (1962, pp. 287–288) revision to frustration–aggression included mediators such as a child's erroneous interpretation of ambiguous social behavior as hostile, and his or her over-readiness to respond aggressively to perceived slights (see also Anderson & Bushman, 2002). Aggressive children (particularly frustrated, reactive aggressive children) reason differently and not as well as their peers. Social-information processing models (e.g., Dodge & Feldman, 1990) extended and elaborated these early notions and have since been widely adopted in social skills training programs for the reduction of school violence (Moeller, 2001). Social modeling and cognitive script theories have been applied to show that aggression and violence in media can be a hazard to children's mental health (Coie & Dodge, 1998; Huesmann, Moise-Titus, Podolski, & Eron, 2003). Taken as a whole, the poor parenting that aggressive children experience in tandem with their biased internalization of social experience, typically buttressed by an extensive constellation of biological and social risks (see Dodge & Pettit, 2003), portray a clear picture of aggression and maladaptation that is strongly communicated in contemporary perspectives on development and psychopathology. For example, Moeller's (2001) synthesis of research at the conclusion of his text on Youth Aggression and Violence incorporates a prenatal stage of "unfavorable innate substrate" and an infancy–toddler stage of "unfavorable psychological substrate." As research on childhood aggression is increasingly interpreted through developmental psychopathology frameworks (Coie & Dodge, 1998), useful questions concerning adaptation and aggression may not come easily to mind.

Ontogeny and Phylogeny

Behavior scientists with a phylogenetic perspective have been particularly likely to stress adaptive functions of aggression because aggressive behavior continues to be with us after a very long time. Zing-Yang Kuo (1922, 1967), a contrarian psychologist from China in the Watsonian tradition, experimented in the field on the development of aggression in birds, cats, and dogs. Kuo was a champion breeder of killer animals. Early isolation, he deduced, was key to the emergence of superior fighting skills; animals that grew up having a variety of social contacts formed sociable and amiable affiliations that disqualified them from main-event fighting. Kuo was always one to stress complexity, scorning those who would simplify behavior just so they could predict it. The "Dr. Jekyll and Mr. Hyde" dogs show the "coexistence of incompatible patterns in the same animal" (Kuo, 1967, p. 169). These dogs were trained to play or sleep with cats when inside their house, but to kill any cat outside, even those with whom previously they were cuddly. Then there was Bobby the smooth-haired Shan Chow, whose fighting behavior exhibited incredible variation in terms of when Bobby would let go versus fight to the death in battle, who he would attack and who he wouldn't, and when he would fight and when he wouldn't (pp. 15–17). Aggressive behavior to Kuo was an adaptational gradient to an environment greatly expanded in context and temporality when compared to the narrow stimuli favored by the preeminent behaviorists of his day (Rodkin, 1996). Iconoclast that he was, Kuo had problems with phylogeny as the behavioral geneticists and evolutionary psychologists saw it. Kuo's suggestions of supragenetic causes of behavioral evolution have retained credibility in the years since his death (Lickliter & Honeycutt, 2003). Kuo was just too concerned with ontogenetic processes to have them overridden by any particular period in the unobserved phylogenetic past. Kuo wished that psychologists would concentrate on creating new behavior patterns that would set the course for future evolution rather than looking backwards, playing a "perpetual guessing game" (p. 202) about what hunter–gatherer civilization was like and how ontogenetic behavior gets linked to it. No intelligent design faker was Zing-Yang Kuo, but he nonetheless had the temerity to close his only book, published at the end of his long career, musing on the "rather dubious twin concepts of 'natural selection' and 'survival value' of behavior for the species" (p. 203).

Kuo's (1967) audacious proposal opened the door to ways of considering the aggression–adaptation relationship in both ontogenetic and phylogenetic time without falling into explanations solely reliant on ancestral origins. Cairns, Gariépy, and Hood (1990) reported on high- and low-aggressive mice bred selectively for 18 generations and studied over the course of their ontogenies in dyadic fighting tests, thus permitting developmental and microevolutionary comparisons. High-aggression mice had increasingly greater attack rates than their low-aggression counterparts for the first five generations, after which differences were maintained. Experiential factors such as group housing versus isolation and expertise with the fighting task, in combination with the age of the mouse when tested, modified the magnitude of genetic differences between high- and low-aggression lines. Ontogenetic trajectories of attack behavior changed most among low-aggressive mice; moreover, these changes appeared to provide a platform for behavioral modifications that endured across generations. Cairns et al. (1990) argued that effects of genetic selection were open to change, and that rapid ontogenetic change supported microevolutionary change patterns, a "dual genesis" proposal where adaptations in ontogeny and phylogeny work in co-incidence (Baldwin, 1895). The question of whether aggression can be adaptive is taken for granted when aggressive behavior is used as an illustrative case for examining adaptation over varying temporal scales. Cairns (1979) was explicit about the adaptability of aggression in his earlier writings:

> Aggressive acts—whether perceived as attacks, punishment, or coercion— are inextricably woven into the patterns of normal interchanges. They constitute a principal means by which organisms control and direct inter- changes. Perhaps the question should not be "Why aggression?" but "Why is there not more aggression?" (p. 185)

Farmer et al. (this volume) feature a detailed review of interactional synchrony patterns, including how aggressive behavior can be at the leading edge of individual adaptation. There is no need to commit the phylogeny fallacy (Lickliter & Honeycutt, 2003) and assume that aggression is adaptive mainly because it worked in the primordial history of hunter–gatherer forebearers, with its adaptiveness essentialized in the genome or any other directing structure. Adaptation, even construed strictly as a central biological principle of organization, is responsive to shifts in time, proximal and distal environments (Gottesman & Hanson, 2005), and behavior (Cairns et al., 1990).

Values and Utility

Irrespective of occupation or specialization, in every age human beings have witnessed aggression against one another, and they have wit- nessed how that aggression can sometimes be effective. This plain, hard truth means that there is less to the debate on the adaptiveness of aggression than meets the eye (cf., Cillessen & Mayeux, this volume). The consensus is clear: aggression can be adaptive (and maladaptive, for the choice is not either/or). It is remarkable that most everywhere that the student of psychology looks, from McDougall to Kuo, Lorenz to Milgram (1976), Dollard to Cairns, there is acceptance of the principle that aggression can be adaptive. On what else could all these behavior scientists agree? It is not a matter of being a nativist, a learning theorist, a sociobiologist, or a social psychologist because obvious phenomena are always accepted by every school of thought.

The real controversy over aggression and adaptation lies in the realm of societal values, not theory (cf., Smith, this volume). The modern research infrastructure that concentrates on aggression and dysfunction has its origins in political events that shaped the social and behavioral sciences, not in a pure scientific breakthrough or paradigm shift. Psychological studies of aggression changed after World War II—they became dominated by American researchers during a period where Americans (and the rest of the world) yearned for quiet, where psychologists and the government found common ground and set a direction.

One danger could be that—in a crass effort to get funding, or as a failure of misguided belief—researchers only allow themselves the freedom to think or say that aggression is maladaptive. The possibility arises that critics of the idea that aggression can be adaptive are softhearted but fuzzy-headed, incapable of staring down the awful truth, fearful of unmasking personal ideology posing as scientific credibility. There is no doubt that developmental researchers need to be more straightforward when dealing with value-laden questions, distinguishing better between objectivity in study design and research procedure and neutrality in interpretation and hypothesis selection. Even logical positivism in psychology was not value-free, but a curious fantasyland of its own with a particular value structure. A value-free discipline can hardly address "'good' or 'bad' parenting, good or bad schooling, good or bad child-care arrangements, good or bad media influences, and good or bad social programs," particularly when researchers and the government must come to agreement on what these terms mean (White & Pillemer, 2005, pp. 2–3; see also Rappaport, 2005). Developmental research naturally exists conjoined to societal concerns and power structures, not apart from them.

Critics of an aggression-as-adaptive perspective (e.g., Aronson, 1995; Staub, 1989) thus legitimately rely on arguments based on value and utility. With respect to value, critics do not deny that aggression was ever adaptive, but instead stress that aggression is not now adaptive, and should not be adaptive in the just societies of tomorrow. Science and ideology have a loose (if dated) interplay in Aronson (1995):

> It may be true that, in the early history of human evolution, highly competitive and aggressive behaviors were adaptive. ... [As we] see a world full of strife, of international and interracial hatred and distrust, of senseless slaughter and political assassination, we feel justified in questioning the current survival value of this behavior. With the major powers in

possession of enough nuclear warheads to destroy the world's population twenty-five times over, I wonder whether building still more warheads might not be carrying things a bit too far. (pp. 257–258)

Aronson (1995) builds on his claim that aggression is unnecessary in today's society by surveying violence-reduction techniques including reason, timely but nonsevere punishment of aggressors (from Olweus, 1991), rewarding prosocial behavior patterns, presenting non-aggressive role models, and building empathy towards others (see also Espelage, Holt, & Henkel, 2003; Mussen & Eisenberg, 2001; Spielman & Staub, 2000). The position that aggression can never be accepted, and should not be part of the just worlds we wish to create, is a powerful moral value and not simply a denial mechanism.

Tremblay and Nagin (2005, p. 100), who also point to the late 20th century as a turning point in societal attitudes towards aggression, have a similar position. Aggression used to be adaptive, and in certain circumstances still is, but: "we are slowly creating a social environment in which the physical aggression solution generally becomes a much less adaptive strategy than its alternatives … in our 21st-century civilization there is an increasing trend to settle conflicts with words." From this perspective, aggression may have been a successful adaptation in the hunter–gatherer psychology of our primordial past, but it has no adaptive place in a civilized world, or in a society where cooperation and empathy are sufficiently important (Staub, 1989). Trajectories of aggression have ontogenetic and microevolutionary temporality and are interdependent (Cairns et al., 1990). The possibility exists that changing societal values may impact the adaptational value of individual aggressive behavior over generational time.

With respect to utility, the preponderance of developmental psychopathology research on childhood aggression may simply mean that developmental psychopathology is a useful framework for understanding and dealing with societal problems like youth violence (Tolan & Dodge, 2005). As reviewed, it is common knowledge that aggression can be an adaptive solution to social problems (Coie & Dodge, 1998, p. 784), but this knowledge has not been consistently accessed to support sustained empirical research. Coie and Dodge focused both on maladaptive aspects of aggression such as poor social cognition (Dodge & Feldman, 1990) and adaptive aspects such as in boys' dominance hierarchies (Coie, Dodge, Terry, & Wright, 1991; Pettit, Bakshi, Dodge, & Coie, 1990). Why did deficit-related phenomena of impaired social reasoning have greater impact than adaptiveness-related phenomena of dominance? Possibly, deficit-related research was more useful to preventionists, educators, and policymakers (e.g., Moeller, 2001).

The real test of the aggression-as-adaptive framework will be its utility in the marketplace of ideas, where many in the audience have a strong interest in reducing aggression within individuals, relationships, between groups, at school, at home, and in the community. Does an aggression-as-adaptive framework spur research into underappreciated dimensions of socialization? Can communicating how aggression can be adaptive be positive for consumers of research? Is it functional to say that aggression can be adaptive? Suggestions from yesteryear, such as McDougall's (1908/1914) exhortation to instill righteous anger in young children, or Dollard et al.'s (1939) recommendation for assertiveness on the playground, will require quite the repackaging to encourage serious, sustained inquiry when contrasting interventions premised on the dysfunctions and deficits of aggressive behavior are easily available. When the adaptational framework proves helpful to those most interested in understanding it, a significant research literature on aggression and adaptation will accumulate.

AGGRESSION AND ADAPTATION IN PEER ECOLOGIES

Aggression is adaptive and maladaptive but it's hard to keep dissonant propositions simultaneously in mind. Can an aggressive boy also enjoy social status at school, adapting well and integrating into his peer culture? Sure, if you think about it, but adults' first idea of a popular child is likely to be an ideal, positive and prosocial, without aggressive behavior (cf., Hawley, this volume). Roger Brown (1986) labeled this habit of human reasoning evaluative consistency: "Good things go together in real people and bad things likewise. It is truly a simple primitive theory, but [it has] ... action consequences" (p. 395). Evaluative consistency is more than an artifice of biased processing. It resembles the social development phenomenon of correlated constraints, where typical correlations between person and environment forces (e.g., good things with other good things) provide redundancy that keeps behavior stable over ontogeny (Farmer et al., this volume; Magnusson & Cairns, 1996). Evaluative consistency also resembles the Lewinian (1951) construct of tension systems, in which people's social environments are conceptualized as charged, multidetermined fields that bring out certain behaviors more than others. Evaluative consistency, correlated constraints, and tension systems help explain why social perception and behavior usually resist change and tend toward distinct configurations of broadly positive and broadly negative life patterns (Cairns & Cairns, 1994). Good-goes-with-good and bad-goes-with-bad development is thus an exaggeration prone to reality.

Phenomena Lost

Although recognized at a conceptual level (e.g., Coie & Dodge, 1998), in everyday life the adaptiveness of aggression remains an unlikely, off-the-diagonal phenomenon: good (adaptive) goes with bad (aggression), and this can fall through interpretative holes despite empirical demonstrations. For instance, studies focusing on aggression as a problem behavior can also give evidence that aggression is normative. An advance of Coie, Dodge, and Copotelli (1982) was the inclusion of "liked least" with "liked most" peer nominations in calculating sociometric status. In that study, "liked least" was necessary to ask because, on its own, being "liked most" and being aggressive were uncorrelated. Social preference needed a dislike dimension to enable the rejection–aggression linkage. An analysis by the NICHD Early Child Care Research Network (2004) uncovered five trajectories of physical aggression from toddlerhood to middle childhood. The most aggressive trajectory, comprising 3% of children, was consistently associated with maladaptive high-risk outcomes. More often than not, children in the two moderate aggression trajectories (one stable, the other declining over time) were similar to their non-aggressive counterparts (e.g., NICHD ECCRN, 2004, Tables 12–13) but differences between aggressive and non-aggressive trajectories were interpreted as the most meaningful.

Unlikely phenomena, like aggression that is adaptive, can have big practical effects. Cairns (1986) put neglect of off-diagonal phenomena, or variation within configurations that are homogeneous only at first glance, at the top of his list for why developmental researchers lose sight of developmental phenomena. The prodigal son, the rare event, the road less traveled, all are critical to a developmental psychology of change and should be subject to intense analysis (Cairns & Rodkin, 1998). The abnormal highlights the normal, the unusual speaks to the usual. Within Lewinian social psychology, small, unlikely circumstances can serve similarly as channel factors that have disproportionately large effects on persons and situations (Ross & Nisbett, 1991). Off-the-diagonal phenomena like the adaptiveness of aggression are practically undervalued as behavioral change agents (Farmer et al., this volume). For example, unpopular-aggressive children fit a stereotype, are socially marginalized, and so are easy to spot as needing intervention. Popular-aggressive children escape identification because they are not easily thought of and because they integrate freely with aggressive and non-aggressive children alike (Farmer et al., 2002). The popular-aggressive child, even when infrequent, can have a huge impact relative to unpopular children in shaping their peer cultures away from learning (McFarland, 2001).

Researchers who point out that aggression is part and parcel of everyday society tend to be in the social critique and reconstruction crowd left behind by the 1950 NSF legislation (Solovey, 2004). The aggression of the rejected child is an aggression of "them," the dysfunctional and at-risk. An aggression of the popular child is an aggression of "us," the adapted, normative culture implicated by McDougall (1908/1914), Murphy et al. (1937), and Dollard et al. (1939). After World War II, aggression–adaptation questions were asked mainly by sociologists who didn't have children's public health as a priority (cf., Smith, this volume). For example, Jack (1999) interviewed 60 women and concluded that their aggression in the context of partner-relationship failures could be positively transformative, realizing potential and enabling survival. This quotation by Jackman (2002) reads much like Cairns (1979, p. 185) in emphasizing how aggression is integrated into social life and should be studied as such.

> Violence incorporates a diverse array of actions that are an integral feature of social life. ... The confinement of the researcher to those injurious actions that are socially deviant ... subverts any attempt to understand why certain forms of violence are tolerated, accepted, endorsed, mandated, or glorified, while others are repudiated or even excoriated, or why some acts of violence erupt only in anger while others occur in tranquility or as an element of recreation. (Jackman, 2002, pp. 389, 403–404)

Jackman (2002, p. 392) points to the importance of funding in determining which forms of violence are most studied and how violence is conceptualized.

Coleman's (1961) *The Adolescent Society* made clear that what adolescents valued wasn't what adults thought they did value, or should value. Coleman's research, sponsored by the educational research arm of the U.S. government to examine high school social climates, found that American high schools oriented youth towards valuing athletic rather than scholastic accomplishment. Youth found characteristics such as strength, beauty, domination, and competitiveness, not academic achievement or scholastics, to rock their world. This is "old hat" today but was an unsettling change in American high schools facing Sputnik. Coleman pointed the finger at adults for this sad state of affairs, criticizing society for failing to construct educational environments that successfully marketed the values of scholarship to the next generation (cf., Erikson, 1950). The adolescent society soon drifted downward into middle childhood. Gary Alan Fine's (1987) *With the Boys* examines preadolescent male culture in little league baseball, a valued societal institution. Fine (1987) observes that little league boys use sexual and aggressive themes in their talk with one another whenever they can, employing it to show off among their peers and act more mature, to declare that they are mastering the imperatives of successful social development (see also Adler & Adler, 1998). Who can argue with them?

Ferguson's (2000) rich ethnography of an urban, multiethnic fourth-through sixth-grade school shows how Black boys, confronted with the superficial morality of an oppressive, aggressive school authority structure, gain self-esteem by causing trouble. Adult authorities are unwittingly implicated in whether and how aggression works for kids (Coleman, 1961; McFarland, 2001). Here is Ferguson's (2000) depiction of 12-year-old Horace:

> Horace's ability and readiness to fight both verbally and physically has garnered a position of authority and respect. ... The fact that [kids in the school] come to Horace for help to sort out difficult situations on the playground is not a signal to the school that he has leadership qualities. ... It indicates just the opposite. Horace becomes an individual to be watched as he gets involved in an alternative authority structure. (p. 126)

Concerned adults should identify the leaders of peer cultures as peers view them, working with peer leaders when possible to restructure social networks, reorient peer values, and redirect social influences (Miller-Johnson & Costanzo, 2004). Aggression can have a constituency, sometimes even a silent majority (Garandeau & Cillessen, in press; Rodkin, Farmer, Pearl, & Van Acker, 2006a).

Children's Peer Ecologies

Bronfenbrenner (1974) wrote that public schools degraded over the '60s into "one of the most potent breeding grounds of alienation in American society" (p. 60) because he believed that unrestrained peer culture became representative of American peer ecologies at school, disconnected from a caring adult environment, and as such inviting "the emergence of egocentrism, aggression, and antisocial behavior" (Bronfenbrenner, 1979, p. 194). This dark view of peer interaction stands in sharp relief to the typical, strong Bronfenbrennian themes of optimism and growth. This may relate to why Bronfenbrenner's (1944) earliest work was devoted to the sociometric mapping and tracking of children's social networks, in particular the correct determination of who, in fact, enjoys high social status in peer cultures. We have also tracked social status and social networks in middle childhood classroom societies. To make children's social relations visible, we have used sociometric and survey techniques to ask children and their teachers to identify peer groups and evaluate children's popularity, prestige, and social behavior. Deriving representations of children's social networks and social centrality provides a layered description of children's peer ecologies. Although individually oriented, trait-like psychological profiles of aggressive children and their targets have utility; identifying how particular aggressive children are networked among their peers provides additional clues as to how aggression can take root and thrive in educational settings (Mulvey & Cauffman, 2001).

To Bronfenbrenner (1996), the peer ecology and other immediate, proximal microsystems were the contexts of paramount importance where development occurs. We suggest that proximal peer ecologies can be organized along correlated horizontal and vertical axes (Rodkin & Fischer, 2003; Rodkin & Hodges, 2003). With respect to the horizontal axis, elementary school children form multiple groups within classrooms that provide them with various opportunities to engage in play, to work, to learn, and to enjoy social support. When a classroom is conceptualized as containing multiple (e.g., four or five) groups, diverse voices— rule-following and oppositional, prosocial and antisocial—can be heard. When group identification is absent from research assessments, or when groups are defined simply as the sum or average of all children in a classroom, only the dominant, rule-following value shines through. The vertical structure of peer ecologies is akin to social power. Children and their groups differ in social status, thereby influencing what peers value and devalue, and what are the norms in different peer ecologies.

As applied to aggression, peer ecologies can assume a variety of forms. Some aggressors are friendless and lonely, reinforcing the classic research portrayals of hostile, rejecting peer ecologies for many externalizing children (e.g., Asher & Coie, 1990). This kind of peer ecology especially relates to bullies who are also victims of repeated aggression. Other aggressors enjoy peer acceptance, but only in small, peripheral social networks composed mainly of unpopular, aggressive children like themselves (Coie & Dodge, 1998; McDougall, Hymel, Vaillancourt, & Mercer, 2001; Rubin, Bukowski, & Parker, 1998; Cillessen & Mayeux, this volume). The peer ecology of such unpopular aggressors may be fertile soil for deviancy to flourish.

Popular-Aggressive Children

Recent research has highlighted peer ecologies in which some aggressive children are popular (LaFontana & Cillessen, 2002; Luthar & McMahon, 1996; Parkhurst & Hopmeyer, 1998; Rodkin, Farmer, Pearl, & Van Acker, 2000), and where some bullies are leaders and expert manipulators who use a network of supporters and affiliates to help accomplish their antisocial endeavors (Salmivalli, Huttunen, & Lagerspetz, 1997; Sutton, Smith, & Swettenham, 1999). The popularity of some aggressive children implies mainstream childhood culture may value aggressive behavior (Rodkin et al., 2000). Aggressors who actively engage peer culture experience a very different, more complicated environment than aggressors whom peers reject. Whereas a tradition that highlights associations between aggression and rejection has led to preventative interventions emphasizing the acquisition of social skills and alleviation of social–cognitive deficits, research on popular aggressors presents a new set of challenges to educators and researchers.

We have performed a series of analyses of a cross-sectional sample of almost 1,000 children (Farmer et al., 2002; Rodkin et al, 2000; Rodkin et al., 2006a, 2006b), with the collective goal of identifying popular-aggressive children and describing their integration within classroom peer ecologies. Our design included measures of teachers' assessments of students, peer assessments, students' self-assessments, as well as social cognitive mapping. Rodkin et al. (2000) focused on the boys in the sample. They concluded that highly aggressive boys sometimes were among the most popular and socially connected children in elementary classrooms. There was not an analogous configuration of popular-aggressive girls (Farmer, Rodkin, Pearl, & Van Acker, 1999). Teachers perceived six behavioral configurations of boys: model, tough, low academic, passive, bright antisocial, and troubled. Of these configurations, teachers and peers nominated model boys (high academic achievement coupled with prosocial attitudes) as being highly popular. Tough boys (aggressive, below-average academically) were also seen as popular. These results show that popular boys are behaviorally heterogeneous. Tough boys saw themselves as most popular and aggressive, suggesting that popular tough boys were well aware of their success at mastering their social environment. But not all types of aggressive boys were popular. For example, although both tough and bright antisocial kids scored above average on aggressiveness, their levels of popularity differed substantially. Teachers ranked tough kids second in popularity only to model kids, but scored bright antisocial kids well below average. Similarly, peers positioned tough kids as the coolest kids in the class, but nominated bright antisocial kids as among the least cool. Troubled kids, with a profile that strongly resembled the classic aggressive-rejected child, were clearly perceived by all as dysfunctional. Children highly esteem some of their aggressive peers, but aggression in and of itself has little significance to social status. Rather, aggressiveness gains meaning when conjoined with other individual characteristics (e.g., athleticism, attractiveness, prosocial behavior) and placed in social context (cf. Magnusson, 1998; Hawley, this volume). Even if a minority of children display a combination of high levels of popularity and antisocial behavior, these children can strongly impact the adjustment of their peers and the overall classroom social dynamic. Rodkin et al. (2000) also stressed the importance of selecting appropriate status measures vis-à-vis aggression, that is, perceived popularity along with social preference (cf. Cilessen & Mayeux, this volume). If we lose sight of the possibility that aggression can be adaptive, we will not capture phenomena pertinent to how aggressors can integrate into and help construct mainstream childhood culture.

Farmer et al. (2002) questioned the deviant peer group hypothesis, which says that aggressive youth are limited to membership in small, peripheral groups situated on the perimeter of conventional social networks. Two thirds of aggressive boys and one half of aggressive girls affiliated with groups who were mostly (more than 50%) non-aggressive. Popular-aggressive boys associated with each other as well as with non-aggressive peers, whereas unpopular-aggressive boys usually associated with only non-aggressive groups. For both boys and girls, youth tended to associate with others who were similar to themselves in socially significant characteristics such as athleticism or popularity, but they did form ties with peers who were both similar and dissimilar in terms of aggressive behavior. These results show that aggressive children, particularly boys, can interact in all types of social spheres and do not always form an easily recognizable, behaviorally homogeneous peer group. Identifying these connections between aggressive and non-aggressive youth, Farmer et al. (2002) recommended that the focus of anti-violence campaigns should also address non-aggressive peers who may support hostile friends.

Rodkin et al. (2006a, 2006b) examined the children who nominated aggressive peers as among the three "coolest" kids in their school. True to the notion that aggression often works via group processes, both aggressive and non-aggressive children who affiliated in aggressive groups nominated aggressive peers as cool. Likewise, children in non-aggressive groups—both aggressive and non-aggressive—were more likely to nominate non-aggressive kids as the coolest. In terms of the correlates of children's nominations of aggressive versus non-aggressive peers as cool, group affiliations trump individual characteristics. These results held for boy and girl same-sex "cool" nominations, although girls disproportionately nominated popular-aggressive boys as cool (see also Bukowski, Sippola, & Newcomb, 2000). Aggressive girls had a narrower base of support that drew more strongly from girls like themselves, as befits a deviant peer group model (e.g., Kiesner & Massimiliano, 2005). One implication of Rodkin et al.'s (2006 a, 2006b) analyses is that children's peer ecologies imbue aggression with meaning, influencing their members' attitudes and behaviors while enabling some aggressive children to have high social status. Another implication is that it is important to study alternatives to peer preference, such as being cool, when considering children's social status. Measures of social centrality, coolness, and popularity, moreso than social preference, reveal that aggression can be proximally adaptive for children, and an integrated part of classroom social networks. Such conclusions have strong implications for educators and other adults concerned with children's welfare.

AGGRESSION, ADAPTATION, AND EDUCATIONAL PROMISE

Given that aggression can be socially adaptive, interventions to limit aggression and violence in schools ought to take an ecological approach that aspires to positively influence the values and norms of all children, including those who are popular and/or aggressive. Rather than attempting primarily to root out evil-doers, a focus on the broader school culture has promise (Mulvey & Cauffman, 2001). A study of school-based violence-prevention interventions found that between 1993 and 1997, elementary schools that focused on improving the school environment achieved success in changing violence-related behavior (Howard, Flora, & Griffin, 1999). Indeed, the power of children feeling accepted and at home while in school should never be underestimated. By as early as third grade, students who express high satisfaction with schooling report supportive interactions with teachers, broad social support, and a positive school climate (Baker, 1999). The dramatic influence of a positive school climate continues as children age. Resnick et al. (1997) found that the most powerful predictor of adolescent well-being is a feeling of connection to school. But how do concerned adults and children create this positive school culture?

Classroom Management Practices

As leaders of the core units of elementary schools, teachers should approach classroom management as an ongoing effort to develop a caring community in the classroom (see Baker, 1998). Holding democratic class meetings, placing emphasis on conflict resolution and empathy, as well as giving attention to moral decision-making and civic responsibility are all approaches that foster a sense of community (Baker, 1998; Kohlberg, 1981). The behaviors and attitudes that teachers model also strongly affect their students. For example, (Chang (2003) found that teachers' aversion to aggression and their empathy toward social withdrawal enhanced the self-perceptions of both aggressive and withdrawn children. Beyond implicit messages, firmly setting high expectations of kindness, cooperation, and social equality help as well; children need adults to tell them that playing fair and respecting all of their peers are worthy, necessary goals to strive for collectively. Integral to an effort to cultivate caring communities is promoting open, honest communication between students and teachers. As Mulvey and Cauffman (2001) caution, reporting threats or scary activities going on in a school environment can occur only if students feel that they are safe and that a reasoned response will result from their reporting. Despite educators' best efforts at developing trusting, open relationships with their students, much information about children and their peer relationships might remain hidden from view.

Sociometry and Social Networks

Primary teachers can use their own classroom-level sociometric measures and social networks analyses to become better attuned to the ways children integrate into their peer ecologies (Blair, Jones, & Simpson, 1968; Gronlund, 1959; Rodkin, 2004). Being armed with information about who is socially isolated or well connected and who is esteemed or undervalued by peers might make teachers more effective at facilitating open communication and mitigating aggression and victimization among their children. Sociometric measures of popularity also might make it easier for teachers to employ direct, proactive interventions with children who play significant roles in the peer ecology. Indeed, the improved group morale derived from satisfying social relationships in the classroom enhances students' attitudes towards learning.

To be sure, teachers are not puppeteers and do not control the social status accorded to all aggressive children, nor do they rein in, at will, the hierarchical structures that facilitate long-term patterns of victimization (see Schafer, Korn, Brodbeck, Wolke, & Schulz, 2005). But through behavior modeling, routine discourse, and an accurate understanding of their classroom social networks, teachers do have the potential to fashion the group ethics of a classroom and orchestrate the interplay of children. Bolstering the self-confidence and visibility of peer-rejected youth by assigning them key classroom responsibilities, publicly praising children for jobs well done, and partnering popular and unpopular children during classroom instruction might moderate classroom hierarchies and promote the positive development of all children in the classroom.

Educators can employ sociometric techniques to identify youth leaders, especially when their leadership qualities escape the attention of school authorities because they counter dominant adult views (Ferguson, 2004; Miller-Johnson, & Costanzo, 2004). By early adolescence, the social context for youth increasingly accepts and reinforces aggression (Cillesson & Mayeux, this volume). As evidence of this developmental trend, Miller-Johnson, Coie, Maumary-Gremaud, Bierman, and the Conduct Problems Prevention Research Group (2002) identified two patterns of leadership among their sample of urban, African American seventh graders: conventional, model leaders (e.g., student government officials) and less mainstream leaders who espoused antisocial attitudes (e.g., trendsetters for norms of dress and speech). Perceived by peers as independent and mature, the unconventional, antisocial leaders may be in stronger positions to shape the value structures of their peer ecologies; indeed, they seem to be responsible for influencing peer orientations that normalize aggression and challenge conventional values during early adolescence (Miller-Johnson & Costanzo, 2004). Teachers can use sociometric measures to identify these unconventional leaders and acknowledge their powers of influence. But as Miller-Johnson and Costanzo (2004) caution, "[t]o intervene successfully, practitioners must also neither implicitly nor explicitly oppose the power of deviant peers or the cliques they lead" (p. 214). Instead, if teachers use sociometric information to ally themselves with aggressive leaders, perhaps they can influence behavior without fomenting oppositional attitudes and resistance among their students (McFarland, 2001).

Valuing Assertiveness, Not Aggression

At first glance, it appears that children's peer ecologies, especially the more hierarchical ones (see Schafer et al., 2005), are prone to having prominent individuals who use their aggression to acquire social status to the psychological and social detriment of some of their peers. But there is hope for more peaceful youth societies that provide opportunities for kids to exert their wills and hone their social skills while respecting the rights of others and honoring a peaceful group ethic. It need not be excruciatingly difficult for the timid to gain confidence, for the isolated to extend their social networks, or for the aggressive, popular kids to lead without damaging their peers. Teaching children assertiveness takes a strong, positive step towards this more harmonious youth culture.

Although assertiveness and aggression are sometimes used interchangeably, the terms connote quite different behavioral meanings. Assertiveness includes proactive attempts to direct or alter another person's activity without the intention to injure (Barrett & Yarrow, 1977). Others cast assertiveness in a more defensive light, defining assertiveness as "[b]ehavior which occurs in response to aggressive behavior of others. It leads to or seeks the maintenance or re-establishment of the realm which the individual controlled at the beginning of the conflict" (Bakker, Bakker-Rabdau, & Breit, 1978, p. 278). Assertiveness, like aggression, gains meaning within ecological and temporal contexts, but unlike aggression, assertiveness tempers personal agency with concern for others' welfare and is characterized by the defense (rather than expansion) of one's rights and privileges. Assertiveness is also distinguished from passivity, or inaction within a social context despite personal needs to acquire social resources. Rotheram, Armstrong, and Booraem (1982) aptly describe the distinctions between assertiveness, aggression, and passivity:

> Although the assertive act is situationally specific, social observers label a number of easily observable behavior patterns as assertive. For example, looking the teacher in the eye or answering a question in 1 to 3 seconds is considered socially assertive. These assertive acts lie on a continuum between passive and aggressive responses. Passive acts are inhibited, self-denying responses which limit contact with others, such as avoiding eye contact. Aggressive acts infringe on others' rights, demanding the person's goals be met, and would be characterized by an aggressive stare towards others. (p. 567)

Although aggression may be adaptive for an individual in the short or long term, assertiveness may be more adaptive for the group. Barrett and Yarrow (1977) found assertiveness to be positively and significantly related to prosocial behaviors such as comforting, sharing, and helping others. If one goal of education is to teach kids how to achieve both personal and group goals while preserving social harmony and personal integrity, then instilling assertiveness is a worthwhile endeavor for schools. Shy, social isolates and victims of peer aggression appear the most obvious beneficiaries of assertiveness training, as they would learn social skills that display personal courage, a stronger sense of self-worth, and a willingness to interact with their peers on egalitarian terms. Assertiveness training might also reshape highly aggressive children's behaviors by teaching them more socially sensitive and self-respecting ways to achieve their goals.

Rotheram et al. (1982) described the effectiveness of one assertiveness training program for fourth- and fifth-grade children. In groups of six, the children learned, via didactic instruction, individual and group problem solving, and assertive behavior rehearsal, how to act assertively instead of aggressively or passively. The intervention was effective in increasing assertiveness as evaluated by teachers and peers. Moreover, children's increased assertiveness was associated with positive social and academic effects. Immediately following the treatment, children who received assertiveness training achieved higher teacher-rated popularity and initiated significantly more contacts with teachers and other children. This is especially good news for timid, unpopular children. More importantly, a year later teachers who were unaware of the children's participation in the study reported higher popularity, better comportment, and higher achievement for the children who underwent assertiveness training. No adverse effect of teachers responding negatively to students' increased assertiveness and activity was found, suggesting the assertiveness training may have reduced at least some undesirable aggression. Another important effect of the assertiveness training program was that it was associated with an improvement in grades 1 year later, an illuminating finding given the correlation between extreme aggression and poor academic achievement.

Psychologists in the generations before World War II (Dollard et al., 1939; McDougall, 1908/1914; Murphy et al., 1937) recognized the merits of developing both children's assertiveness as well as their cooperative behavior. Can we, in today's world, promote children being assertive without running the risk of having assertive exchanges frequently escalate into negative, explosive aggressive interchanges? An aggression-as-adaptive framework enables renewed consideration of long-forgotten strategies such as assertiveness training. The challenges of future research in this area are to map the social relations and dynamics of assertive children, and to design interventions that sensitize children and adults to distinctions between constructive assertiveness and destructive aggression. Of course, what is constructive and destructive can be a matter of perspective. Questions of value—for instance, those posed by Staub (1989) and Aronson (1995)—are pertinent. Would it be desirable to expend resources trying to promote an assertive society, even if we could? The utility of work in assertiveness and the value others place on it will determine its future direction and success.

CONCLUSIONS

Major social-developmental scientists have recognized that aggression can be adaptive or maladaptive. Aggression can happen in all kinds of ways, whether among children in a classroom or in the abstract theories of scholars. There emerged in the societal and social scientific zeitgeist of post-World War II America a set of dominant ideas about how to handle a pervasive problem: the challenge of ameliorating the risk and danger to themselves and others of reactively aggressive, often rejected children with a multisystemic profile of dysfunction. As encompassing a problem as this is, other questions pertaining to how children socialize aggression among themselves and use aggression to organize peer ecologies have not been asked enough. An aggressive-as-adaptive framework is valuable once attention is focused on how aggression is integrated into children's peer ecologies. Teachers need to understand their classrooms' social dynamics from the perspective of their students and to have insight into how their teaching practices influence the social status of antisocial behavior among students. Systematic use of sociometric and emerging social network technologies can help educators and scientists track, manage, and influence peer ecologies in which aggression is deeply rooted. Guided by a more accurate understanding of children's social networks and social status, educators can then cultivate assertiveness as one way to positively influence the values and behaviors of such peer ecologies and to enhance the quality of school climates. It is completely fitting that one critical test of an aggression-as-adaptive approach shall lie in its actualized potential for making schools more positive places for more children.

REFERENCES

Adler, P. A., & Adler, P. (1998). *Peer power: Preadolescent culture and identity.* New Brunswick, NJ: Rutgers University Press.

Allport, F. H. (1924). *Social psychology.* New York: Houghton Mifflin.

Allport, G. W. (1954). *The nature of prejudice.* Cambridge, MA: Addison-Wesley.

Anderson, C. A., & Bushman, B. J. (2002). Human aggression. *Annual Review of Psychology, 53,* 27–51.

Aronson, E. (1995). *The social animal* (7th ed.). New York: W.H. Freeman and Company.

Asher, S. R., & Coie, J. D. (1990). Peer rejection and loneliness in childhood. In S. R. Asher & J. D. Coie (Eds.), *Peer rejection in childhood* (pp. 253–273). New York: Cambridge University Press.

Baker, J. E. (1998). Are we missing the forest for the trees? Considering the social context of school violence. *Journal of School Psychology, 36,* 29–44.

Baker, J. E. (1999). Teacher–student interaction in urban at-risk classrooms: Differential behavior, relationship quality, and student satisfaction with school. *Elementary School Journal, 100,* 57–70.

Bakker, C. B., Bakker-Rabdau, M. K., & Breit, S. (1978). The measurement of assertiveness and aggressiveness. *Journal of Personality Assessment, 42,* 277–284.

Baldwin, J. M. (1895). *Social and ethical interpretations in mental development.* London: Macmillan.

Bandura, A. (1969). *Principles of behavior modification.* New York: Holt, Rinehart and Winston.

Bandura, A., & Walters, R. H. (1959). *Adolescent aggression.* New York: Ronald Press.

Barker, R. T., Dembo, T., & Lewin, K. (1941). Frustration and aggression: An experiment with young children. *University of Iowa Studies in Child Welfare, 18,* 1.

Barrett, D. E., & Yarrow, M. R. (1977). Prosocial behavior, social inferential ability, and assertiveness in children. *Child Development, 48,* 475–481.

Berkowitz, L. (1962). *Aggression: A social psychological analysis.* New York: McGraw-Hill.

Bierman, K. L., Smoot, D. L., & Aumiller, K. (1993). Characteristics of aggressive-rejected, aggressive (nonrejected), and rejected (non-aggressive) boys. *Child Development, 64,* 139–151.

Blair, G. M., Jones, R. S., & Simpson, R. H. (1968). *Educational psychology* (3rd ed.). New York: Macmillan.

Bowlby, J. (1950). *Attachment.* New York: Basic Books.

Bowlby, J. (1966). *Maternal care and mental health* (2nd ed.). New York: Shocken Books.

Bronfenbrenner, U. (1944). A constant frame of reference for sociometric research: II. Experiment and inference. *Sociometry, 7,* 40–75.

Bronfenbrenner, U. (1974). The origins of alienation. *Scientific American, 231,* 53–61.

Bronfenbrenner, U. (1979). *The ecology of human development: Experiments by nature and design.* Cambridge, MA: Harvard University Press.

Bronfenbrenner, U. (1996). Foreword. In R. B. Cairns, G. H. Elder Jr., & E. J. Costello (Eds.), *Developmental science* (pp. ix–xvii). New York: Cambridge University Press.

Brown, R. (1965). *Social psychology.* New York: The Free Press.

Brown, R. (1986). *Social psychology: The second edition.* New York: The Free Press.

Bukowski, W. M. (2003). What does it mean to say that aggressive children are competent or incompetent? *Merrill-Palmer Quarterly, 49,* 390–400.

Bukowski, W. M., Sippola, L. K., & Newcomb, A. F. (2000). *Developmental Psychology, 36,* 147–154.

Cairns, R. B. (1979). *Social development: The origins and plasticity of social interchanges.* San Francisco: Freeman.

Cairns, R. B. (1986). Phenomena lost: Issues in the study of development. In J. Valsiner (Ed.), *The individual subject and scientific psychology* (pp. 87–111). New York: Plenum.

Cairns, R. B., & Cairns, B. D. (1994). *Lifelines and risks: Pathways of youth in our time.* Cambridge, UK: Cambridge University Press.

Cairns, R. B., & Cairns, B. D. (2001). Aggression and attachment: The folly of separatism. In A. C. Bohart & D. J. Stipek (Eds.), *Constructive and destructive behavior: Implications for family, school, and society* (pp. 21–47). Washington, DC: American Psychological Association.

Cairns, R. B., Gariépy, J. L., & Hood, K. E. (1990). Development, microevolution, and social behavior. *Psychological Review, 97,* 49–65.

Cairns, R. B., & Rodkin, P. C. (1998). Phenomena regained: From configurations to pathways. In R. B. Cairns, L. R. Bergman, & J. Kagan (Eds.), *Methods and models for studying the individual: Essays in honor of Marian Radke-Yarrow* (pp. 245–266). Thousand Oaks, CA: Sage.

Chang, L. (2003). Variable effects of children's aggression, social withdrawal, and prosocial leadership as functions of teacher beliefs and behaviors. *Child Development, 74,* 535–548.

Coie, J. D., & Dodge, K. A. (1998). Aggression and antisocial behavior. In W. Damon (Gen. Ed.) & N. Eisenberg (Series Ed.), *Handbook of child psychology: Vol. 3. Social, emotional, and personality development* (5th ed., pp. 779–862). New York: Wiley.

Coie, J. D., Dodge, K. A., & Coppotelli, H. (1982). Dimensions and types of social status: A cross-age perspective. *Developmental Psychology, 18*, 557–570.

Coie, J. D., Dodge, K. A., Terry, R., & Wright, V. (1991). The role of aggression in peer relations: An analysis of aggression episodes in boys' play groups. *Child Development, 62*, 812–826.

Coleman, J. S. (1961). *The adolescent society: The social life of the teenager and its impact on education* (2nd ed.). New York: The Free Press.

Courtwright, D. T. (1996). *Violent land: Single men and social disorder from the frontier to the inner city*. Cambridge, MA: Harvard University Press.

Dishion, T. J., Patterson, G. R., & Griesler, P. C. (1994). Peer adaptations in the development of antisocial behavior: A confluence model. In L.R. Huesmann (Ed.), *Aggressive behavior: Current perspectives* (pp. 61–95). New York: Plenum.

Dodge, K. A., & Feldman, E. (1990). Issues in social cognition and sociometric status. In S. R. Asher & J. D. Coie (Eds.), *Peer rejection in childhood* (pp. 119–155). New York: Cambridge University Press.

Dodge, K. A., & Pettit, G. S. (2003). A biopsychosocial model of the development of chronic conduct problems in adolescence. *Developmental Psychology, 39*, 349–371.

Dollard, J., Doob, Miller, Mowrer, Sears, Ford, et al. (1939). *Frustration and aggression*. New Haven, CT: Yale University Press.

Erikson, E. (1950). *Childhood and society*. New York: Norton.

Eron, L. D. (1994). Theories of aggression: From drives to cognitions. In L.R. Huesmann (Ed.), *Aggressive behavior: Current perspectives* (pp. 3–11). New York: Plenum.

Espelage, D. L., Holt, M. K., & Henkel, R. R. (2003). Examination of peer-group contextual effects on aggression during early adolescence. *Child Development, 74*, 205–220.

Farmer, T. W., Leung, M., Rodkin, P. C., Cadwaller, T. W., Pearl, R., & Van Acker, R. (2002). Deviant or diverse peer groups? The peer affiliations of aggressive elementary students. *Journal of Educational Psychology, 94*, 611–620.

Farmer, T. W., Rodkin, P. C., Pearl, R., & Van acker, R. (1999). Teacher-assessed behavioral configurations, peer-assessments, and self-concepts of elementary students with mild disabilities. *Journal of Special Education, 33*, 66–80.

Ferguson, A. A. (2004). *Bad boys: Public schools in the making of black masculinity*. Ann Arbor, MI: University of Michigan Press.

Fine, G. A. (1987). *With the boys: Little league baseball and preadolescent culture*. Chicago: The University of Chicago Press.

Freud, S. (1930/1961). *Civilization and its discontents*. New York: Norton.

Garandeau, C. F., & Cillessen, A. H. N. (in press). From indirect aggression to invisible aggression: A conceptual view on bullying and peer group manipulation. *Aggression and Violent Behavior*.

Goodenough, F. L. (1931). *Anger in young children*. Minneapolis: University of Minnesota Press.

Gottesman, I. I., & Hanson, D. R. (2005). Human development: Biological and genetic processes. *Annual Review of Psychology, 56*, 263–286.

Gronlund, N. (1959). *Sociometry in the classroom*. New York: Harper and Brothers.

Hartup, W. W. (2005). The development of aggression: Where do we stand? In R. E. Tremblay, W. W. Hartup, & J. Archer (Eds.), *Developmental origins of aggression* (pp. 3–22). New York: Guilford.

Holt, M. K., & Espelage, D. L. (2003). A cluster analytic investigation of victimization among high school students: Are profiles differentially associated with psychological symptoms and school belonging? *Journal of Applied School Psychology, 19*, 81–98.

Howard, K., Flora, J., & Griffin, M. (1999). Violence-prevention programs in schools: State of the science and implications for future research. *Applied and Preventive Psychology, 8*, 197–215.

Huesmann, L. R., Moise-Titus, J., Podolski, C., & Eron, L. D. (2003). Longitudinal relations between children's exposure to TV violence and their aggressive and violent behavior in young adulthood: 1977–1992. *Developmental Psychology, 39*, 201–221.

Jack, D. C. (1999). *Behind the mask: Destruction and creativity in women's aggression*. Cambridge, MA: Harvard University Press.

Jackman, M. R. (2002). Violence in social life. *Annual Review of Sociology, 28*, 387–415.

Juvonen, J., & Graham, S. (Eds.). (2001). *Peer harassment in school: The plight of the vulnerable and victimized*. New York: Guilford.

Kohlberg, L. (1981). *Essays on moral development, Volume I: The philosophy of moral development*. San Francisco: Harper & Row.

Kiesner, J., & Massimiliano, P. (2005). Differences in the relations between antisocial behavior and peer acceptance across contexts and across adolescence. *Child Development, 76*, 1278–1293.

Kuo, Z. -Y. (1922). How are our instincts acquired? *Psychological Review 29*, 344–365.

Kuo, Z. -Y. (1960). Studies on the basic factors in animal fighting: IV. Developmental and environmental factors affecting fighting in quails. *Journal of Genetic Psychology, 96*, 225–239.

Kuo, Z. -Y. (1967). *The dynamics of behavior development: An epigenetic view*. New York: Random House.

LaFontana, K. M., & Cillessen, A. H. N. (2002). Children's perceptions of popular and unpopular peers: a multimethod assessment. *Developmental Psychology, 38*, 635–647.

Lehrman, D. S. (1953). A critique of Konrad Lorenz's theory of instinctive behavior. *The Quarterly Review of Biology, 28*, 337–363.

Lewin, K. (1951). *Field theory in social science: Selected theoretical papers* (D. Cartwright, Ed.). New York: Harper.

Lewin, K., Lippitt, R., & White, R. (1939). Patterns of aggressive behavior in experimentally created "social climates." *Journal of Social Psychology, 10*, 271–299.

Lickliter, R., & Honeycutt, H. (2003). Developmental dynamics: Toward a biologically plausible evolutionary psychology. *Psychological Bulletin, 129*, 819–835.

Lippitt, R., Polansky, R., Redl, F., & Rosen, S. (1952). The dynamics of power: A field study of social influence in groups of children. In G. E. Swanson, T. M. Newcomb, & E. L. Hartley (Eds.), *Readings in school psychology* (rev. ed., pp. 623–636). New York: Holt.

Lorenz, K. (1963). *On aggression.* New York: Harcourt.

Luthar, S. S., & McMahon, T. J. (1996). Peer reputation among inner-city adolescents: Structure and correlates. *Journal of Research on Adolescence, 6,* 581–603.

Magnusson, D. (1998). The logic and implications of a person-oriented approach. In R. B. Cairns, L. R. Bergman, & J. Kagan (Eds.), *Methods and models for studying the individual* (pp. 33–64). Thousand Oaks, CA: Sage.

Magnusson, D., & Cairns, R. B. (1996). Developmental science: Toward a unified framework. In R. B. Cairns, G. H. Elder Jr., & E. J. Costello (Eds.), *Developmental science* (pp. 7–30). New York: Cambridge University Press.

McDougall, W. (1908/1914). *An introduction to social psychology.* Boston: John W. Luce & Co.

McDougall, W. (1920). *The group mind.* London: Cambridge University Press.

McDougall, W. (1926). Men or robots? In C. Murchison (Ed.), *Psychologies of 1925* (pp. 273–305). Worcester, MA: Clark University Press.

McDougall, P., Hymel, S., Vaillancourt, T., & Mercer, L. (2001). The consequences of childhood peer rejection. In M. Leary (Ed.), *Interpersonal rejection* (pp. 213–250). New York: Oxford University Press.

McFarland, D. A. (2001). Student resistance: How the formal and informal organization of classrooms facilitate everyday forms of student defiance. *American Journal of Sociology, 107,* 612–678.

Milgram, S. (1976). *Human aggression* [Motion picture]. University Park, PA: Pennsylvania State University Audio-Visual Services.

Miller-Johnson, S., Coie, J. D., Maumary-Gremaud, A., Bierman, K., & the Conduct Problems Prevention Research Group. (2002). Peer rejection and aggression and early starter models of conduct disorder. *Journal of Abnormal Child Psychology, 30,* 217–230.

Miller-Johnson, S., & Costanzo, P. (2004). If you can't beat 'em ... induce them to join you: Peer-based interventions during adolescence. In J. B. Kupersmidt & K. A. Dodge (Eds.), *Children's peer relations: From development to intervention* (pp. 209–222). Washington, DC: American Psychological Association.

Mintz, S. (2004). *Huck's raft: A history of American childhood.* Cambridge, MA: Harvard University Press.

Moeller, T. G. (2001). *Youth aggression and violence.* Mahwah, NJ: Lawrence Erlbaum Associates.

Moffitt, T. E. (2005). The new look of behavioral genetics in developmental psychopathology: Gene–environment interplay in antisocial behaviors. *Psychological Bulletin, 131,* 533–554.

Mulvey, E. P., & Cauffman, E. (2001). The inherent limits of predicting school violence. *American Psychologist, 56,* 797–802.

Murchison, C. (Ed.). (1926). *Psychologies of 1925.* Worcester, MA: Clark University Press.

Murphy, G., Murphy, L. B., & Newcomb, T. M. (1937). *Experimental social psychology.* New York: Harper & Brothers.

Mussen, P., & Eisenberg, N. (2001). Prosocial development in context. In A. C. Bohart & D. J. Stipek (Eds.), *Constructive & destructive behavior: Implications for family, school, & society* (pp. 103–126). Washington, DC: American Psychological Association.

NICHD Early Child Care Research Network. (2004). Trajectories of physical aggression from toddlerhood to middle childhood: Predictors, correlates, and outcomes. *Monographs of the Society for Research in Child Development, 69*(4, Serial No. 278).

Olweus, D. (1991). Bully/victim problems among schoolchildren: Basic facts and effects of a school-based intervention program. In D. Pepler & K. Rubin (Eds.), *The development and treatment of childhood aggression* (pp. 411–448). Hillsdale, NJ: Lawrence Erlbaum Associates.

Parkhurst, J. T., & Hopmeyer, A. (1998). Sociometric popularity and peer-perceived popularity: Two distinct dimensions of peer status. *Journal of Early Adolescence, 18,* 125–144.

Patterson, G. R., & Bank, C. L. (1989). Some amplifying mechanisms for pathologic processes in families. In M. Gunnar & E. Thelen (Eds.), *Systems and development: Symposia on child psychology* (pp. 167–210). Hillsdale, NJ: Lawrence Erlbaum Associates.

Pettit, G. S., Bakshi, A., Dodge, K. A., & Coie, J. D. (1990). The emergence of social dominance in young boys' play groups: Developmental differences and behavioral correlates. *Developmental Psychology, 26,* 1017–1025.

Rappaport, J. (2005). Community psychology is (thank God) more than science. *American Journal of Community Psychology, 35,* 231–238.

Resnick, M. D., Bearman, P. S., Blum, R. W., Bauman, K. E., Harris, K. M., Jones, J. et al. (1997). Protecting adolescents from harm: Findings from the National Longitudinal Study on Adolescent Health. *Journal of the American Medical Association, 278,* 823–832.

Rodkin, P. C. (1996). A developmental, holistic, future-oriented behaviorism: Kuo's *The Dynamics of Behavior Development* revisited. *Contemporary Psychology, 41,* 1085–1088.

Rodkin, P. C. (2004). Peer ecologies of aggression and bullying. In D. L. Espelage & S. M. Swearer (Eds.), *Bullying in American schools: A social-ecological perspective on prevention and intervention* (pp. 87–106). Mahwah, NJ: Lawrence Erlbaum Associates.

Rodkin, P. C., Farmer, T. W., Pearl, R., & Van Acker, R. (2000). Heterogeneity of popular boys: Antisocial and prosocial configurations. *Developmental Psychology, 36,* 14–24.

Rodkin, P. C., Farmer, T. W., Pearl, R., & Van Acker, R. (2006a). They're cool: Ethnic and peer group supports for aggressive boys and girls. *Social Development, 15,* 175–204.

Rodkin, P. C., Farmer, T. W., Van Acker, R., Pearl, R., Thompson, J. H., & Fedora, P. (2006b). Who do students with mild disabilities nominate as cool in inclusive general education classrooms? *Journal of School Psychology, 44,* 67–84.

Rodkin, P. C., & Fischer, K. (2003). Sexual harassment and the cultures of childhood: Developmental, domestic violence, and legal perspectives. *Journal of Applied School Psychology, 19*, 177–196.

Rodkin, P. C., & Hodges, E. V. (2003). Bullies and victims in the peer ecology: Four questions for psychologists and school professionals. *School Psychology Review, 32*, 384–400.

Ross, L., & Nisbett, R. E. (1991). *The person and the situation: Perspectives of social psychology.* New York: McGraw-Hill.

Rotheram, M. J., Armstrong, M., & Booraem, C. (1982). Assertiveness training in fourth- and fifth-grade children. *American Journal of Community Psychology, 10*, 567–582.

Rubin, K. H., Bukowski, W. M., & Parker, J. G. (1998). Peer interactions, relationships, and groups. In W. Damon (Series Ed.) & N. Eisenberg (Vol. Ed.), *Handbook of child psychology: Social, emotional, and personality development* (5th ed., Vol. 3, pp. 619–700). New York: Wiley.

Rudolph, K. D., & Asher, S. R. (2000). Adaptation and maladaptation in the peer system: Developmental processes and outcomes. In A. J. Sameroff, M. Lewis, & S. Z. Miller (Eds.), *Handbook of developmental psychopathology* (pp. 157–175). New York: Kluwer Academic/Plenum.

Salmivalli, C., Huttunen, A., & Lagerspetz, K. M. (1997). Peer networks and bullying in schools. *Scandinavian Journal of Psychology, 38*, 305–312.

Salmivalli, C., Lagerspetz, K., Björkqvist, K., Osterman, K., & Kaukiainen, A. (1996). Bullying as a group process: Participant roles and their relations to social status within the group. *Aggressive Behavior, 22*, 1–15.

Salmivalli, C., & Nieminen, E. (2002). Proactive and reactive aggression among school bullies, victims, and bully-victims. *Aggressive Behavior, 28*, 30–42.

Salmivalli, C., & Voeten, M. (2004). Connections between attitudes, group norms, and behaviour in bullying situations. *International Journal of Behavioral Development, 28*, 246–258.

Schafer, M., Korn, S., Brodbeck, F. C., Wolke, D., & Schulz, H. (2005). Bullying roles in changing contexts: the stability of victim and bully roles from primary to secondary school. *International Journal of Behavioral Development, 29*, 323–335.

Sears, R. R. (1959). Foreward. In A. Bandura & R. H. Walters (Eds.), *Adolescent aggression: A study of the influence of child-training practices and family interrelationships* (pp. iii–v). New York: Ronald Press.

Sears, R. R. (1961). Relation of early socialization experiences to aggression in middle childhood. *Journal of Abnormal and Social Psychology, 63*, 466–492.

Sears, R. R., Maccoby, E. E., & Levin, H. (1957). *Patterns of child rearing.* Evanston, IL: Row, Peterson.

Sherif, M. (1956). Experiments in group conflict. *Scientific American, 195*, 54–58.

Skinner, B. F. (1985). Toward the cause of peace: What can psychology contribute? In S. Oskamp (Ed.), *International conflict and national public policy issues* (pp. 21–25). Beverly Hills, CA: Sage.

Solovey, M. (2004). Riding natural scientists' coattails onto the endless frontier: The SSRC and the quest for scientific legitimacy. *Journal of the History of the Behavioral Sciences, 40*, 393–422.

Spielman, D. A., & Staub, E. (2000). Reducing boys' aggression: Learning to fulfill basic needs constructively. *Journal of Applied Developmental Psychology, 21,* 165–181.

Staub, E. (1989). *The roots of evil: The origins of genocide and other group violence.* New York: Cambridge University Press.

Sutton, J., Smith, P. K., & Swettenham, J. (1999). Social cognition and bullying: Social inadequacy or skilled manipulation? *British Journal of Developmental Psychology, 17,* 435–450.

Tolan, P. H., & Dodge, K. A. (2005). Children's mental health as a primary care and concern: A system for comprehensive support and service. *American Psychologist, 60,* 601–614.

Tremblay, R. E., & Nagin, D. S. (2005). The developmental origins of physical aggression in humans. In R. E. Tremblay, W. W. Hartup, & J. Archer (Eds.), *Developmental origins of aggression* (pp. 83–106). New York: Guilford.

Watson, J. B. (1926). What the nursery has to say about instincts. In C. Murchison (Ed.), *Psychologies of 1925* (pp. 1–35). Worcester, MA: Clark University Press.

White, S. H., & Pillemer, D. B. (2005). Introduction: What kind of science is developmental psychology? In D. B. Pillemer & S. H. White (Eds.), *Developmental psychology and social change: Research, history, and policy* (pp. 1–7). Cambridge, UK: Cambridge University Press.

Author Index

276   AUTHOR INDEX

Subject Index

A

abuse, 67, 157, 158, 175, 223
academic achievement, 4, 112, 114, 121, 167, 186, 214, 250, 253, 259
action-control theory, 122, 123, 127
adolescence-limited trajectory, 138
advice book, 164
affiliation, 5, 18, 46, 147, 213–215, 220, 244, 252, 254
agency, 8, 9, 123, 167, 258
agonism, 2, 7, 11, 12, 15, 17, 19, 44–46, 88, 93, 94, 100, 107, 109
alliance building, 12, 18, 90, 95, 101, 200, 215, *see also* coalition building
allomothering, 67
alpha member, 44
alternative school, 225
altruism, 2, 9, 10, 71, 187
ambiguity, 97, 191, 192, 243
anger, 120, 127, 146, 160, 164, 177, 192, 236, 248, 250
animal behavior, 2, 6, 7, 11, 15, 37, 67, 70, 71, 86, 244
antipathy, 128, 173
antisocial behavior, xi, 77, 260
  benefits, 71, 72, 214
  causes, 4, 12, 54
  condemned, 75, 242, 251
  link to aggression, 5, 66, 120
  link to peer rejection, 15, 72, 139, 150, 204

link to popularity, 143–145, 153, 252, 253, 257
anxiety, 126, 189, 192, 202, 205, 241
ascendance, 5–7, 17
assertiveness training, 257–260
athletes, 216, 250, 253, 254
attachment theory, 1, 239, 242
attention, 7, 45, 51, 137, 157, 159, 162, 163, 168, 170, 172, 173, 198, 199
attractor state, 141, 142
attribution bias, 111, 146, 192
authoritarian personality, 242
authority, 32, 139, 211, 239–242, 251, 256
autonomy, 8, 9, 187
avoidance, 50, 93, 95, 162, 167, 169, 190, 193, 199, 258

B

beauty, 14, 21, 22, 100, 101, 162, 164, 173–175, 250, 253
behavioral contagion, 225
behaviorism, 3, 237–239, 244
bistrategic controller, 14, 15, 17, 18, 20–22, 42, 43, 46, 72, 73, 149
boredom, 200, 201
boundary, 213, 216, 217, 222, 223, 226
Buffy the Vampire Slayer, 171–175
bullies, 12, 20, 40, 66, 79, 188, 223
  and social skills, 71, 73, 218
  and their victims, 50, 152, 174, 193, 212, 216, 221, 227, 252